CONTEMPORARY TOPICS
IN IMMUNOBIOLOGY
VOLUME 6

Contemporary Topics in Immunobiology

A Continuation Order Plan is available for this series. A continuation order will bring delivery of each new volume immediately upon publication. Volumes are billed only upon actual shipment. For further information please contact the publisher.

CONTEMPORARY TOPICS IN IMMUNOBIOLOGY

VOLUME 6

Immunobiology of Oncogenic Viruses

EDITED BY

MICHAEL G. HANNA, JR.

Frederick Cancer Research Center
Frederick, Maryland

and

FRED RAPP

The Pennsylvania State University College of Medicine
Hershey, Pennsylvania

PLENUM PRESS • NEW YORK AND LONDON

Library of Congress Cataloging in Publication Data

Main entry under title:

Immunobiology of oncogenic viruses.

   (Contemporary topics in immunobiology; v. 6)
   Includes bibliographies and index.
   1. Viral carcinogenesis. 2. Cancer—Immunological aspects. 3. Oncogenic viruses. I.
Hanna, Michael G., 1936-   II. Rapp, Fred. III. Series. [DNLM: 1. Oncogenic
viruses—Immunology. W1 CO77 v. 6/QW160.05 I33]
QR180.C632 vol. 6 [RC268.57] 574.2'9'08s   76-54885
ISBN 978-1-4684-3053-0   ISBN 978-1-4684-3051-6 (eBook) [616.9'94'0194]
DOI 10.1007/978-1-4684-3051-6

© 1977 Plenum Press, New York
Softcover reprint of the hardcover 1st edition 1977
A Division of Plenum Publishing Corporation
227 West 17th Street, New York, N.Y. 10011

Contributors

Stuart A. Aaronson

Laboratory of RNA Tumor Viruses, Viral Carcinogenesis Branch
National Cancer Institute
Bethesda, Maryland 20014

P. Bentvelzen

Radiobiological Institute TNO
Rijswijk, The Netherlands

Maurice M. Black

New York Medical College
Flower & Fifth Avenue Hospitals
New York, New York 10029

Paul H. Black

Infectious Disease Unit
Massachusetts General Hospital and Department of Medicine
Harvard Medical School
Boston, Massachusetts 02114

Dani P. Bolognesi

Duke University Medical Center
Department of Surgery
Durham, North Carolina 27710

P. C. Creemers

Radiobiological Institute TNO
Rijswijk, The Netherlands

Bert C. Del Villano

Department of Immunopathology
Scripps Clinic and Research Foundation
La Jolla, California 92037

M. Essex

Department of Microbiology
Harvard University School of Public Health
Boston, Massachusetts 02115

M. G. Hanna, Jr.

Basic Research Program
NCI Frederick Cancer Research Center
Frederick, Maryland 21701

Martin S. Hirsch

Infectious Disease Unit
Massachusetts General Hospital and Department of Medicine
Harvard Medical School
Boston, Massachusetts 02114

James N. Ihle

Basic Research Program
NCI Frederick Cancer Research Center
Frederick, Maryland 21701

Stephen J. Kennel

Department of Immunopathology
Scripps Clinic and Research Foundation
La Jolla, California 92037

Richard A. Lerner   *Department of Immunopathology*
                        Scripps Clinic and Research Foundation
                        La Jolla, California 92037

Paul H. Levine   *Laboratory of Viral Carcinogenesis*
                        National Institutes of Health
                        National Cancer Institute
                        Bethesda, Maryland 20014

Max R. Proffitt   *Infectious Disease Unit*
                        Massachusetts General Hospital and Department of Medicine
                        Harvard Medical School
                        Boston, Massachusetts 02114

Fred Rapp   *Department of Microbiology*
                        and Specialized Cancer Research Center
                        The Milton S. Hershey Medical Center
                        The Pennsylvania State University
                        College of Medicine
                        Hershey, Pennsylvania 17033

Werner Schäfer   *Max-Planck-Institut für Virusforschung*
                        Tübingen, Germany

John R. Stephenson   *Laboratory of RNA Tumor Viruses, Viral Carcinogenesis Branch*
                        National Cancer Institute
                        Bethesda, Maryland 20014

Satvir S. Tevethia   *Department of Pathology and Cancer Research Center*
                        Tufts University School of Medicine
                        Boston, Massachusetts 02111

Preface

It has long been suspected, and recently confirmed, that there is an etiologic relationship between several viruses and naturally occurring neoplasias. Virus precursors in the form of nucleic acids or antigens have consistently been associated with certain neoplasias. However, the role of these virus-specified precursors in etiology remains obscure. Recent studies of virus-associated neoplasias have led to advances in molecular techniques, which have yielded increasingly sensitive assays for detection of virus-specific nucleic acids, and which have enabled the disruption of virus particles without concomitant loss in antigenicity of the components. These procedures have, in turn, resulted in molecular probes that allow more definitive evaluation of the host response to its virus and to the tumor cell with which the virus or its precursors are associated. Evaluations of the immune response and status of the host have provided important information about carcinogenesis and the tools for seroepidemiological studies of a variety of cancers. These seroepidemiological studies have demonstrated that several human cancers, e.g., Burkitt's lymphoma and nasopharyngeal carcinoma, are probably virus-induced, and that antibodies that are diagnostic and prognostic for these diseases are detectable. The conclusion that feline leukemia is a disease transmitted horizontally by a virus resulted primarily from immunological experiments. The important corollary to this conclusion is that the disease can be prevented by removal of diseased animals from the population or by antivirus vaccines; the latter approach has already been proven effective in preventing the naturally occurring Marek's disease of chickens.

There is considerable evidence that the immune response plays a role in neoplasia. Experimental studies indicate that, just as antigenic stimulation causes activation of type C viruses, the graft-vs.-host reaction may result in a similar phenomenon. Do such observations have a bearing on the increased incidence of neoplastic disease in humans receiving organ transplants? It is tempting to speculate that they do. Studies on natural immunity of lower animals to oncornaviruses are providing data for similar studies in the human population. The latter have been badly hindered by lack of appropriate reagents, but these should soon be available.

The authors of chapters in this book have attempted to summarize the status of research in the various areas of immunology concerned with virus-associated and virus-induced tumors. The results are often exciting and have led to a far better understanding of the role of the immune response in governing the onset and spread of virus-associated neoplasia. Extrapolation of the experimental results to the human population will be intellectually and practically rewarding. Interruption of the neoplastic process, at present, can only primarily be achieved by combined modalities of treatment, including surgical and radiological procedures to reduce total tumor burden, and chemotherapy and immunotherapy to eliminate residual tumor cells and to prevent their dissemination. It is hoped that continued progress in the area of virus-associated neoplasias will result in prevention, by direct vaccination or increase in immunologic capability, or detection of cancer cells prior to development of a clinically detectable mass.

Frederick Cancer Research Center   M. G. Hanna, Jr.

The Pennyslvania State University,   Fred Rapp
  College of Medicine

Contents

Chapter 2
Immunity to Leukemia, Lymphoma, and Fibrosarcoma in Cats: A Case for Immunosurveillance
M. Essex

Chapter 3
Intracellular and Systemic Regulation of Biologically Distinguishable Endogenous Type C RNA Viruses of Mouse Cells
Stuart A. Aaronson and John R. Stephenson

Chapter 7
Autoimmunity, Oncornaviruses, and Lymphomagenesis
Martin S. Hirsch, Max R. Proffitt, and Paul H. Black

Chapter 8
Natural Immunity to Murine Mammary Tumor Viruses
P. Bentvelzen and P. C. Creemers

Chapter 9
Immunogenicity and MuMTV-like Antigenicity of Human Breast Cancer Tissues
Maurice M. Black

Chapter 10
Clinical Implications of Immunity to Oncogenic Viruses
   Paul H. Levine

Chapter 1

Comparative Immunology of Carcinogenesis by DNA Viruses

Satvir S. Tevethia

Department of Pathology and Cancer Research Center
Tufts University School of Medicine
Boston, Massachusetts 02111

and

Fred Rapp

Department of Microbiology
and Specialized Cancer Research Center
The Milton S. Hershey Medical Center
The Pennsylvania State University
College of Medicine
Hershey, Pennsylvania 17033

I. INTRODUCTION

Investigations during the last decade have established a definitive role for certain viruses in the induction and maintenance of neoplasia under natural and laboratory conditions. Although the causal relationship between viruses and neoplasia in animals is well established, no viruses have yet been demonstrated to be the direct cause of human cancer. A close association, however, has been made between the DNA-containing herpesvirus, Epstein-Barr virus (EBV), and Burkitt's lymphoma (BL) and nasopharyngeal carcinoma (NPC) in the human population. DNA-containing tumor viruses differ from one another in morphology, nucleic acid content, host range, mode of replication, and ability to undergo latency and to cause neoplasia in their natural host. These include viruses that cause neoplasia in the host in which they replicate (herpes-, pox-, and papovaviruses) and viruses that induce tumors in heterologous hosts in which they undergo abortive infection (papovaviruses and adenoviruses). These

1

viruses invariably transform both permissive and nonpermissive cells in culture to malignancy. One of the consequences of viral transformation of mammalian cells both *in vitro* and *in vivo* is the synthesis of macromolecules by the transformed cells, which are distinctly antigenic in the autochthonous or syngeneic host and to which the host makes both a cellular and a humoral immune response. The new antigens expressed in virally transformed cells may be directly coded by the viral genome integrated into the host chromosome or they may be of cellular origin. The synthesis of these antigens, both virion and nonvirion, and the immune response of the host to these antigens have been used to associate a DNA tumor virus with a particular tumor. These antigens tend to possess virus specificities and are also induced during the virus cytolytic cycle. These properties of the antigens have made them valuable markers in studies on the mechanism of transformation by DNA viruses, on mapping of the viral genome, and on the role of virus-specific antigens in the initiation and maintenance of the transformed state. The specific antigens associated with DNA-virus-transformed cells, especially those expressed at the cell surface, induce cellular and humoral immune responses in the autochthonous and syngeneic host which influence the growth of the virus-induced tumors. The immune response, depending upon its nature and magnitude, may either inhibit or enhance tumor growth. The type of immune response, whether cellular or humoral, will be influenced by the strength and nature of antigens associated with the virus-transformed cells. Therefore, a clear understanding of the biological and biochemical nature of these antigens and of the immune response of the host is needed in order to control tumorigenesis by immunological means.

Our review will focus on the properties of antigens associated with cells transformed by various DNA viruses, their genetic origins, and their roles in the inhibition or enhancement of tumor growth. Emphasis will be placed on the reaction of the host to specific and cross-reactive antigens and the factors that might affect the immune response.

II. PROPERTIES OF ONCOGENIC DNA VIRUSES

DNA tumor viruses differ from one another in many respects. Papovaviruses are widespread in nature and contain a supercoiled circular DNA of approximately 3×10^6 daltons. These viruses replicate in the nucleus of the host cell and invariably induce host cell DNA synthesis. Only the papilloma viruses in the papova group produce self-limiting benign tumors in the natural host. The other papovaviruses induce tumors in a heterologous host and transform mammalian cells in culture. Papovaviruses generally are not related to each other and thus demonstrate no cross-reactivity, except for newly isolated human papovaviruses, which show considerable cross-reactivity with simian papovavirus SV40.

The adenoviruses comprise a large group of viruses that cause respiratory disease in the natural host and have been isolated from avian, murine, canine, bovine, simian, and human species. Adenoviruses are nonenveloped icosahedral viruses containing linear double-stranded DNA of $20-25 \times 10^6$ daltons; they replicate in the nuclei of permissive host cells. There are 31 human serotypes that have been classified into three subgroups based on the guanine and cytosine (GC) content of the DNA and oncogenicity in rodents. Adenoviruses are capable of transforming a wide variety of mammalian cells in culture. However, unlike the papovaviruses, the rescue of infectious virus from the transformed cells has not been accomplished. Both adenoviruses and papovaviruses generate defective variants during replication in permissive cells.

Herpesviruses are enveloped icosahedral viruses of 150 nm in diameter containing a linear double-stranded DNA of approximately 100×10^6 daltons; these viruses replicate in the nucleus of the infected cell. Several herpesviruses have been associated with neoplasia in the natural host, including man. Simian herpesviruses (*Herpesvirus saimiri* and *Herpesvirus ateles*) have been demonstrated to cause lymphoproliferative disease in nonhuman primates (for review, see Deinhardt *et al.*, 1974). The Lucke frog virus has been associated with adenocarcinoma in frogs. Marek's disease virus causes a lymphoma of thymus-derived cells in susceptible chickens, and, similarly, a herpesvirus of rabbits also causes lymphoproliferative disease in that species. Several human herpesviruses have been associated with neoplasia in humans. Most notable among these is EBV, which causes infectious mononucleosis in young adults and may be the etiological agent of BL and NPC in certain human populations. The genome of EBV is present in the tumor cells; and the virus can transform human B lymphocytes *in vitro*. EBV also induces a lymphoproliferative disease in marmosets. EBV, although a herpesvirus, is not related to the other subgroups of human herpesviruses. Cytomegalovirus (CMV), and herpes simplex virus type 1 (HSV-1) and type 2 (HSV-2) transform rodent cells in culture. The transformed cells are malignant *in vivo*, with persistence of the virus genome in the transformed cells. Epidemiological evidence associates carcinoma of the cervix and HSV-2. All herpesviruses generate natural defective viruses.

III. ONCOGENIC POTENTIAL OF DNA VIRUSES *IN VIVO*

The oncogenic potential of a DNA tumor virus *in vivo* either in a permissive or in a nonpermissive host is determined by (1) the ability of the virus to transform normal cells to malignancy and (2) proliferation of the transformed cells into a tumor. The progressive growth of the transformed focus *in vivo* will be influenced by the immune response of the host to antigens expressed in the transformed cells. The immune response, depending upon its nature and magnitude, can be either inhibitory or stimulatory to the developing tumor. Thus, the immune response to tumor-associated cell-surface antigens plays a very important role in the growth of tumors and provides us with a means of manipulating tumor growth. In this section, we will analyze the oncogenic potential of DNA tumor viruses in permissive and nonpermissive hosts and the effect of the immune response on tumor development.

A. Papovaviruses

1. Simian Virus 40 (SV40)

The most studied papovaviruses are SV40 and polyoma viruses; these viruses will, therefore, be dealt with in greater detail than other members of the papovavirus group.

SV40 induces tumors readily in newborn hamsters (Eddy, 1964). The latent period for tumor induction by SV40 ranges from 3 months to more than a year, depending upon virus concentration and the age of the animal at the time of inoculation. Newborn hamsters are susceptible to the oncogenic effects of SV40 whether inoculated by the subcutaneous, intracerebral, intraperitoneal, or intrathoracic route. DNA isolated from SV40-infected monkey cells is also oncogenic in hamsters (Boiron et al., 1965).

Histologically, SV40-induced tumors in subcutaneous tissues, lungs, and kidneys have been designated as undifferentiated sarcomas (Eddy, 1964). Intracerebral inoculation of the virus into newborn hamsters resulted in the development of ependymomas (Kirschstein and Gerber, 1962).

The age-dependent tumor induction by SV40 in hamsters indicates that resistance might be mediated by the immune response of the host. This possibility was indicated in experiments of Allison et al. (1967), who demonstrated that adult hamsters inoculated with SV40 directly into the cheek pouch, an immunologically privileged site, developed tumors at the site within 90 days, as compared to 490 days when animals of the same age were inoculated by the subcutaneous route. Additionally, X-irradiation of adult animals prior to virus inoculation enhanced their susceptibility to tumor induction. Adult animals inoculated with SV40 develop a specific transplantation immunity to specific antigens at the surfaces of SV40-transformed cells (Khera et al., 1963; Defendi, 1963; Zarling and Tevethia, 1973a). The development of such a response could be prevented by treatment of the host with antithymocyte sera during virus inoculation, suggesting that adult hamster cells are susceptible to virus infection or transformation in vivo. However, in the adult animal, the potential transformed cells are inhibited from proliferation by the host's immune response.

Recently, Diamandopoulos (1973) has demonstrated that adult hamsters are susceptible to SV40 oncogenesis if inoculated via the intravenous route. Surprisingly, nearly 85–95% of the virus-inoculated animals developed tumors which were lymphocytic leukemias, lymphosarcomas, osteogenic sarcomas, reticulum cell sarcomas, and anaplastic sarcomas. The etiological role of SV40 in these tumors was confirmed by the presence of SV40-specific tumor (T) antigen in the nuclei of tumor cells. Later studies demonstrated that the development of these lymphoid neoplasms in adult animals, when administered SV40 via the intra-venous route, was dependent upon the concentration of the virus and the age of the animals (Diamandopoulos and McLane, 1974). The possibility was con-sidered that the lymphoid neoplasms were induced by a variant of SV40 that was defective in the synthesis of specific transplantation antigen at the cell surface. However, this was found not to be the case as two of the lymphoid neoplasms (lymphocytic leukemia and lymphosarcoma) were shown to possess specific SV40 transplantation antigens (Tevethia, 1974). The lymphosarcoma (GD-36) was, however, weakly immunogenic as compared to the lymphocytic leukemia (GD-248). These results clearly indicate that papovaviruses are capable of inducing not only solid tumors but lymphoid neoplasms as well.

SV40 has generally been demonstrated to be oncogenic in hamsters only. Other species are normally resistant to the oncogenic effects of this virus. However, Allison and Taylor (1967) have demonstrated the induction of tumors in thymectomized random-bred and inbred rats by SV40. Within 8 months after virus inoculation, 80% of the virus-inoculated thymectomized animals had devel-oped subcutaneous neoplasms. Only 20% of the nonthymectomized animals developed tumors. A recent report (Hargis and Malkiel, 1975) has described the development of tumors in mice inoculated at birth with SV40 via the intra-venous route.

The rhesus monkey is the natural host for SV40; the virus produces a latent infection in this species. However, neither SV40-natural nor SV40-induced tumors have ever been reported in this species.

It is becoming clear that SV40 produces tumors in nonpermissive hosts and that the oncogenic potential of SV40 in different species is determined by the immunocompetence of the host and its capacity to mount an immune response resulting in the elimination of the potentially tumorigenic clones. It is con-ceivable that SV40 may be potentially oncogenic in the natural host but the oncogenic potential is not expressed due to strong immunosurveillance. As we will demonstrate in a later section, monkey cells which replicate virus also synthesize specific transplantation antigens at the cell surface; these would induce a very strong immune response in the natural host.

2. Polyoma Virus

The polyoma virus of mice is endemic in populations of wild and laboratory mice and produces tumors in newborn mice inoculated with the virus. The resistance of certain strains of mice to polyoma virus oncogenesis is mediated by the host's immune defenses, as polyoma-virus-inoculated mice develop virus-induced tumors after thymectomy (Law and Ting, 1965). Mice treated with anti-mouse-thymocyte sera also became susceptible to virus oncogenesis (Allison and Law, 1968). Additionally, nude mice that lack T-cell functions have been shown to develop tumors upon virus inoculation (Vandeputte *et al.,* 1974; Allison *et al.,* 1974; Stutman, 1975).

Polyoma virus also produces tumors in nonpermissive hosts. Newborn hamsters, rats, and rabbits are susceptible to polyoma virus oncogenesis. Treatment of rats with antithymocyte sera or thymectomy enhances susceptibility to virus oncogenesis (Vandeputte, 1969), indicating the role of cellular immune response of the host in resistance to polyoma virus oncogenesis.

3. Human Papovaviruses

Recently, several new human papovaviruses have been isolated from brains of patients with progressive multifocal leukoencephalopathy (PML), a rare demyelinating disease, and from urine of immunosuppressed patients who had undergone renal transplants or chemotherapy for malignant diseases. The DAR and EK viruses from PML cases (Weiner *et al.,* 1972) seem identical to SV40, whereas JC and BK viruses appear to be distinct from SV40. These human papovaviruses cross-react with SV40 antigenically (Penny and Narayan, 1973). Both EK and JC viruses from PML cases induce the development of gliomas in hamsters inoculated intravenously at birth (Walker *et al.,* 1973). Infectious virus was isolated when virus-free tumor cells were fused with susceptible cells. BK virus, however, produces tumors only infrequently.

Seroepidemiological studies have indicated that antibody to BK and PML viruses is common in man. By 10 years of age nearly 100% of the population has developed antibody to BK virus.

The oncogenic potential of these human papovaviruses in hamsters raises the possibility of their oncogenicity in the natural host, the human. Recently, Weiss *et al.* (1975) have demonstrated the presence of specific tumor or T antigen in the cells which are derived from human meningiomas. The T antigen could be detected by using sera reactive with SV40 T antigen. The tumor cells were free of infectious virus, but synthesis of virus could be induced by the fusion of human meningioma cells containing specific T antigen with African green monkey kidney cells. Accidental contamination of cultures by SV40 was ruled out. These human viruses have also been shown to transform hamster cells *in vitro* (Major and Di Mayorca, 1973). The presence of persisting T antigen in these human tumors may indicate a causal role of human papovaviruses in the development of meningiomas. It would be interesting to test the presence of papovavirus DNA sequences in the meningioma cells that do not express SV40 T antigen. A demonstration of the specific transplantation antigens at the surface of meningioma cells that are positive for T antigen would definitely be of interest, as this would indicate a positive role for the immune response in the inhibition of neoplasia induced by these viruses.

4. Papilloma Viruses

The papilloma viruses have been shown to cause tumors in the permissive host under natural conditions. In man, human papilloma virus causes skin warts, which rarely become malignant and have a tendency to undergo spontaneous regression. Infectious virus is associated with the keratinized cells of the skin. The papilloma virus most studied is the rabbit papilloma virus, which is widespread among cottontail rabbits and causes tumors of the skin. The benign skin lesions have been shown to develop into squamous cell carcinomas even under natural conditions (Syverton et al., 1950) and to contain virus antigens but not infectious virus (Evans et al., 1962).

B. Adenoviruses

Trentin et al. (1962) were the first to demonstrate the oncogenic potential of adenovirus type 12 in newborn hamsters. A number of human adenoviruses since then have been demonstrated to possess oncogenic potential in hamsters, mice, and rats. Based on this property, the 31 human adenoviruses were classified into three groups. Types 12, 18, and 31, which are highly oncogenic in hamsters, comprise group A, whereas group B viruses consist of types 3, 7, 11, 14, 16, and 21 and are weakly oncogenic in hamsters. Group C viruses (types 1, 2, 5, and 6), although nononcogenic, can transform cells in vitro. Recently, however, adenovirus type 9, which was previously shown to be nononcogenic in hamsters, has now been shown to induce fibroadenomas in female rats (Ankerst et al., 1974).

Tumors induced by human adenoviruses are mostly undifferentiated sarcomas that often resemble lymphomas (Larson et al., 1965; Trentin et al., 1968). Yohn (1973) has summarized the role of intrinsic factors that determine adenovirus type 12 oncogenesis in hamsters. It was demonstrated that adenovirus 12 oncogenesis was more efficient in females than in males. The incidence of tumors decreased in ovariectomized animals and increased in castrated males. Additionally, treatment of animals with estradiol resulted in significant increase in tumor incidence.

Tumors induced by adenoviruses as a rule do not undergo spontaneous regression, although in one report regression of tumors induced by adenovirus type 12 was observed (Yohn, 1973). The regression of tumors in hamsters by adenovirus type 12 could be prevented by treatment of the recipient with 2–5 mg of cortisone, which depresses the cellular immune responses. Similarly, thymectomy of 1-week-old hamsters inoculated with adenovirus type 12 resulted in enhanced tumor production, indicating that the immune response of the host plays a determining role in resistance to adenovirus oncogenesis. Allison *et al.* (1967) provided further evidence for the role of the cellular immune response in resistance to adenovirus oncogenesis in inbred mice. Inbred CBA mice are susceptible to a high dose of virus but are resistant to a low virus dose. CBA mice inoculated at birth with low doses of adenovirus type 12 and thymectomized at 2 days of age developed tumors, whereas the nonthymectomized mice inoculated with the same virus dose failed to develop tumors. Treatment of virus-inoculated mice with antilymphocyte serum yielded similar results. These authors further demonstrated that C3H mice, which are completely resistant to adenovirus oncogenesis, will develop tumors upon treatment with antithymocyte sera.

Several simian adenoviruses (SA7, SV20, and SV25), canine adenovirus, avian adenovirus (CELO), and bovine adenovirus type 3 have demonstrated oncogenicity in newborn hamsters. The tumors induced were undifferentiated sarcomas. CELO virus has also been shown to induce hepatomas and adenocarcinomas in hamsters (Anderson *et al.*, 1971).

C. Herpesviruses

1. Human Herpesviruses

Herpesviruses are endemic in human populations, commonly produce mild or subclinical infections in the children, and persist in the host in a latent state until they are activated by changes in the environment. Herpesviruses are often lytic to the host cell but are able to establish latency *in vivo* in some cells. Although no virus particles can be detected in this state, the virus can be activated to replicate, which indicates that the intact virus genome has been retained (Rapp, 1974). Herpesviruses generate defective particles during replication, and it is postulated that these defective viruses may initiate transformation without producing cytopathology.

Of the human herpesviruses, herpes simplex virus (HSV) types 1 and 2, CMV, and EBV have been implicated in human neoplasia. At the present time, there is no direct evidence that HSV-1 or HSV-2 cause tumors either in humans or in experimental animals. Indirect evidence, however, exists for the involvement of HSV in human neoplasia. HSV-2 (the major cause of genital lesions) has been associated with cervical cancer by seroepidemiology; a higher number of patients with cervical cancer have neutralizing antibodies to HSV-2 than do matched controls (Rawls *et al.*, 1969). The DNA of cervical carcinoma cells has been shown to contain HSV sequences (Frenkel *et al.*, 1972). Cervical carcinoma cells have also been shown to possess HSV-specific antigens (Royston and Aurelian, 1970). Infectious HSV-2 was isolated from a neoplastic cell line derived from a carcinoma of the cervix (Aurelian *et al.*, 1971). HSV-1 and HSV-2 have been shown to transform hamster cells *in vitro* to malignancy (Rapp, 1974). The cells transformed by HSV produced adenocarcinomas and fibrosarcomas (Rapp and Duff, 1973). The transformed cells contain a partial genome of HSV (Frenkel *et al.*, 1975), and HSV-specific antigens have been demonstrated in these transformed cells (Rapp, 1974).

Attempts to induce tumors in laboratory animals by HSV-1 and -2 have been largely unsuccessful. However, in one report (Nahmias *et al.*, 1970*b*) a few animals developed tumors after inoculation of hamsters with HSV-2. No evidence was presented for the presence of HSV genome in the hamster tumor cells.

Another human herpesvirus, CMV, has been shown to transform hamster cells *in vitro* (Albrecht and Rapp, 1973). These *in-vitro*-transformed hamster cells produce tumors *in vitro* and have been shown to contain CMV-specific antigens. Human cell-retaining antigens and virus DNA have also been transformed by this virus (Rapp *et al.*, 1975).

Epstein-Barr virus (EBV) was first discovered in lymphoblastoid cell lines from a Burkitt's tumor (Epstein *et al.*, 1964). The virus causes infectious mononucleosis (Henle and Henle, 1973), a benign lymphoproliferative disease that is self-limiting in young adults. The virus has been associated with BL and NPC. Burkitt's tumor cells and cells derived from NPC contain EBV DNA (Wolf *et al.*, 1973). Early antigen (EA) and virus capsid antigen (VCA) are generally absent, however. Cells from biopsy material contain EBV-specific nonvirion antigen (EBNA) in the nucleus of the tumor cells. The cells also contain EBV-specific membrane antigen (MA). EBV can transform normal human lymphocytes *in vitro*. The transformed cells have the properties of cells derived from BL.

Shope *et al.* (1973) were successful in inducing malignant lymphomas and reticulum cell sarcomas with EBV in cottontop marmosets. The latent period for the development of lymphomas after virus inoculation was 31–46 days. It is interesting that immunosuppressive therapy enhanced tumor production, thus indicating the role of immune response in the resistance of host to virus-induced neoplasia. Similarly, owl monkeys inoculated with cells from Burkitt's tumor (EB-3) died of lymphoproliferative malignancy 14 weeks later.

2. Primate Herpesviruses

Herpesvirus saimiri (HVS) and herpesvirus ateles (HVA), isolated from squirrel and spider monkeys (Melendez *et al.*, 1968, 1972), respectively, produce fatal lymphomas and leukemias in a variety of species but produce only milk infections in their natural hosts (Melendez *et al.*, 1972). HVS induced lymphomas in marmosets; the lymphomas were free of virus particles but infectious virus could be isolated by cocultivation with permissive monkey cells. HVS also produces lymphomas in owl and spider monkeys and a lymphomalike disease in rabbits. HVA produces lymphoproliferative disease in marmosets only (Melendez *et al.*, 1972; Deinhardt *et al.*, 1974). Since these two viruses do not appear to be oncogenic in their natural host, it is probable that this nononcogenicity may be due to the immune response of the host to these viruses. Recent evidence suggests that the squirrel monkey's resistance to oncogenic properties of HVS may derive from the rapid development of antibodies after infection (Klein, 1973).

3. Marek's Disease Virus (MDV) of Chickens

Marek's disease (Marek, 1907) is a lymphoproliferative disorder endemic in chicken populations. Although chickens are the natural host, turkeys, pheasants, and quail may also harbor the virus (Purchase, 1974; Nazerian, 1973). The virus is transmitted horizontally and infection via the respiratory tract appears most likely. The incubation period for the induction of lymphomas by a high dose of virus is about 2 weeks and clinical symptoms appear in about 3 weeks (Payne and Biggs, 1967). Clinical signs include paralysis of legs, wings, and eyelids. Pathologically, affected nerves are enlarged and gonads, liver, lungs, heart, muscle, and skin have lymphoid tumors along with atrophy of the thymus and bursa of fabricius (Purchase and Biggs, 1967). The lymphoid tumors consist of lymphocytes. The tumor cells are of thymic origin since bursectomy has no effect on the disease (Payne and Rennie, 1970). Also, the lymphoma cells themselves were shown to be of T-cell origin (Hudson and Payne, 1973) and continuous cell lines have been established from MD lymphomas which are clearly of T-cell origin (Powell *et al.*, 1974). The tumor cells have been shown to contain viral DNA (Nazerian *et al.*, 1973). It has been further demonstrated that in susceptible chickens subjected to thymectomy and γ-radiation the tumor incidence dropped to 9% as compared to 80% in intact chickens, indicating that the multiplication of virus *in vivo* is not related to the development of neoplasia (Sharma, 1975).

4. Herpesviruses of Rabbits and Guinea Pigs

A herpesvirus of rabbits has been shown to induce lymphomas in wild cottontail rabbits (Hinze, 1971). Herpesvirus from strain-2 guinea pigs has been isolated from lymphoblasts of the affected animals. The virus replicated in the presence of an immune response (Tenser and Hsiung, 1973).

IV. ONCOGENIC POTENTIAL OF DEFECTIVE GENOMES

Viruses generate defective particles that are incapable of completing the cycle of replication under certain conditions. Defective genomes of a tumor virus may be incorporated into the genome of an unrelated nononcogenic virus and may depend on the helper nononcogenic virus for replication. Since DNA tumor viruses transform nonpermissive cells more efficiently than permissive cells, the defective particles may be potentially oncogenic in a permissive host or transform permissive cells *in vitro* more efficiently. Defective viruses may also induce neoplasia more efficiently by virtue of the duplication of transforming genes in the defective genomes. Defective genomes of both naturally occurring deletion mutants and deletion mutants created in the laboratory are also useful in studying the function of a particular segment of a viral genome.

A. Oncogenicity of Defective Viruses Produced by Exogenous Treatment

Defendi and Jensen (1967) demonstrated that tumors were induced by SV40 with a higher frequency in newborn hamsters after the virus had been inactivated by ultraviolet (UV) or by γ-irradiation. Most of the virus in the irradiated stock had been inactivated. Enhanced oncogenicity of hydroxylamine-treated SV40 was also demonstrated by Altstein *et al.* (1967*a*) in newborn hamsters. Oncogenesis by apparently nononcogenic defective SV40 (PARA) upon irradiation has been demonstrated by Duff *et al.* (1972). Defendi and Jensen (1967) explained their results on the basis of increased concentration of defective particles after irradiation. This, however, may not be the only explanation for oncogenicity because fully infectious particles can also induce neoplasia (revealed by isolation of complete genomes from some SV40-transformed cells). Defective SV40 (PARA) populations with reduced oncogenic potential *in vivo* (Rapp *et al.*, 1969) have been described. A likely possibility might be that the transplantation rejection antigen induced by the irradiated virus is able to immunize hosts as efficiently as the nonirradiated virus.

HSV-1 and HSV-2 are lytic to a large number of mammalian cells *in vitro* and pathogenic in a variety of hosts *in vivo*. Duff and Rapp (1971, 1973) have demonstrated the oncogenic potential of HSV-1 and -2 in hamsters by transforming hamster cells to malignancy *in vitro* with UV-irradiated HSV-1 and -2. However, the direct oncogenic potential of irradiated HSV has not been demonstrated in newborn hamsters except in one case (Nahmias, 1970*b*), and no evidence was presented that the tumors were induced by the herpesvirus. Another herpesvirus, CMV, has also yielded transformants after inactivation by UV light (Albrecht and Rapp, 1973; Rapp and Li, 1974).

Viral infectivity of DNA viruses may also be inactivated by treating the virus with heterocyclic dyes followed by exposure to white light. Photodynamically inactivated viruses (SV40 and HSV) have been shown to transform mammalian cells in culture (Rapp *et al.*, 1973; Seemayer *et al.*, 1973). Recently, defective SV40 particles have been created in the laboratory, but the oncogenic potential of these is unknown (Mertz *et al.*, 1974; Davoli and Fareed, 1974).

B. Oncogenic Potential of Naturally Occurring Defective Genomes

Defective SV40 genomes (PARA) and E46+, which are encased in adenovirus 7 capsids, are oncogenic in newborn hamsters (Huebner *et al.*, 1964*a*; Rowe and Baum, 1964; Rapp *et al.*, 1964*c*). SV40 and adenovirus 7 DNA in the PARA particle are covalently linked (Baum *et al.*, 1966). The hybrid DNA contains 75% of the complete SV40 DNA, and approximately 12% of the adenovirus 7 DNA is deleted (Kelly and Rose, 1971). The SV40 genome in the hybrid particle does not induce the synthesis of SV40 coat protein but does induce SV40 early antigens (EA) (Huebner *et al.*, 1964*a*; Rapp *et al.*, 1964*c*, 1966).

Adenovirus 7–SV40 hybrid virus, or -PARA, induced tumors in newborn hamsters that were the SV40 type, since the tumors contained SV40 T and transplantation antigens (Huebner *et al.*, 1964*a*; Rapp *et al.*, 1966; Lausch *et al.*, 1968; Jensen and Defendi, 1968). The tumors induced by the original PARA-adenovirus 7 population had latent periods similar to those induced by the parental SV40. Transcapsidation of the defective SV40 genome carried in the PARA-adenovirus 7 to adenovirus types 1, 2, 3, 5, and 6 conferred oncogenicity in newborn hamsters. Transcapsidants of adenovirus types 14, 16, and 21 were nononcogenic (Rapp *et al.*, 1968). Both nononcogenic and oncogenic PARA-adenoviruses induced specific SV40 transplantation immunity in hamsters and SV40 T antigen *in vitro;* when PARA was transcapsidated from nononcogenic adenovirus 21 to adenovirus 6, it remained nononcogenic. PARA from the PARA-adenovirus 6 population, which was oncogenic upon transcapsidation to adenovirus 21, remained oncogenic (Rapp *et al.*, 1968), indicating that variants of PARA that differed in oncogenicity were present in the original population of PARA-adenovirus 7. Such variants were subsequently isolated by plaque purification in monkey cells and 20 of 112 viruses were nononcogenic in newborn hamsters (Rapp *et al.*, 1969). However, the nononcogenic variants were capable of transforming cells *in vitro* (Butel *et al.*, 1971; Rapp and Duff, 1971). Transcapsidation of PARA from adenovirus 7 to highly oncogenic adenovirus type 12 resulted in a population that induced tumors containing SV40 T antigen in hamsters in a significantly shorter period than the parental SV40. Artificial mixtures of SV40 and adenovirus were unable to induce SV40 tumors with a short latent period. Early tumors induced by PARA-adenovirus 12 contained SV40 transplantation antigens (Butel *et al.*, 1971).

Several other adenovirus 2–SV40 hybrid viruses have been isolated from a strain of Ad2^{++}, which was adapted to grow in monkey cells. Two of the defective hybrid viruses (Ad2^{++}HEY and Ad2^{++}LEY) yielded infectious SV40 with different efficiencies and contained differing amounts of complete SV40 genome integrated with Ad2 DNA (Lewis and Rowe, 1970; Kelly *et al.*, 1974). However, the oncogenic potential of these viruses has not been determined *in vivo*.

In addition, five nondefective Ad2^{+}-SV40 hybrids (which are capable of replication independently of helper adenovirus) have been isolated (Lewis *et al.*, 1969, 1973). The five nondefective hybrid viruses (Ad2^{+}ND1, Ad2^{+}ND2, Ad2^{+}ND3, Ad2^{+}ND4, and Ad2^{+}ND5) contain 0.18, 0.32, 0.06, 0.43, and 0.28 of SV40 genome integrated at the same site in the adenovirus 2 molecule. Despite induction of SV40 transplantation antigens by only two of the hybrid viruses (Ad2^{+}ND2 and Ad2^{+}ND4), all five hybrid viruses including Ad2^{+}ND4 virus, which contains 0.43 unit of SV40 genome and induced both SV40 T and transplantation rejection antigen (TrAg), are nononcogenic in newborn hamsters (Lewis *et al.*, 1974*a,b*).

All five hybrid viruses will, however, transform hamster cells *in vitro;* only the cells transformed by Ad2^{+}ND4 contained SV40 T and TrAg (Lewis *et al.*, 1974*a,b*). The reasons for the nononcogenicity of independently replicating hybrid viruses are not known.

Other hybrid virus populations have been isolated in which a portion of simian adenovirus 7 (SA7) genome is incorporated into an adenovirus type 2 genome. Ad2-SA7 populations in monkey cells were capable of inducing SA7 T antigen but not SA7 viral antigen. These hybrid viruses were nononcogenic in newborn hamsters, although the parental SA7 from which they were derived was highly oncogenic. The Ad2-SA7 populations remained nononcogenic even upon transcapsidation to other adenovirus serotypes. Interestingly, Ad2-SA7 populations that were nononcogenic in newborn hamsters were capable of inducing specific transplantation immunity in adult hamsters against a challenge of SA7 hamster tumor cells (Kaplan *et al.*, 1971).

Naturally occurring SV40 particles, which are defective in the synthesis of late viral proteins and infectious virus but which are able to induce the synthesis of SV40 T antigen, have been described (Sauer *et al.*, 1967; Altstein *et al.*, 1967*b*; Uchida *et al.*, 1968). During undiluted serial passage in monkey cells, SV40 DNA undergoes genetic reassortment resulting in the formation of heterogeneous circular DNA molecules shorter than those of wild-type SV40. After serial passage, cellular DNA sequences are incorporated into defective SV40 genomes in place of viral DNA sequences (Yoshiike, 1968; Tai *et al.*, 1972; Lavi and Winocour, 1972). The naturally occurring defective particles in preparations of SV40 were oncogenic in newborn hamsters and the resulting tumors contained SV40 T antigen (Uchida and Watanabe, 1969).

Naturally occurring defective particles have also been documented for adenovirus type 12 and simian adenovirus 7. The defective particles had the same oncogenic potential in newborn hamsters as the parental virus (Schaller and Yohn, 1974). Defective particles also accumulate when HSV is passaged serially in cell culture (Roizman and Kieff, 1975); however, no information is available regarding their oncogenic potential.

V. NEOPLASTIC TRANSFORMATION *IN VITRO* BY DNA VIRUSES

The earlier findings that the *in vitro* interaction of papovavirus SV40 with nonpermissive cells would lead to heritable changes similar to ones observed in cells derived from hamster tumors induced by SV40 led to the widely believed (though not always correct) conclusion that *in vitro* transformation of cells by a DNA virus represents the oncogenic potential of the virus *in vivo*. The interaction of a DNA tumor virus with a cell may be either (1) productive, resulting in the synthesis of new virus and cell death, or (2) abortive, often leading to cell transformation. The criteria for transformation of cells by a DNA tumor virus generally include the following: (a) loss of contact inhibition, (b) altered morphology, (c) growth to high saturation density, (d) growth in low-serum medium, (e) increased capacity to persist in serial subculture, (f) anchorage-independent growth, (g) membrane changes which include transport or permeability, (h) impaired intercellular communication and junction, (i) changes in agglutinability by lectins, (j) changes in electrophoretic mobility, and (k) biochemical changes involving glycoproteins and glycolipids. Transformed cells, in addition, retain either a complete or incomplete viral genome in integrated or plasmid form. Generally, the cells will synthesize virus-coded or virus-specific products located intracellularly or at the cell membrane.

The central question that needs to be answered is the mechanism by which a cell infected and transformed *in vivo*, either in a heterologous or natural host, undergoes proliferation to establish a tumor, since a greater understanding of the factors that affect the growth of the transformed cells *in vivo* would be of immense help in controlling tumor growth.

It is not our intention to review all aspects of transformation since excellent reviews have already been published (Black, 1968; Butel *et al.*, 1972; Sambrook, 1973; Klein, 1973; Tooze, 1973; Rapp, 1974). We will examine those aspects of transformation by DNA viruses which deal with the malignant potential of transformed cells and their antigenicity.

A. Papovaviruses

Even though SV40 produces tumors consistently only in hamsters, it can transform a wide variety of cells *in vitro* (for reviews, see Butel *et al.*, 1972;

Sambrook, 1973; Tevethia and Tevethia, 1975a). The virus can transform human, monkey, bovine, rabbit, mouse, rat, and reptile cells, in addition to hamster cells. The virus can transform cells from a wide variety of organs and tissues. Cells from kidney, lung, liver, heart, skin, lens epithelium, brain, prostate, and pituitary can be transformed by SV40. Lymphoid cells have also been shown susceptible to transformation by SV40 (Collins et al., 1974).

Since in vitro transformation of mammalian cells by SV40 results in the integration of viral genome into the host cell DNA, and since the transformed cells synthesize early SV40 antigens and acquire the ability to grow indefinitely in vitro, it has been assumed that the transformation observed in vitro is analogous to tumor induction in vivo. This analogy is valid for hamster cells, which upon transformation by SV40 are invariably transplantable in the syngeneic host (Duff and Rapp, 1970b). However, variation in transplantability has been reported (Butel et al., 1971). Mouse cells which are more susceptible to transformation by SV40 in vitro than hamster cells become transplantable only after the transformed cells have been cultivated in vitro for a prolonged period of time (Takemoto et al., 1968; Kit et al., 1969; Wesslen, 1970; Tevethia and McMillan, 1974). A similar situation holds true for rat cells. This apparent lack of transplantability of inbred mouse transformed cells even in immunosuppressed mice raises the question of the role of the viral genome in malignancy. Recent studies (Tevethia and McMillan, 1974) have shown that freshly derived BALB/c embryo cells upon transformation with SV40 failed to produce tumors in immunocompetent or immunosuppressed syngeneic newborn or adult mice, thus ruling out the possibility that the lack of tumor induction by these transformed cells was due to the immune response of the host to SV40 transplantation antigens present at the cell surface. The cells did become transplantable in immunosuppressed hosts only after prolonged in vitro cultivation. Thus, at least in the case of mouse cells, morphological transformation (synthesis of virus-specific antigens, integration of viral genome, and other cellular changes) can be separated from malignant transformation, and the malignant property might be acquired independently. Recent studies by Risser et al. (1974) and Shin et al. (1975) have shown that the ability of the SV40-transformed cells to grow in soft agar and to synthesize plasminogen activator correlated with their ability to form tumors in nude mice which lack T-cell function. It is conceivable that previous findings (Takemoto et al., 1968; Kit et al., 1969; Tevethia and McMillan, 1974), in which prolonged cultivation of transformed cells was necessary for the cells to form tumors in syngeneic hosts, can be explained on the basis that the prolonged cultivation in vitro selected those transformed cells which were capable of anchorage-independent growth.

Other experimental evidence also indicates that mere integration of the viral genome in infected cells does not confer upon them the properties of malignancy. Smith et al. (1971) isolated abortively SV40-transformed mouse cells. Most of the abortive transformants reverted back to the normal cell phenotype and no viral genome was demonstrated in these cells. However, in one case (Smith *et al.*, 1972) it was shown that cryptic transformants with normal cell phenotype contained several copies of viral DNA. No viral functions or viral RNA was demonstrated, and no infectious virus was recovered from these cells by fusion with susceptible cells.

The transplantability of these cryptic or flat transformants was tested in CBF1 hybrid mice which had been thymectomized, lethally irradiated, and reconstituted with bone marrow cells. The results (Wright *et al.*, 1973) showed that cryptic transformants also produced tumors, but after a long latent period. The tumor cells were negative for SV40 T antigen, but the presence of the SV40 genome in these cells was not investigated. The study was inconclusive as the parental line (BALB/3T3) from which the transformed cells were derived produced tumors itself.

Other recent evidence that integration of virus-specific sequences in host cells does not always convert these cells to malignancy comes from the work of Jaenisch and Mintz (1974), who demonstrated that when mouse blastocysts were infected with SV40 DNA and implanted into the uterine horns of a pseudopregnant recipient, mature and healthy mice developed. Various tissues from the adult mice were shown to contain SV40 sequences by hybridization techniques. Interestingly, no tumors have developed in these mice over a 1-year period. The presence of SV40 sequences in the adult mouse tissue indicates that the cells containing the viral genome have not been eliminated by the immune response of the host to specific transplantation antigens. If the transcription or the translation of the viral genome can occur in the infected mice, then it should be possible to demonstrate the presence of lymphocytes immune to SV40 transplantation antigens in these mice. The likelihood of tumor induction in mice by SV40 DNA-infected blastocysts would be increased if the blastocysts of mice of nude background were infected with SV40 DNA and implanted into pseudopregnant mice, since nude mice lack T-cell functions and would not be able to reject the developing tumor. Another possibility is that the SV40 genes are silent in the tissues of the infected animals. This possibility is quite likely in light of recent evidence gathered by Kelly and Sambrook (1974), who isolated transformed cells resistant to cytochalasin B from the SVT2 line of SV40-transformed mouse cells. The resistant cells showed no SV40 T antigen in the nucleus, and there was a quantitative and qualitative loss in integrated viral DNA sequences. It would be interesting to know if the cytochalasin B-resistant clones became nontumorigenic concomitant with the loss of SV40 T antigen.

The transformation of a normal cell into a cancer cell has generally been regarded as an irreversible change. However, there are several reports that indicate the transformed cells may revert back to the normal cell phenotype. Pollack *et al.* (1968) selected variants from SV40- and polyoma-virus-transformed 3T3 mouse cells and cells from a polyoma-virus-induced hamster tumor by treatment of the cells with FUdR. The variant clones contained virus-specific

T antigens but had reduced tumorigenicity. Hamster embryo fibroblasts transformed by polyoma virus have been reported to undergo reversion of properties characteristic of transformation (Rabinowitz and Sachs, 1968, 1969, 1970; Inbar *et al.*, 1969). The variant cells were not agglutinable by plant lectins and were less tumorigenic than the parental transformed cells. Several of the cell lines were shown to lack polyoma-virus-specific cell-surface transplantation antigens.

However, whether the revertant cell lines had actually lost the polyoma-virus-specific transplantation antigens or had become immunoresistant was not tested. Immunoresistant cells, although possessing specific transplantation antigens, cannot be rejected by the immunized host (Tevethia *et al.*, 1971).

B. Adenoviruses

As do papovaviruses, adenoviruses transform mammalian cells in culture (reviewed by Casto, 1973). Human adenoviruses have been classified into highly, weakly, and nononcogenic groups based on the frequency of tumors induced in hamsters. Viruses belonging to group C, which do not produce tumors in newborn hamsters, have now been shown to transform hamster (Finkelstein and McAllister, 1969; Lewis *et al.*, 1974*a*; Goldman *et al.*, 1974) and rat (Freeman *et al.*, 1967; Van Der Noorda, 1968; McAllister *et al.*, 1969; McDougall *et al.*, 1974; Graham *et al.*, 1974*a,b*) cells. The adenovirus 2-transformed rat cells induced tumors only in immunosuppressed animals (Gallimore, 1972; McDougall *et al.*, 1974). The transformation of rat cells by nononcogenic human adenoviruses (which are transplantable under certain conditions in the syngeneic animals) indicates that the apparent nononcogenicity of these transforming human adenoviruses may be due to a strong immunological reactivity of the host to antigens associated with these transformed cells.

Transformation of hamster or rat cells by highly or weakly oncogenic human adenoviruses often leads to tumor production by the transformed cells in the appropriate host (for reviews, see Casto, 1973; Tooze, 1973). Transformation of hamster cells by adenoviruses other than those of human origin has also been demonstrated (see Casto, 1973).

C. Herpesviruses

1. Herpes Simplex and Cytomegaloviruses

Confirmed reports (see Nazerian, 1973) of herpesviruses as etiological agents of naturally occurring lymphomas in chickens, the very strong association of EBV to BL (Epstein, 1970; Klein, 1973, 1974), and the association of HSV to carcinoma of the cervix by seroepidemiological evidence (Rawls *et al.*, 1969; Nahmias *et al.*, 1970*a*) led Duff and Rapp (1971, 1973) to demonstrate the *in vitro* transforming potential of HSV-2 and -1, respectively. CMV was also soon added to the list of transforming viruses (Albrecht and Rapp, 1973). One problem in demonstrating the transforming potential of HSV has been its lytic activity in most mammalian cells. HSV stocks were therefore inactivated by ultraviolet irradiation and exposed to hamster embryo fibroblasts in culture. Foci of transformed cells appeared in the culture 3–4 weeks after exposure to irradiated HSV-2 (Duff and Rapp, 1971). The evidence that the cells were transformed by HSV-2 was as follows: (1) transformed cells produced tumors in hamsters, and tumor cell metastases were observed in the lungs, kidneys, and liver of tumor-bearing animals (Rapp and Duff, 1973); (2) tumors induced by HSV-2-transformed cells were classified as fibrosarcomas; (3) virus-specific antigens located at the cell surface and intracellularly were present in the transformed cells; (4) tumor-bearing hamsters responded by making neutralizing antibodies to HSV-2, suggesting the presence of a HSV glycoprotein at the surface of the tumor cells; (5) although no infectious virus was recovered from the transformed cells, synthesis of HSV-specific messenger RNA was demonstrated (Collard *et al.*, 1973); and (6) the viral genome in the transformed cells complemented HSV temperature-sensitive (*ts*) mutants at nonpermissive temperatures (Kimura *et al.*, 1974).

Similar results were obtained with cells transformed by HSV-1 and CMV (see reviews by Rapp, 1974; Rapp and Li, 1974). HSV-1-transformed cells induced adenocarcinomas (Rapp and Duff, 1973). The transformation of hamster cells by HSV was subsequently confirmed by Kutinová *et al.* (1973) and by others (for review, see Rapp and Westmoreland, 1976).

2. Epstein-Barr Virus

As previously mentioned, the association between EBV and BL is very strong (for reviews, see Epstein, 1970; Klein, 1973, 1974; Henle and Henle, 1974). Biopsy specimens from BL have been shown to contain EBV DNA (zur Hausen *et al.*, 1970; Nonoyama *et al.*, 1973), specific membrane antigens (MA) (Klein *et al.*, 1967), and an EBV-specific nonvirion intranuclear antigen (EBNA) (Reedman and Klein, 1973). Cells cultured from the BL biopsy may synthesize other virus-specific products in addition to EBNA and MA. These may include, depending upon the cell line, an early antigen (EA) which may be diffuse (D) or restricted (R) (G. Henle *et al.*, 1971; W. Henle *et al.*, 1970), virus capsid antigen (VCA) (G. Henle and W. Henle, 1966; Nadkarni *et al.*, 1970), or even virus particles (Epstein *et al.*, 1964).

The first indication that EBV was capable of transforming human lymphocytes came from the studies of G. Henle *et al.* (1968), who demonstrated that permanent lymphoblastoid cell lines could be established from a person with infectious mononucleosis. The established cell lines contained EBV antigens. Transformation of normal lymphocytes into lymphoblastoid cell lines was accomplished by exposing peripheral leukocytes of newborn female children to lethally X-irradiated cells from an EBV-producing cell line derived from BL. The transformed cell line contained EBV and had a female karyotype (W. Henle *et al.*, 1967). Transformation was also demonstrated by using cell-free medium from EBV-producer lines (Nilsson *et al.*, 1971; Pope *et al.*, 1969), concentrated virus (Gerber *et al.*, 1969), and throat washings from infectious mononucleosis patients (Gerber *et al.*, 1972; Miller *et al.*, 1973). The target cell from transformation by EBV has been shown to be a B lymphocyte (Pattengale *et al.*, 1974).

Recently, Shope *et al.* (1973) have been able to transform peripheral blood leukocytes from cottontop marmosets after exposure to EBV. The resulting transformed cells contained EBV antigens and released EBV particles *in vitro* (Miller *et al.*, 1973). A common step in the transformation of leukocytes by EBV into permanent cell lines is the stimulation of host cell DNA synthesis (Gerber and Hoyer, 1971). During productive infection of lymphoid cells by EBV, the following sequence of events may be visualized (Klein, 1973; Hampar *et al.*, 1974). Following virus infection there is a stimulation of host-cell DNA synthesis with the synthesis of EBNA in the nucleus of infected cells. This is followed by the synthesis of EA for which no viral DNA synthesis is required (Gergely *et al.*, 1971*b*). The synthesis of EA is followed by the inhibition of host DNA synthesis and commitment of the cells to a productive infection resulting in synthesis of viral DNA, virus capsid antigen, and virus particles. MA is a complex of several antigenicities (Klein *et al.*, 1971) and appears early in the course of viral infection; its synthesis is not inhibited by inhibitors of DNA synthesis. In the abortive infection, only EBNA is synthesized and the appearance of EA is blocked.

Two strains of EBV, which differ in their transforming properties, have been described. EBV isolated from the P3HR-1 clone of JiJoye, a cell line derived from BL by Hinuma and Grace (1967), produces productive infection in cord blood lymphocytes. Strain B95-8, isolated from a patient with infectious mononucleosis, induces extensive infection of cord blood lymphocytes (Miller *et al.*, 1974; Klein, 1974). Strain B95-8 stimulates host-cell DNA synthesis and the synthesis of EBNA but no EA, whereas P3HR-1 virus does not stimulate host-cell DNA synthesis and does not transform cord blood lymphocytes. This property of stimulation of host-cell DNA synthesis by the transforming strains of EBV has been used successfully to classify EBV isolates into transforming and nontransforming viruses (Robinson and Miller, 1975).

The EBV genome is also present in biopsy material from NPC (zur Hausen *et al.*, 1970; Nonoyama *et al.*, 1973) and cells derived from NPC have been shown to contain EBNA (Klein *et al.*, 1974). However, direct transformation of epithelial cells by EBV has not yet been demonstrated *in vitro*.

VI. ROLE OF VIRUS GENOME IN CELL TRANSFORMATION

Three main approaches have been taken to determine the role of viral information in the establishment and maintenance of transformation by oncogenic DNA viruses. These approaches include (1) analysis of the specific viral sequences present in transformed cells, (2) transformation of cells by restriction nuclease cleavage fragments of viral DNA, and (3) determining the ability of *ts* mutants to transform cells at temperatures that are nonpermissive for replication of the mutants, as well as the ability of the cells transformed by its mutants to maintain characteristics of the transformed state at elevated temperatures. The first approach has been most extensively applied to adenovirus-transformed cells. Sambrook *et al.* (1974), using defined segments of adenovirus DNA produced by cleavage with restriction nucleases *Eco*RI and *Hpa*I as probes in kinetic hybridization experiments, have determined that ten lines of rat embryo cells which have been transformed by adenovirus 2 contain several copies of the same set of viral sequences comprising 14% of the adenovirus genome. All of the viral sequences present in these cells map at the left-hand end of the viral genome. In six of the cell lines these are the only sequences present. None of the cell lines tested contained a complete set of viral genes. As all of the cell lines tested were T-antigen positive, the sequences coding for or responsible for the induction of this antigen as well as functions required for the maintenance of transformation must also be contained within the left-hand 14% of the viral genome. Similarly, hamster cells transformed by adenovirus 5 contain several copies of the extreme left-hand segment of viral DNA comprising 35–40% of the total viral genome (Sambrook *et al.,* 1974) and adenovirus 7-transformed hamster cells contain several hundred copies of 10–20% of the viral genome (Fujinaga *et al.,* 1974). These results strongly indicate that the left-hand ends of these adenovirus genomes provide functions which are necessary and sufficient for *in vitro* transformation. The viral sequences required for transformation by adenoviruses were further localized by Graham *et al.* (1974 *a,b*) by testing the ability of specific restriction endonuclease fragments to transform human and rodent cells *in vitro.* The G fragment of both adenovirus 2 and 5 DNA produced after cleavage of the DNA with a restriction enzyme from *Haemophilus suis* (R·*Hsa*1) has a molecular weight of 1.6×10^6 and represents the left-hand 7% of the genome. These fragments alone are capable of transforming rodent cells. Transforming activity of adenovirus DNA was significantly reduced by treatment with exonuclease III and S_1 nuclease only after 1% of the terminal DNA sequences had been removed, indicating that the terminal 1% of sequences in adenovirus DNA are not essential for transformation.

Although these studies serve to locate the DNA sequences required for the initiation and maintenance of transformation, they are not sufficient to determine the functions required for *in vitro* transformation. An answer to this question requires both characterization and mapping of *ts* mutants which are defective in aspects of *in vitro* transformation. One *ts* mutant of adenovirus 5 has been recently mapped at the left-hand end of the viral genome (Sambrook *et al.* 1975). This mutant fails to synthesize viral DNA or to transform rat embryo cells at temperatures which are nonpermissive for viral replication (Wilkie *et al.*, 1973; Williams *et al.*, 1974). Mutants in a second complementation group of DNA-minus *ts* mutants transform rat embryo cells more efficiently than the wild type at elevated temperatures (Ginsberg *et al.* 1974). This result suggests that a viral gene product normally prevents transformation. This possibility and the observation that no adenovirus–transformed cells containing the entire genome have been identified suggest that transformation may require the integration of the left-hand end of the viral genome and the selective loss of other viral sequences. Further characterization of this and other mutants of adenoviruses is needed in order to establish relationships between specific viral gene products and transformation.

Considerable progress has been made toward determining viral sequences, gene products, and functions required for transformation by papovavirus SV40. By using renaturation kinetics to measure the amounts of each of four fragments produced by the sequential cleavage of SV40 DNA by *Eco*RI and *Hpa*I restriction endonucleases in the SV40-transformed cell lines (SVT2), Sambrook *et al.* (1974) have determined that the late-transcribing region is present approximately once per diploid quantity of cell DNA, whereas the early region of the SV40 genome is represented about six times. Since infectious virus can be easily rescued from SVT2 cells following formation of heterokaryons with permissive green kidney cells, it is presumed that one complete copy of the SV40 genome is integrated with the early and late sequences in tandem. Although many SV40-transformed cells contain the entire viral genome, not all of the SV40 sequences are required for the initiation and maintenance of transformation. Both defective SV40 viruses, which are missing viral sequences, and heavily irradiated SV40 can transform cells efficiently.

In order to determine which viral sequences are required for transformation, Abrahams *et al.* (1975) transformed baby rat kidney cells with specific fragments of SV40 DNA prepared by the combined action of restriction endonucleases. Linear molecules of genome length prepared with endonucleases R·*Eco*RI and R·*Hpa*II, each of which make one break at a different site in the late-transcribing region, transform as efficiently as circular SV40 DNA.

The smallest fragment capable of transforming was a 59% fragment produced by cleavage with R·*Bam*HI and R·*Hap*IIA which contains the entire early region. Treatment of SV40 DNA with R·*Hpa*I endonuclease yields three fragments of 42%, 38%, and 20% of the genome in size, none of which transforms baby rat kidney cells. R·*Hpa*I introduces one break in the early portion of the

SV40 genome at a site where SV40 *tsA* mutants have been mapped. These results indicate that at least part of the early sequences must remain intact in order for transformation to occur.

SV40 has been subjected to intensive genetic studies with the aim of clarifying the role of specific SV40 gene products in the initiation and maintenance of transformation. Temperature-sensitive mutants of SV40 have been classified into complementation groups representing three cistrons *A, B-C,* and *D.* The product of the *A* cistron is essential for the initiation of SV40 DNA replication (Tegtmeyer, 1972; Chou and Martin, 1975). Mutants in the *B-C* group are defective in capsid synthesis (Tegtmeyer and Ozer, 1971, 1972; Dubbs *et al.,* 1974; Chou and Martin, 1974, 1975). Mutants in the *D* complementation group produce an altered protein late in the infectious cycle which becomes part of the virion and which apparently cannot be removed during uncoating at elevated temperatures (Robb and Martin, 1972; Chou and Martin, 1974, 1975). As removal of the protein is required in order for transcription of the SV40 genome to be initiated, *tsD*-infected cells at nonpermissive temperatures behave as uninfected cells.

None of the *tsD* or *tsA* mutants transforms any of a variety of rodent or primate cells at temperatures which are nonpermissive for replication of the mutants (Martin and Chou, 1975; Tegtmeyer, 1975; Brugge and Butel, 1975; Osborn and Weber, 1975; Kimura and Itagaki, 1975). When cells are transformed *in vitro* by *tsD* mutants at a permissive temperature and are then shifted to a nonpermissive temperature, the cells maintain all aspects of their transformed phenotype (Martin and Chou, 1975). However, a variety of cells transformed by *tsA* mutants at a permissive temperature lose one or more characteristics of a transformed phenotype when passaged at a nonpermissive temperature (Martin and Chou, 1975; Tegtmeyer, 1975; Brugge and Butel, 1975; Osborn and Weber, 1975; Kimura and Itagaki, 1975). This revision of the transformed phenotype depends both on the transformed cell line and on the particular *tsA* mutant in question. Thus rabbit kidney cells transformed by *tsA30* at 33°C produce colonies readily at both permissive and nonpermissive temperatures, whereas Syrian hamster embryo cells transformed by the same mutant show a marked reduction in the ability to replicate at elevated temperatures. A second mutant, *tsA57,* had no effect on the ability of either type of cell to form colonies at the nonpermissive temperature (Tegtmeyer, 1975). Interestingly, cells transformed by one *tsA* mutant, *tsA28,* consistently were unable to form clones at elevated temperatures regardless of whether the cell lines were of rabbit, hamster, human, or rat origin (Tegtmeyer, 1975; Brugge and Butel, 1975; Osborn and Weber, 1975). Although many aspects of the transformed state were monitored for reversion to normal at high temperature, the ability to form colonies on plastic, in soft agar, or on monolayers of normal cells most consistently fluctuated with the temperature of growth. Microscopic examination of *tsA*-transformed cells plated at low density and incubated at a nonpermissive temperature suggests that these cells do not divide normally (Tegtmeyer, 1975). The requirement of the *A*-gene function for the initiation of transformation was shown in temperature shift experiments. When rat embryo cells infected with a *tsA* mutant were held for a short time at a high temperature and then shifted to permissive temperature, the number of transformants produced was no higher than that observed when the cells were held at high temperature throughout the experiment (Kimura and Itagaki, 1975).

Thus, at least one specific SV40 gene product is required for the initiation and maintenance of some features of the transformed state. The precise function of this product in transformation or its interaction with cellular products which lead to the transformed state remains to be determined.

VII. ANTIGENS ASSOCIATED WITH DNA-VIRUS-TRANSFORMED CELLS

The antigens present in transformed cells or in tumors induced by DNA tumor viruses either are nonvirion in nature or are components of the virus particle itself. The nonvirion antigens are as a rule specific for the transforming virus. The antigens in the tumor cells can be classified into two categories based on location within the transformed cells: (1) intracellular antigens that are located either in the nucleus or cytoplasm of the transformed cells, and (2) cell-surface antigens. The intracellular antigens are antigenic in the autochthonous or syngeneic host and induce a humoral immune response only. They do not play any role in the rejection of tumors because of their location in the tumor cells. Cell-surface antigens, on the other hand, induce both humoral and cellular immune responses and presumably participate in the rejection of tumors. In this section, we will review comparative properties of DNA-virus-induced antigens.

A. Intracellular Antigens

1. Papovaviruses (SV40)

a. Tumor or T Antigen. The tumor or T antigen in SV40 tumor or transformed cells was first demonstrated by means of the complement-fixation (CF) test using sera from hamsters bearing SV40-induced tumors (Black *et al.*, 1963). The nuclear localization of T antigen was later demonstrated by the indirect immunofluorescence test (Pope and Rowe, 1964; Rapp *et al.*, 1964*a*). The demonstration of the synthesis of an antigenically similar T antigen during productive infection by SV40 in monkey cells provided evidence for associating the virus with the virus-free transformed cells (Rapp *et al.*, 1964*b*). The T antigen induced by SV40 is specific for SV40, but recently an antigenically similar T antigen has been demonstrated in tumors induced by human papovaviruses (Walker *et al.*, 1973; Takemoto and Mullarkey, 1973). The T antigen has also been localized in the cytoplasm of cells infected with, or transformed by, mutants of defective SV40 populations (Butel *et al.*, 1969). The cytoplasmic localization of T antigen as detected by the indirect immunofluorescence technique did not alter its antigenic properties or the malignant behavior of the tumor cells. Kinetic studies have shown that T antigen appears 12–24 hr after infection of monkey cells by SV40. The synthesis of T antigen is inhibited by actinomycin D but not by inhibitors of DNA synthesis, showing that T-antigen synthesis is dependent upon an early viral function and that the synthesis of viral DNA is not required for its expression (Rapp *et al.*, 1965). It is also susceptible to inhibition by interferon during the infectious cycle (Oxman and Black, 1966). T antigen is heat labile and resistant to deoxyribonuclease and ribonuclease, but it is susceptible to trypsin. It has a molecular weight of about 70,000 (Del Villano and Defendi, 1973). The biological function of T antigen is unknown; however, the recent findings that T antigen binds to double-stranded DNA (Carroll *et al.*, 1974; Jessel *et al.*, 1975) and binds preferentially to SV40 DNA at the origin of replication (S. Reed *et al.*, 1975) suggest an important role in DNA regulation. This possibility is strengthened by the fact that T antigen is not produced at normal levels by virus mutants which are defective in viral DNA synthesis (Tegtmeyer and Ozer, 1971).

The presence of T antigen in the transformed cells has been used to follow the development of SV40-induced tumors *in vivo*. By using the indirect immunofluorescence test, Diamandopoulos (1973) was able to demonstrate the development of SV40-induced lymphocytic leukemia, lymphosarcoma, and reticulum cell sarcomas in adult hamsters inoculated intravenously with SV40. The presence of T antigen was demonstrated in the nucleus of cells in imprints made from lymph nodes of animals inoculated with SV40. Even when only rare cells containing T antigen were present, they were easily demonstrated in the tissue imprint.

Animals bearing tumors induced either by the virus or by transformed cells develop antibody to T antigen. In hamsters, the antibody to T antigen is located in γ_2 fraction of 7 S immunoglobulin (Tevethia, 1967). The presence of antibody to T antigen in animals inoculated with the virus has generally been correlated with the presence of a virus-induced tumor. Recently, however, it has been demonstrated that a certain percent of virus-inoculated hamsters develop T antibody in the absence of neoplasia (Diamandopoulos and McLane, 1974). Also, the development of T antibody has been demonstrated in animals (rabbits and monkeys) which support virus replication but do not develop neoplasia (Rapp *et al.*, 1967; Tevethia, 1970). SV40 T antigen, because of its location in the nucleus of tumor cells, does not play a role in the rejection of SV40 tumor cells by virus-immunized animals. This conclusion is supported by the observation that hamsters bearing tumors induced by one of the lines of SV40-transformed cells do not synthesize antibodies to SV40 T antigen but are still capable of rejecting a transplant of syngeneic SV40 tumor cells (Lausch *et al.*, 1970).

When the presence of SV40 T antigen was first demonstrated, it was thought to be specific for SV40 virus, a unique property in light of observations with T antigens induced by various adenoviruses. Cross-reaction between T antigens of human and simian adenoviruses has also been demonstrated (Riggs *et al.*, 1968). Recently, viruses of papovavirus morphology have been isolated from human cases of progressive multifocal leukoencephalopathy and from the urine of patients who had undergone renal transplantation (Padgett *et al.*, 1971; Gardner *et al.*, 1971; Weiner *et al.*, 1972; Dougherty and DiStefano, 1974). These human viruses grow in human cells, can transform hamster cells, and can induce tumors in hamsters. The human papovaviruses, although distinct, are antigenically related to SV40. These viruses induce a T antigen in the nucleus of infected cells which is antigenically similar to SV40 T antigen. Hamsters with tumors induced by the JC human papovavirus develop antibodies cross-reactive with the T antigen of JC and SV40 viruses (Walker *et al.*, 1973).

b. U Antigen. U antigen is specific for SV40. Several lines of evidence also indicate that U may be antigenically distinct from T antigen (Lewis and Rowe, 1971). Like the T antigen, it is located in the nucleus of cells infected or transformed by SV40. In cells infected by $Ad2^+ND_1$ virus, which contains a portion of SV40 DNA covalently linked to human adenovirus 2 DNA, U antigen is located at the nuclear membrane. The synthesis of U antigen by SV40 is not inhibited by ara C and, as with T antigen, appears 12–24 hr after virus infection. In the case of $Ad2^+ND_2$ virus, however, U-antigen synthesis is diminished in the presence of ara C, whereas T-antigen synthesis is unaffected. U antigen is more heat stable than is T antigen and can be distinguished from T by using *ts* mutants of SV40. The mutant *tsB11* induces T but not U antigen at the nonpermissive temperature (Robb *et al.*, 1974). Hamsters bearing tumors induced by SV40 develop antibodies to U antigen in addition to T antigen; the antibody to T antigen is present in higher titer than is the antibody to U antigen. Recently, it has been reported that U antigen cannot be demonstrated in mouse cells transformed by SV40 (Robb *et al.*, 1974). There is a possibility that U represents a cleavage product of T.

2. Other Papovaviruses

The T antigen induced by polyoma virus in the cytolytic cycle and in transformed cells has properties similar to SV40 T antigen, but does not cross-react with it antigenically. However, the T antigen induced by human papovaviruses is antigenically indistinguishable from SV40 T antigen. Paradoxically, the regions of the genome of SV40 and the human papovaviruses that hybridize are the late regions (Khoury et al., 1975). This forces the conclusion that the molecular hybridization technique is not sufficiently sensitive to pick up a small region of homology which confers T-antigen reactivity or that the T antigen represents a virus-modified host protein.

3. Adenoviruses

Tumors induced by adenovirus type 12 were shown to contain tumor or T antigen (Huebner et al., 1963). T antigen was detected by both complement-fixation and immunofluorescence tests using sera from animals bearing adenovirus 12 tumors (Pope and Rowe, 1964). The antigen was located in both the nucleus and cytoplasm of cells transformed or infected with adenovirus 12. In addition to T antigen, adenovirus 12-transformed cells also contained an antigen associated with the adenovirion, referred to as the C antigen (Huebner et al., 1964b). In the immunofluorescence test, sera from adenovirus 12 tumor-bearing animals reacted with cells infected by either adenovirus 2 or adenovirus 7 (Pope and Rowe, 1964; Feldman et al., 1966). Unlike the antigen in adenovirus 12-infected cells, the T antigen in cells infected with adenovirus 2 or 7 was localized predominantly in the nucleus of infected cells. Other studies with adenovirus 12 tumor-bearing hamster sera demonstrated that at terminal dilution the sera reacted with antigens in cells infected with adenovirus types 12, 18, and 31, but not with cells infected with adenovirus types 1–3, 5–7, 14, 16, or 21 (Riggs et al., 1968). At lower dilutions, however, the sera reacted with the T antigens of all group A, B, and C adenoviruses. Sera from adenovirus 7 tumor-bearing animals reacted with T antigens of group A and B adenoviruses but not with cells infected with group C adenoviruses in the complement-fixation tests. Huebner et al. (1965) found no cross-reactivity between T antigens of group A and B adenoviruses.

Tumors induced by simian adenoviruses, like those induced by human adenoviruses, contained T antigen that could be detected by immunofluorescence and complement-fixation tests using sera from tumor-bearing animals. Simian adenoviruses have been placed into three groups based on the serological reactivity of their T antigens using CF tests (Gilden et al., 1968). Group I includes SV1, SV11, SV25, SV34, and SV38. Group II includes SV20 and SV23. SA7 is the sole member of group III. Using CF tests, the simian adenovirus T antigens did not cross-react with either group A or B human adenoviruses. In contrast, sera from animals bearing adenovirus 7 or 12 tumors reacted in immunofluorescence tests with T antigen of group I and III simian adenoviruses (Riggs et al., 1968).

The T antigen of adenoviruses is a mixture of several components with reported sedimentation coefficients of 5.9, 3.9, 3.1, and 2.2 S (Tockstein *et al.,* 1968). However, Gilead and Ginsberg (1968) were able to demonstrate only one 2.6 S component in purified preparations of adenovirus T antigen.

4. Herpesviruses

a. Epstein-Barr Virus. Cells derived from biopsies of BL may possess both nonvirion and virion intracellular antigens induced by EBV. These intracellular antigens can be demonstrated by the IF test and include EBNA (Reedman and Klein, 1973), EA which may be diffuse (D) or restricted (R) (Henle *et al.,* 1971), or VCA (Henle and Henle, 1966). In addition, soluble antigens have been described in BL nonproducer cell lines by the complement-fixation test (Pope *et al.,* 1969; Vonka *et al.,* 1970).

Cell lines derived from BL that contain EBV DNA are of two types: (1) producers which synthesize viral DNA and late viral antigens, and may release infectious virus, and (2) nonproducer lines in which virus DNA may be synthesized but which do not produce infectious particles. During the nonproductive infection, the only intracellular antigen induced is EBNA. EBNA is present in the nucleus of all lymphoblastoid cell lines carrying EBV DNA from BL and infectious mononucleosis (IM) patients and cell lines derived by *in vitro* transformation of lymphoid cells (Reedman and Klein, 1973). EBNA can be detected by an anticomplement fluorescence technique by using fluorescein-labeled anti-$B_1 C/B_1 A$. The EBNA is associated with chromosomes during metaphase and is similar to the T antigens specified by papovaviruses as it is present only in cells that contain EBV DNA (Klein, 1974); its synthesis does not depend upon viral DNA replication. The soluble antigens associated with nonproducer cell lines carrying the EBV genome have recently been shown to be identical to EBNA (Klein and Vonka, 1974).

Another intracellular antigen, EA, is synthesized during the virus lytic cycle. No viral DNA synthesis is required for its expression (Gergely *et al.,* 1971 *a,b*). EA may be of the D or R type. Antibodies to the D type are most prevalent in IM patients, whereas antibodies to R occur in BL patients. EA is a nonvirion antigen.

The only intracellular virion antigen synthesized during the productive cycle of EBV is the VCA. The presence of VCA correlates with the presence of virus particles (zur Hausen *et al.,* 1967). Not surprisingly, synthesis of VCA can be blocked by inhibitors of DNA synthesis.

b. Herpes Simplex Virus. When hamster cells were transformed *in vitro* to malignancy (Duff and Rapp, 1971, 1973), the transformed cells demonstrated cytoplasmic antigens by the indirect immunofluorescence test using sera prepared against HSV-1 or -2 in weanling hamsters. The fluorescence was detected in only 5—10% of the transformed cells. Similar results were also reported by Kimura *et al.* (1975), who transformed hamster cells by HSV-2 and demonstrated the localization of herpes virion antigens in the cytoplasm of the transformed cells. The expression of the antigen is dependent upon the cell cycle (Schaffer, unpublished observations). HSV virion antigens have also been demonstrated in the cytoplasm of rat cells transformed by UV-irradiated HSV-1 and -2 or by *ts* mutants of both viruses (Macnab, 1974). Thus far, nonvirion antigens have not been demonstrated in HSV-transformed cells.

Cytoplasmic antigens, which are probably virion antigens, have also been associated with CMV-transformed cells (Albrecht and Rapp, 1973; Rapp and Li, 1974).

B. Antigens Associated with the Surface of DNA-Virus-Transformed Cells

1. Papovaviruses (SV40)

In this section, we will review the cell-surface antigens associated with cells transformed by the oncogenic DNA virus, SV40. We will examine in detail the properties of SV40-specific TrAg. TrAg is one of the most important antigens present at the surface of all cells transformed by SV40 because it mediates the development of a cellular immune response in the host which leads to the rejection of tumor cells carrying the same antigen. The presence of cell-surface antigens detected by serological means and embryonic antigens will also be discussed.

a. SV40 Transplantation Rejection Antigen. The presence of TrAg in SV40-transformed cells has been demonstrated by transplantation rejection tests. Syngeneic adult animals immunized either with the virus or with transformed cells are able to specifically reject a transplant of SV40-transformed or tumor cells (Khera *et al.*, 1963; Defendi, 1963). TrAg is not a virion antigen. Antiviral antibodies have no effect on the growth of SV40 tumor cells (Khera *et al.*, 1963), and the tumor cells themselves have been shown to be free of infectious virus and of virion antigens (Butel *et al.*, 1972; Tevethia and Tevethia, 1975*a*).

The TrAg present in cells transformed *in vitro* is identical to the antigen in tumor cells; immunization of animals with *in vitro* transformed cells can protect hamsters against a challenge of cells derived from a tumor induced by SV40 and vice versa (Khera *et al.*, 1963). The cross-reactivity of SV40 TrAg is not limited to tumors induced by SV40 within the same animal species. TrAg in SV40-transformed cells of one species cross-reacts with the TrAg in SV40-transformed cells from another species (Girardi, 1965). TrAg is synthesized during the virus cytolytic cycle in monkey cells (Girardi and Defendi, 1970; Tevethia and Tevethia, 1976). The TrAg in transformed cells remains stable during the growth of tumor cells either *in vitro* or *in vivo*. However, it has been shown that in the SV40 system the expression of TrAg at the surface of tumor cells can be altered in such a way that immunoresistant cells escape rejection by an immunized host. The immunoresistant cells, however, retain immunogenicity (Tevethia *et al.,* 1971).

SV40 TrAg is located at the cell surface and has been isolated in "soluble" form by using 3 M KCl and by limited papain digestion. The activity of soluble SV40 TrAg was monitored by the *in vitro* macrophage migration-inhibition test (Blasecki and Tevethia, 1973, 1975*a*) and has also been shown to be immunogenic in a syngeneic host (Drapkin *et al.,* 1974). The biochemical nature of TrAg remains unknown.

In addition to transplantation rejection and the macrophage migration—inhibition tests, the presence of TrAg can also be measured by using the *in vivo* tumor cell neutralization test. In this test, lymphoid cells from syngeneic animals (which have rejected a transplant of SV40 tumor cells) when mixed with the tumor cells in a ratio of 100 lymphocytes to one tumor cell and inoculated into a normal adult recipient will inhibit tumor formation by SV40 tumor cells (Zarling and Tevethia, 1973*a;* Howell *et al.,* 1974). This cellular reactivity of lymphoid cells to SV40 TrAg has been correlated with the *in vivo* rejection phenomenon.

b. Surface (S) Antigens Detected by Serological Means. Tevethia *et al.* (1965) first demonstrated specific antigens at the surface of SV40-transformed hamster cells using the indirect IF test with sera from SV40-vaccinated hamsters that had rejected a transplant of virus-free tumor cells. The reaction was specific for SV40-transformed cells since antibody against S antigen did not react either with normal hamster cells or with cells transformed by unrelated viruses. Tevethia *et al.* (1968*a*) later demonstrated that hamsters synthesized S antibody when immunized with SV40 virus alone, thereby ruling out the participation of isoantigens in the membrane reaction. The presence and specificity of S antigen in SV40-transformed cells were later confirmed and extended (Kluchareva *et al.,* 1967; Girardi, 1967). Specific antigens at the surface of SV40-transformed cells were also demonstrated *in vitro* by the mixed hemadsorption test (Hayry and Defendi, 1968; Metzgar and Oleinick, 1968), the colony inhibition test (Tevethia *et al.,* 1970), the isotopic antiglobulin test (Ting and Herberman, 1971), and the cytotoxic test using ^{51}Cr-labeled target cells (Wright and Law, 1971) and *in vivo* by inhibition of transformed cell replication in diffusion chambers implanted in the peritoneal cavity of immune hamsters (Coggin and Ambrose, 1969). Additional studies using antisera to syngeneic SV40-transformed cells have also indicated that specific antigens can be detected by the *in vitro* microcytotoxicity test. All of these studies showed that antigen(s) detected at the surface of SV40-transformed cells with humoral antibodies are specific for SV40.

c. Embryonic Antigens. Serological evidence has also been presented which supports the presence of fetal antigens at the surface of SV40-transformed cells using either sera from pregnant hamsters (Duff and Rapp, 1970*a*; Coggin *et al.,* 1970) or anti-mouse-egg sera prepared in guinea pigs (Baranaska *et al.,* 1970; Koprowski *et al.,* 1971). Ting *et al.* (1972) prepared antisera to fetal antigens by immunizing male C3H mice with X-irradiated syngeneic minced fetal tissue. These sera reacted with all the tumors tested irrespective of the transforming agent. The antibody activity could be absorbed with any of the tumor types or with fetal tissues. The antibody prepared against the tumor cells themselves in the syngeneic host reacted specifically only with the tumor type used for immunization. Immunization with fetal tissue failed to provide protection against challenge by virus-transformed cells. On the other hand, work carried out by Coggin and Anderson (1974) indicates that the cross-reacting antigens present in embryonic cells may be capable of inducing resistance to a challenge of SV40-transformed cells.

d. Normal Cell Antigens. Hayry and Defendi (1970), using the mixed hemadsorption test, suggested that S antigen may be a normal cell antigen that is specifically unmasked during SV40 transformation. This conclusion was based on the observation that after brief treatment with trypsin, spontaneously oncogenic or polyoma-virus-transformed cells reacted with SV40 S antibody. The normal cell antigen described by Hayry and Defendi (1970) is not involved in tumor rejection by immunized animals since SV40 and polyoma virus TrAg do not cross-react. Collins and Black (1973 *a,b*), in a comprehensive study, claimed that each SV40-transformed cell possesses a unique antigen which is masked and can only be uncovered by treatment of the cells with phospholipase *c.* Whether these unique antigens are capable of inducing resistance in the syngeneic host was not elucidated. These findings remain unconfirmed.

2. Other Papovaviruses

The first evidence for TrAg in cells transformed by papovaviruses was demonstrated in the polyoma virus tumor system independently by Sjögren *et al.* (1961) and Habel (1961, 1962) using the transplantation rejection test in syngeneic mice. The nonvirion nature of the antigen was later demonstrated (Habel, 1962; Sjögren, 1964). Polyoma-virus-induced TrAg has many properties in common with SV40 TrAg.

Specific surface antigens present in polyoma-virus-transformed cells have been detected with antisera made in syngeneic animals against polyoma tumor cells using the IF test (Irlin, 1967; Lherisson *et al.,* 1967), the colony inhibition test (Hellstrom and Sjögren, 1965), and the isotopic antiglobulin test (Ting *et al.*, 1972; Volkers and Pitts, 1973). Specific antigens in polyoma-virus-transformed cells have also been demonstrated by methods which measure cellular immunity (Habel, 1962; Sjögren, 1964; Datta and Vandeputte, 1971; Sjögren and Bansal, 1971). Polyoma-specific surface antigens have also been demonstrated during the virus cytolytic cycle (Irlin, 1967; Malmgren *et al.*, 1968; Meyer and Birg, 1970; Volkers and Pitts, 1973).

3. Adenoviruses

Tumors induced by adenovirus type 12 also possess specific TrAg at the cell surface which have been detected by the transplantation rejection test in syngeneic mice (Trentin and Bryan, 1966; Sjögren *et al.*, 1967; Berman, 1967).

Specific cell-surface antigens in adenovirus-transformed cells have also been detected *in vitro* by the colony inhibition test using lymphocytes from immune or tumor-bearing animals (Hellstrom and Sjögren, 1967; Ankerst and Sjögren, 1970). The transplantation antigens induced by group A and B human adeno-virus types cross-reacted in the *in vitro* colony inhibition test. Adenovirus types 1 and 5 induce a common antigen that did not cross-react with antigens induced by adenoviruses belonging to groups A and B.

Other adenoviruses (SA7 and CELO) have also been demonstrated to induced specific transplantation antigens at the surface of transformed cells (Kaplan *et al.*, 1971; Pauluzzi and Rapp, 1969).

4. Herpesviruses

a. Herpes Simplex and Cytomegalovirus. Hamster cells transformed *in vitro* by HSV-1 or -2 which become transplantable in the syngeneic host were shown *not* to contain TrAg by the classical transplantation rejection test. Adult hamsters immunized by HSV were unable to reject or delay the development of tumors induced by HSV-2 tumor cells (Rapp and Duff, 1973). Similar results were obtained with CMV-transformed cells. The presence of specific surface antigens in CMV- or HSV-transformed cells was demonstrated by the indirect IF test using antisera against the respective viruses (Rapp, 1974). Also, the tumor-bearing animals developed virus-neutralizing antibodies, suggesting that the antigens at the surface of HSV- or CMV-transformed cells are virion in nature.

The presence of HSV- and CMV-specific antigens on cells transformed by the respective viruses was also demonstrated by *in vitro* techniques which measure cellular immunity (Lausch *et al.*, 1975*b*). Spleen cells from tumor-bearing animals or animals immunized with the virus demonstrated specific cytotoxicity to the appropriate target cells. The cytotoxic activity of the spleen cells was blocked by sera from tumor-bearing animals. That the sera contained antibodies to specific antigens was indicated by the observation that the lymphocyte-blocking activity of the sera was absorbed only by the specific target cells. The exact nature of the antigens present at the surface of HSV- or CMV-transformed cells remains unknown. However, at least one HSV-1-transformed cell line contains a virus-specific glycoprotein at the surface (C. Reed *et al.*, 1975).

There is some evidence that HSV-2-transformed cells possess cross-reactive antigens that might be embryonic in origin. Rapp and Duff (1973) demonstrated that HSV-2 tumor cells have the capacity to metastasize to lungs. The number of lung metastases was actually enhanced rather than inhibited by immunization of the animals with HSV prior to challenge with HSV-2-transformed cells. The development of metastases in the lungs of tumor-bearing hamsters was inhibited by prior immunization of animals with papovavirus SV40, thus indicating that the animals might be responding to antigens common to SV40- and HSV-transformed cells which might be embryonic in nature.

b. Marek's Disease and Epstein-Barr Viruses. Membrane-associated antigens in cells infected by MDV have been demonstrated by the membrane IF test (Chen and Purchase, 1970; Ahmed and Schidlovsky, 1972; Nazerian and Chen, 1973). Cell-surface antigens have also been demonstrated on the surface of MDV tumor cells and the lymphoblastoid lines which carry the viral genome. This antigen does not seem to be a part of the virion and can be demonstrated in nonproducer lymphoblastoid cell lines (Witter *et al.*, 1975).

Cells derived from BL biopsy or established cell lines releasing EBV carry membrane-associated antigens (MA) which are specific for EBV (Klein *et al.*, 1966, 1967). MA can be induced in EBV-negative lines upon infection with EBV (Gergely *et al.*, 1971a). MA consists of three antigenic entities which are located on the same molecule (Svedmyr *et al.*, 1970; Klein *et al.*, 1971). The synthesis of MA in EBV-infected cells is not blocked by inhibitors of DNA synthesis (Gergely *et al.*, 1971a) and appears to be a glycoprotein, which is also found in the virion envelope (Silvestre *et al.*, 1971).

VIII. GENETIC ORIGIN OF DNA-VIRUS-SPECIFIED ANTIGENS

Antigens present in DNA-virus-transformed cells have been used to follow *in vitro* and *in vivo* transformation of mammalian cells. Their presence on the cell membrane has provided immunologists and virologists alike with a handle to regulate the growth of tumors as these antigens tend to induce an immune response in the autochthonous or syngeneic host. Initially, both intracellular and membrane antigens were demonstrated to be specific for the transforming virus (Sjögren, 1965; Klein, 1966, 1969; Deichman, 1969; Hellström and Hellström, 1969), but there are recent reports that cross-reactive antigens are present in tumors induced by different DNA tumor viruses or chemical carcinogens (Coggin and Anderson, 1974; Baldwin *et al.*, 1974). The simultaneous presence of virus-specific and cross-reactive antigens in cells transformed by DNA tumor viruses has raised questions about the role of these antigens in tumor rejection. In order to utilize these antigens as a diagnostic tool or in immunotherapy, it is important to understand their nature and genetic origin since these proteins, although antigenic in the autochthonous or syngeneic host, may have other cell regulatory functions, such as maintenance of the transformed state.

The intracellular and cell membrane antigens, which are constituents of the virion, will not be discussed in this section as they are almost certainly coded by the viral genome. These virion antigens include MA of EBV- and HSV-transformed cells. However, there is a considerable argument concerning the origin of nonvirion antigens in DNA-virus-transformed cells. Two schools of thought have developed: (1) that the antigens are derepressed host cell proteins, and (2) that antigens are coded by the virus genome.

A. Origin of Intracellular Antigens

There is evidence suggesting that the nonvirion T antigen present in SV40-transformed or tumor cells and produced during the virus cytolytic cycle is coded by the virus genome. The fact that antigenically identical T antigen is produced in all transformed and infected cells regardless of species of origin is indicative of the role of the virus genome in the synthesis of T antigen. Another line of evidence (Oxman and Black, 1966) showing that the synthesis of SV40 T antigen is inhibited by interferon suggested that a prereplicative SV40 gene product is required for the production of T antigen during the viral lytic cycle. Along the same lines, the synthesis of T antigen was induced in permissive cells upon microinjection with RNA complementary to SV40 DNA transcribed *in vitro*. The synthesis could, however, be blocked by prior treatment of cells with interferon (Graessmann *et al.*, 1974).

Recently, evidence has been presented which more strongly suggests that T antigen is coded by the virus genome. It has been demonstrated that SV40 A gene is involved in the initiation of DNA synthesis in permissive cells (Tegtmeyer, 1972) and is involved in the maintenance of the transformed-cell phenotype. Cells transformed by the *tsA* mutants show a transformed cell phenotype at the permissive temperature. However, at nonpermissive temperatures, the transformed cells revert back to the normal cell phenotype (Brugge and Butel, 1975; Kimura and Itagaki, 1975; Martin and Chou, 1975; Osborn and Weber, 1975; Tegtmeyer, 1975). Concomitant with the reversion of the transformed cell to a normal state, the T antigen in the nucleus of cells transformed by *tsA* mutants is not detected at a normal level at the nonpermissive temperature (Osborn and Weber, 1975). Additionally, the T antigen isolated from permissive cells infected by *tsA* mutants has a differing sedimentation value at the permissive and nonpermissive temperatures (Osborn and Weber, 1975). Recently, Tegtmeyer *et al.* (1975) have isolated a protein of 100,000 molecular weight from *tsA*-infected and -transformed cells at nonpermissive temperature by precipitation with sera from tumor-bearing hamsters which contain activity against the T antigen. This 100,000 dalton protein is overproduced in cells infected or transformed by *tsA* mutants at nonpermissive temperature and is rapidly degraded in the transformed or infected cells. Since the protein is large enough to account for the entire coding capacity of the early region of the SV40 genome and since the *tsA* mutants have been mapped in this region (Lai and Nathans, 1974), the obvious conclusion is that it is coded by the *tsA* gene. Its precipitation by antibodies to SV40 T antigen indicates that T antigen is the product of the *tsA* gene. However, the possibility (Osborn and Weber, 1975) exists that gene A may code for a protein that modifies or induces a host-cell protein that has the antigenicity of T antigen.

T antigen induced by DNA viruses has been thought to be specific for the transforming virus. Thus, the SV40 T antigen failed to cross-react with T antigen induced by other DNA viruses until recently, when it was shown to cross-react with T antigens induced by the newly isolated human papovaviruses. Besides T antigen, viral antigens of the human papovaviruses (EK, JC, and BK) also cross-react with SV40 virion antigens. A study (Khoury *et al.,* 1975) has demonstrated that SV40 and BK virus DNA share 10–20% of their nucleotide sequences. The shared nucleotide sequences were found to be located exclusively in the late region of the genome, which might account for the cross-reactivity of virion proteins between BK and SV40 but does not explain the strong cross-reactivity between the T antigens of two viruses (which is determined by the early region of the genome). The authors raise several possibilities: (1) T antigen is not virus coded but is induced as a result of virus–host-cell interaction and (2) the hybridization technique used was not sensitive enough to detect a limited homology in the early regions of SV40 and BK virus genomes, which may account for the antigenic cross-reactivity.

T antigen from cells transformed by the *tsA* mutant of polyoma virus has also been demonstrated to be temperature sensitive by the complement-fixation test (Paulin and Cuzin, 1975) and by the IF test in polyoma *tsA*-infected permissive cells at the nonpermissive temperature (Oxman *et al.,* 1972).

No information is available at this time concerning whether or not EBNA, which is a nonvirion EBV-induced antigen and is present in all cell lines containing EBV DNA, is coded by the viral genome.

B. Origin of Cell-Surface Antigens

Those DNA viruses that are released from cells by budding modify the plasma membrane of infected cells. Herpesviruses, among DNA tumor viruses, fall into this category (Klein, 1973; Roizman and Kieff, 1975). The altered antigenicity of the plasma membrane of herpesvirus-infected cells is due to the virion glycoproteins synthesized in the infected cells (Roizman and Kieff, 1975). Thus, the virion glycoproteins act as transplantation antigens in cells transformed by herpesviruses and the host responds by making either a cellular or a humoral immune response to these antigens on the membrane of transformed cells. It is now clear that the membrane antigens in EBV-transformed or HSV-transformed cells are virion in nature (Klein, 1973; Rapp, 1974). The only exception may be the cell membrane antigen described in Marek's-disease-virus-induced lymphoma cell lines (Witter *et al.*, 1975). Preliminary evidence indicates that this might be a nonvirion antigen. However, since MD virion glycoproteins have not been as extensively characterized as those of HSV, the possibility that the membrane antigen on MD lymphoma cells is a virion antigen cannot be ruled out.

Papovaviruses and adenoviruses, on the other hand, are nonenveloped viruses and thus are not released from productively infected cells by budding; yet cells infected or transformed abortively or permanently by these DNA viruses undergo cell membrane changes which confer new antigenicity upon the infected or transformed cells (for reviews, see Sambrook, 1973; Tevethia and Tevethia, 1975*a,b*). The origin of the antigens in SV40-transformed cells has been a subject of controversy. The early region of SV40 DNA can code for 100,000-dalton protein, and the nonvirion T antigen, if it is assumed to be coded solely by the viral genome, might account for at least 70,000 daltons (Tegtmeyer *et al.*, 1975). One still needs to account for the SV40 TrAg which is present at the surface of all transformed cells that contain SV40 DNA and U antigen associated with the nuclear membrane.

The TrAg in SV40-transformed cells is specified by the early region of the virus genome. The evidence for this statement comes from the studies with adenovirus–SV40 hybrid viruses which contain varying amounts of early SV40 DNA (Lewis and Rowe, 1973). None of these viruses induces SV40 virion antigens. The hybrid viruses (Ad2$^+$ND4 and E46$^+$) contain 43% and 75% of the SV40 genome and induce SV40 TrAg in hamster cells (Rapp *et al.*, 1966; Lewis and Rowe, 1973). The SV40 DNA in the hybrid virus (Ad2$^+$ND4) can be localized in the early region of the SV40 genome (Kelly and Lewis, 1973). Since the entire early SV40 region may code for T antigen, it is possible that TrAg specific for SV40 may be a glycosylated T antigen. Several lines of evidence indicate that this may not be the case: (1) a nondefective adenovirus–SV40 hybrid virus (Ad2$^+$ND2) which contains 32% of the SV40 genome induces SV40 TrAg and U antigen but does not induce the synthesis of SV40 T antigen, whereas Ad2$^+$ND4 induces both T and TrAg, suggesting that the regions of SV40 which specify T and TrAg may be different, and (2) a cell line transformed by PARA-12 has been described which contains both SV40 T and TrAg. However, hamsters bearing tumors induced by this cell line become immunologically tolerant to T antigen and yet develop a good immune response to SV40 TrAg (Lausch *et al.*, 1970). It will be important to test the ability of the *tsA* mutant of SV40 for the synthesis of SV40 TrAg at the nonpermissive temperature, as the *tsA* gene product has been shown to be involved in the maintenance of the transformed state and may be the T antigen.

Since the TrAg and the S antigen(s) are both present at the cell surface, it has been tempting to assume that the *in vitro* serological tests are actually measuring TrAg. Tevethia *et al.* (1968*b*) demonstrated the lack of relationship between TrAg and S antigen in certain hamster cell lines that became oncogenic after exposure to SV40 (Diamandopoulos *et al.*, 1968). Some of these cell lines, although positive for S antigen, were found to be negative for detectable TrAg. The S^+TrAg^- cells were later shown to lack detectable amounts of both SV40 messenger RNA (Levin *et al.*, 1969) and SV40 DNA (Levine *et al.*, 1970), suggesting that the S antigen in these cells may not be coded by a persisting viral genome.

The possibility has been considered that SV40 TrAg is coded by the host-cell genome and represents a derepressed host protein (Coggin and Anderson, 1974). This conclusion was based on the following observations: (1) immunization with fetal tissue from midgestational period interrupts primary SV40 tumorigenesis in hamsters and also elicits a state of resistance in adult male hamsters against a challenge of SV40 tumor cells (Coggin *et al.*, 1971; Girardi *et al.*, 1973); (2) pregnant hamsters develop antibody which is cytostatic for SV40 tumor cells and also develop sensitized lymphocytes reactive with SV40 tumor cells (Coggin and Anderson, 1974); (3) the fetal antigen from hamster embryos capable of inducing tumor resistance was found not to be species-specific as mouse and human embryo cells could also elicit resistance (Ambrose *et al.*, 1971).

The data published so far suggest that during transformation of cells by SV40 an embryonic antigen appears at the cell surface. Indeed, more than one embryonic antigen may be present (Ting *et al.*, 1973). The data also suggest that the embryonic antigens under certain circumstances induce a cellular immune response in the host which may delay the appearance of either primary or transplanted SV40 tumors. The published data strongly suggest, however, that the weakly immunogenic embryonic antigens are distinct from the virus-specific transplantation antigen: (1) immunization of an adult host with either live virus or irradiated tumor cells results in the development of specific cellular immune responses to the TrAg specified by the particular virus (Zarling and Tevethia, 1973*a*); (2) specific immunity *in vivo* using irradiated tumor cells is stronger than the immunity induced by the fetal cells (Girardi *et al.*, 1973); (3) only male hamsters develop a detectable rejection response upon immunization with fetal cells, whereas both males and females can be immunized rather easily to TrAg (Dierlam *et al.*, 1971), either with live virus or with irradiated tumor cells (Girardi *et al.*, 1973).

The evidence discussed above indicates that embryonic antigens as well as specific TrAg are present at the surface of SV40-transformed cells. The origin of TrAg is still unresolved. The finding that TrAg appears during the infectious cycle (Girardi and Defendi, 1970; Tevethia and Tevethia, 1976) indicates that SV40 plays an active role in the production of TrAg. Several possibilities as to the genetic origin of TrAg exist: (1) TrAg may be a host protein which is derepressed by an SV40 gene product; (2) an SV40 gene product may modify a normal cell protein, thereby converting it to TrAg; (3) TrAg may be a protein translated from a heterogenomic messenger RNA, a product of the integrated SV40 DNA containing both host and viral sequences; or (4) TrAg may itself be the product of an SV40 gene. The use of *ts* and deletion mutants of SV40, which are defective in the synthesis of TrAg, may be needed to resolve the role of the viral genome in the production, maintenance, and expression of TrAg in transformed cells.

IX. IMMUNE RESPONSE OF THE HOST
TO DNA-TUMOR-VIRUS-INDUCED ANTIGENS

Hosts undergoing spontaneous or induced neoplasia by DNA tumor viruses under natural or experimental conditions respond immunologically to the antigens (intracellular and cell surface) associated with transformed or tumor cells. Depending upon the nature and magnitude, the immune response will greatly influence the neoplastic growth. In this section, we review the role of immune response to tumor-associated antigens in the progression and regression of DNA-virus-induced tumors.

A. Papovaviruses (SV40 and Polyoma)

1. Intracellular Antigens

Two major distinct antigens (T and U) are located intracellularly in SV40-transformed or tumor cells. Hamsters bearing tumors induced either by SV40 or virus-free SV40 tumor or transformed cells develop antibodies to intranuclear T and U antigens. The amount of antibody to T antigen, located in the γ_2 fraction of 7 S immunoglobulins (Tevethia, 1967) does not correlate with the tumor mass. However, animals bearing tumors usually develop antibody to T antigen. Not all animals which bear large tumors develop T antibody, however. It was demonstrated (Lausch *et al.,* 1970) that hamsters bearing tumors induced by a particular line of SV40 tumor cells did not develop antibodies to T antigen

during the entire course of tumor development. This immunological unresponsiveness to T antigen was shown to be due to the immunological tolerance to T
antigen which could be terminated by tumor resection and reimmunization with
tumor homogenate in Freund's complete adjuvant. The antibodies to T antigen
in hamsters have also been shown to develop in the absence of a visible tumor
(Diamandopoulos and McLane, 1974).

Antibodies to SV40 T antigen also develop in the permissive natural host in
the absence of a detectable tumor (Rapp *et al.*, 1967; Vonka *et al.*, 1967). The
synthesis of antibodies to T antigen in a semipermissive host (rabbit) was
demonstrated to depend upon the dose of infecting virus. Using a rabbit as a
model animal, in which the virus both replicates and transforms cells, it was
demonstrated (Tevethia, 1970) that infection of adult rabbits with a low dose of
SV40 resulted in the synthesis of antibodies to virion antigens only, whereas the
inoculation of rabbits via the intravenous route with a high dose of SV40
particles resulted in the synthesis of antibodies to T and V antigens. The
antibodies to T and V antigens fix complement (for review, see Butel *et al.*,
1972; Tevethia and Tevethia, 1975a; Tevethia, 1975).

2. Cell-Surface Antigens

Adult animals immunized by either live virus or virus-free tumor or transformed cells become resistant to the transplantation of syngeneic virus-free
tumor cells (Sjögren *et al.*, 1961; Habel, 1962; Khera *et al.*, 1963; Defendi,
1963; Habel and Eddy, 1963; Deichman and Kluchareva, 1964). Similarly,
hamsters undergoing primary SV40 tumorigenesis can be immunized by inoculation during the latent period with live virus (Goldner *et al.*, 1964) or with
virus-transformed cells (Girardi, 1965; Tevethia *et al.*, 1968b; Coggin *et al.*,
1970). Syngeneic animals bearing tumors induced by SV40- or polyoma-virus-
transformed cells also develop concomitant immunity to the transplantation of
syngeneic tumors at sites other than the site of primary tumor growth (Lausch
and Rapp, 1971; Sjögren and Bansal, 1971; Zarling and Tevethia, 1973a).

The rejection of papovavirus-induced tumors by the immunized syngeneic
host is mediated by the lymphoid cells (for review, see Hellström and Hellström,
1974; Tevethia and Tevethia, 1975a; Tevethia *et al.*, 1976). The cellular basis of
resistance to DNA-virus-induced tumors has been demonstrated by showing the
ability of lymphoid cells from SV40-virus- or tumor-cell-immunized mice to
protect against the transplantation of syngeneic SV40 tumor cells. The immune
lymphoid cells have been demonstrated to be present in the spleen, lymph
nodes, and peritoneal cavity of virus-immunized and tumor-bearing mice (Zarling
and Tevethia, 1973a). The reactivity of lymphocytes immune to SV40 TrAg was
specific in nature since neither adenovirus 7-induced tumors nor a spontaneously
oncogenic cell line were inhibited. Inhibition of tumor growth by polyoma

tumor cells was also shown to be inhibited by lymphocytes which were immune to polyoma-specific TrAg (Habel, 1962; Sjögren, 1964). Kinetics studies have shown that the immune lymphocytes, which are capable of inhibiting SV40 tumor cells *in vivo,* appear between 7 and 14 days after virus immunization and between 5 and 11 days after tumor transplantation (Zarling and Tevethia, 1973*a*; Tevethia and Tevethia, 1976).

A cellular immune response of the host to SV40- and polyoma-virus-induced tumors has also been demonstrated by the *in vitro* colony inhibition test (Smith *et al.,* 1970; Datta and Vandeputte, 1971; Coggin *et al.,* 1974; Sjögren and Borum, 1971; Howell *et al.,* 1974) and by the *in vitro* macrophage migration inhibition test (Blasecki and Tevethia, 1973, 1975*a*). The data obtained in the macrophase migration inhibition test correlated with the *in vivo* tumor inhibitory activity of lymphoid cells. Polyoma virus oncogenesis could also be interrupted by the adoptive transfer of immune lymphocytes to susceptible animals (Law *et al.,* 1967).

The nature of the cellular immune response to SV40- and polyoma-virus-specific cell-surface transplantation antigens has been elucidated by the use of thymectomized animals. The thymus plays a determining role in resistance to viral carcinogenesis. Neonatal thymectomy of the resistant strains of mice has been shown to increase the incidence of virus-induced tumors in mice (Vandeputte *et al.,* 1963; Law, 1966; Allison and Taylor, 1967). Similarly, mice which lack T-cell functions are more susceptible to polyoma virus oncogenesis as compared to their immunocompetent littermates (Vandeputte *et al.,* 1974; Allison *et al.,* 1974; Stutman, 1975). The susceptibility of nude mice to polyoma virus oncogenesis is, however, age dependent. It has also been demonstrated that SV40-inoculated hamsters thymectomized at 7 days of age cannot be immunized during the latent period with SV40-transformed cells carrying SV40 TrAg (Girardi and Roosa, 1967). Further, treatment of the host with antithymocyte serum resulted in enhanced susceptibility to viral oncogenesis (Allison and Law, 1968; Vandeputte, 1969), and sensitization of adult hamsters to TrAg by SV40 could be prevented by treatment of animals with antithymocyte serum (Tevethia *et al.,* 1968*c*).

These studies have indicated that thymus-derived lymphocytes play a determining role in resistance to SV40 and polyoma virus oncogenesis. The role of T cells in the cellular immune response to SV40 tumors has been demonstrated by Tevethia *et al.* (1974), who showed that BALB/c mice (thymectomized, lethally irradiated, and reconstituted, TIR, with bone marrow cells) did not develop sensitized lymphocytes in the spleens upon SV40 immunization. The absence of sensitized lymphocytes in the spleens of SV40-immunized TIR mice was demonstrated by their inability to inhibit tumor development by SV40 tumor cells *in vivo.* The immunized TIR mice did lack θ-positive cells in their spleens. Further, the activity of spleen cells which are capable of inhibiting tumor cells *in vivo* from SV40-immunized mice could be abolished by treatment with anti-θ sera and complement, indicating that T cells are essential for inhibition of SV40 tumor cells *in vivo*. Similar data have been reported by Howell *et al.* (1974).

Although there is overwhelming evidence available for the role of T cells in the cellular immune response to SV40 and polyoma tumor cells, some evidence for the involvement of non-T cells in tumor inhibition is also available. First the susceptibility of nude mice which lack T cells to polyoma virus oncogenesis was found to be age dependent (Vandeputte *et al.,* 1974; Stutman, 1975). The resistance to polyoma virus oncogenesis could be transferred with B cells (Stutman, 1975). Further evidence for the participation of B cells was demonstrated by Sjögren and Borum (1971), who showed that lymph node cells from thymectomized animals bearing polyoma-virus-induced tumors were reactive against polyoma-virus-transformed cells *in vitro*. It is not clear at this time whether the B-cell killing of target cells was mediated by antibody. In a recent report, Lausch *et al.* (1975a) have demonstrated killing of SV40 hamster tumor cells *in vitro* by normal hamster lymphoid cells in the presence of sera from animals immunized with SV40 tumor cells.

Evidence is quite clear that T cells alone may bring about the rejection of allogeneic tumors both *in vitro* and *in vivo* (Cerottini and Brunner, 1974) and of some syngeneic tumors (Röllinghoff and Warner, 1973). However, there is increasing evidence for the participation of macrophages as effector cells in the rejection of antigenic tumors in syngeneic animals (for review, see Levy and Wheelock, 1974; Tevethia *et al.,* 1976).

Evidence has been gathered which shows that uncommitted bone-marrow-derived cells, probably macrophages, cooperate with sensitized T lymphocytes *in vivo* in the inhibition of SV40 tumor cells in BALB/c mice. This conclusion was based on the following observations: (1) a low number of sensitized lymphocytes, when mixed with syngeneic SV40 tumor cells in a ratio of 1:1 and inoculated into young adult BALB/c mice, prevented tumor formation by the SV40 tumor cells; (2) irradiated, sensitized lymphocytes, which were unable to replicate, inhibited tumor growth; (3) tumor growth inhibition by immune lymphocytes was less efficient in irradiated and in newborn mice; (4) bone marrow cells, after differentiation in irradiated (700 R) syngeneic hosts, provided the cells necessary for tumor-cell neutralization by immune T lymphocytes; and (5) tumor-cell inhibition by immune lymphocytes was diminished in animals pretreated with silica, a specific macrophage toxin (Tevethia and Zarling, 1972; Zarling and Tevethia, 1973b). Further, the presence of macrophages in tumors undergoing rejection has been demonstrated by histological and electron microscopic techniques (Tevethia *et al.,* 1976). The requirement for host cells in the inhibition of SV40 tumors in mice by sensitized lymphocytes has also been reported by Howell *et al.* (1974). *In vitro* studies by Zembala *et al.* (1973) have also demonstrated the requirement of normal macrophages for the destruction of polyoma-virus-induced tumors in the presence of sensitized lymphocytes. Thus it would appear that the efferent limb of cellular immunity to syngeneic SV40 and polyoma tumor cells may be more like that of delayed hypersensitivity reaction, in which macrophages have been assigned an unequivocal role (Mackaness, 1971; Tubergen and Feldman, 1971; Volkman and Collins, 1971). Macrophages also have been demonstrated to be involved in the rejection of chemically induced tumors (Zbar *et al.,* 1970; Evans and Grant, 1972; Nelson, 1974).

Animals bearing tumors induced by either the virus or virus-induced tumor cells have been demonstrated to develop resistance to the transplantation of syngeneic tumor cells; however, the primary tumor continues to grow (Zarling and Tevethia, 1973*a*). Tumor-bearing animals also possess lymphocytes capable of inhibiting the growth of syngeneic tumor cells *in vitro* (Sjögren and Borum, 1971; Datta and Vandeputte, 1971; Dierlam *et al.,* 1971) and *in vivo* (Zarling and Tevethia, 1973*a*). However, the presence of immune lymphocytes capable of inhibiting tumor cells *in vivo* may not always be detected at all stages of tumor growth in the tumor-bearing host (Mikulska *et al.,* 1966; Barski and Youn, 1969). In the SV40 tumor system, immunologically reactive lymphocytes were shown to be present in all anatomical locations in BALB/c mice bearing tumors induced by the SV40-transformed MKS-TU5 line (Zarling and Tevethia 1973*a*; Howell *et al.,* 1975), whereas in BALB/c mice bearing tumors induced by another line of SV40-transformed cells (VLM), immunologically active lymphocytes could not be demonstrated by the *in vivo* tumor-cell neutralization test (Blasecki and Tevethia, 1975*b*). In animals bearing very small tumors induced by VLM cells, immune lymphocytes were shown to be present by the macrophage migration inhibition test (Blasecki and Tevethia, 1975*a*). No cellular immune response could, however, be detected in BALB/c mice bearing large tumors induced by either of the two lines of SV40-transformed cells (TU-5 and VLM) until the tumors were removed by surgery (Blasecki and Tevethia, 1975*a,b*). By using the macrophage migration inhibition test, Blasecki and Tevethia (1975*a*) demonstrated that peritoneal cells from BALB/c mice bearing large VLM tumors, which were not inhibited by SV40-specific soluble TrAg, were capable of specifically blocking the migration inhibition of PE cells from mice immune to SV40 TrAg. Both the unresponsiveness and blocking capacity of cells from tumor-bearing mice could be abolished by culturing the PE cells *in vitro* for 4–5 days, thus suggesting that the sensitized lymphocytes are present in the tumor-bearing animals; however, the activity of these lymphocytes might be blocked. In a later study, Blasecki and Tevethia (1975*b*) demonstrated that lymphocytes from VLM-tumor-bearing mice which were shown to be unresponsive in the tumor-cell neutralization test could be specifically activated by brief treatment with proteolytic enzymes. Specific activation of lymphocytes from tumor-bearing animals has also been shown to occur after repeated washings (Coggin *et* *al.*, 1974) and after culturing *in vitro* for short (Laux and Lausch, 1974) and long (Blasecki and Tevethia, 1975*b*) periods.

The presence of blocking factors in the sera of animals bearing tumors induced by the polyoma virus has been demonstrated by the *in vitro* test (Sjögren and Borum, 1971; Sjögren and Bansal, 1971). The blocking activity in the serum of animals correlated with the status of the tumor-bearing host, being absent in immune or tumor-free animals and present in high amounts in animals bearing large tumors (Sjögren and Bansal, 1971). Further, the tumor growth was facilitated by the sera from tumor-bearing animals shown to contain blocking factors (Bansal *et al.*, 1972). The action of the blocking factors in the sera of tumor-bearing animals could be neutralized by "unblocking" sera made in rats or rabbits immunized with BCG and polyoma tumor cells (Bansal and Sjögren, 1971). It was further demonstrated that the inoculation of unblocking sera into rats transplanted with syngeneic polyoma-virus-induced tumors prevented the appearance of blocking activity in the sera of the recipient and also induced regression of the transplanted tumor (Bansal and Sjögren, 1971). Unblocking sera were also shown to inhibit the development of primary polyoma virus-induced kidney sarcomas in splenectomized rats (Bansal and Sjögren, 1972). The nature of the blocking and unblocking factors remains unknown.

B. Other Papovaviruses and Adenoviruses

Rabbit papilloma virus induces papillomas in rabbits which, as a rule, regress spontaneously but occasionally go on to develop into carcinomas. The spontaneous regression of papillomas is immunologically mediated since the animals in which the papillomas have regressed are immune to the development of further papillomas (Evans *et al.*, 1962; Evans and Ito, 1966). Hellström *et al.* (1969) were able to demonstrate sensitized lymphocytes in rabbits in which papillomas had regressed spontaneously, as well as in rabbits with persistent papillomas. These sensitized lymphocytes were able to inhibit cells derived either from papillomas or from carcinomas in a colony inhibition test. Sera from persistent animals but not from regressor animals abrogated the lymphocyte-mediated cytotoxicity, suggesting the presence of blocking factors in the sera of tumor-bearing rabbits.

Warts in humans are viral in origin and also regress spontaneously. A correlation between antibodies to virion antigen and the regression of warts has been made (Pyrhönen and Johansson, 1975). Not much information is available with regard to the existence of a nonvirion TrAg in wart-virus-induced papillomas because of the unavailability of cell cultures derived from wart tissue.

Studies similar to those on the immune response of the host to SV40- and polyoma-virus-induced tumors have also been reported in adenovirus tumor systems. Cells transformed or tumors induced by adenoviruses contain virus-specific transplantation antigens which induce a rejection response in the immunized host (Trentin and Bryan, 1966; Sjögren et al., 1967; Berman, 1967; Kaplan et al., 1971). The rejection response is cell mediated (Berman, 1967; Sjögren et al., 1967; Hellström and Sjögren, 1967).

C. Herpesviruses

1. Herpes Simplex and Cytomegalovirus

HSV-1 and HSV-2 induce transformation in vitro of hamster cells after inactivation with ultraviolet light or after photodynamic inactivation (Duff and Rapp, 1971, 1973; Rapp et al., 1973). These in vitro transformed cells produce progressively growing tumors at the site of inoculation which metastasize to the lung and other organs. HSV-transformed cells have also been demonstrated to possess a virion antigen at the cell surface which is an HSV-specific glycoprotein (C. Reed et al., 1975). The ability of the cell-surface antigen in HSV-transformed cells to act as transplantation rejection test was tested in syngeneic hamsters. It was reported (Duff et al., 1973) that immunization of adult hamsters with HSV or HSV-transformed cells did not affect the growth of subcutaneous tumors. The results on the incidence of metastasis in the lungs of HSV-2-tumor-bearing hamsters which were preimmunized with HSV-2 or with transformed cells indicated that the preimmunization of hamsters by HSV resulted in an enhancement of metastasis in these animals. Significant decrease in the incidence of metastasis was observed in animals preimmunized with UV-irradiated HSV-2-transformed or normal hamster embryo fibroblasts. Immunization of hamsters with SV40 completely inhibited metastases by HSV-transformed cells (Rapp and Duff, 1973; Duff et al., 1973). The authors interpreted their results to indicate that HSV-transformed cells contain cell-surface antigens which are unable to function as rejection antigens and the inhibition of metastases after preimmunization with SV40 might be due to a common embryonic antigen. The alternate explanation by the authors (Rapp and Li, 1974) was that the inhibition of metastases after preimmunization with SV40 might be due to the nonspecific resistance induced in the immunized animals. A recent study (Sadowski and Rapp, 1975) showed that the incidence of metastases to lung by HSV-transformed cells could be inhibited by Levamisole, an immunopotentiator. These studies have indicated that antigens associated with HSV-1- and -2-transformed cells are not strong enough to induce transplantation immunity in hamsters. Hamsters immunized by HSV or animals bearing tumors induced by HSV-1- and -2-transformed cells, however, do develop cellular immunity which can be demonstrated by the in vitro microcytotoxicity assay (Lausch et al.,

1975*b*). Spleen cells from tumor-bearing hamsters killed homologous tumor cells but not normal hamster cells or cells transformed by SV40. Sera from tumor-bearing hamsters blocked the lymphocyte-mediated cytotoxicity.

Studies similar to those on the immune response of hamsters to antigens associated with HSV-transformed cells have also been carried out in hamsters bearing tumors induced by CMV-transformed cells. Spleen cells from hamsters bearing tumors induced by CMV-transformed cells specifically inhibited CMV-transformed cells *in vitro* and sera from tumor-bearing hamsters blocked lymphocyte-mediated cytotoxicity. The surface antigens in CMV-transformed cells are too weak to act as rejection antigens (Murasko and Lausch, 1974; Murasko, 1975).

2. Marek's Disease Virus

Chickens infected with MDV develop antibodies to the virus which can be detected by the indirect immunofluorescence, virus neutralization, immunodiffusion, and complement-fixation tests (for review, see Nazerian, 1973; Biggs, 1973; Purchase, 1974). The magnitude of the antibody response correlates with the age of birds when infected by MDV (Witter *et al.*, 1971). However, a deficiency in the humoral immune response of naturally resistant chickens did not alter their resistance to MDV (Sharma and Witter, 1975). It is becoming evident that cell-mediated immunity plays a determining role, since the chickens which are deficient in T-cell functions do not resist MDV-induced tumors. MD can be successfully prevented by vaccination of susceptible chickens with a herpesvirus of turkeys (HVT) (Okazaki *et al.*, 1970). HVT is apathogenic for turkeys and is nononcogenic for avian and mammalian species (Witter, 1972). Chickens vaccinated with HVT at the time of hatching develop a lifelong resistance to MDV-induced neoplastic disease. However, vaccinated chickens that are resistant to lymphoma development by MDV still support the replication of MDV (Purchase and Okazaki, 1971). The mechanism of protection by vaccination of MDV-induced lymphoma is not clear. However, it has been demonstrated that cell-mediated immunity plays a determining role in the protection of vaccinated chickens, since cyclophosphamide-treated chickens cannot be vaccinated by HVT against MD (Purchase and Sharma, 1974). The observation that bursectomy did not prevent the protecting effect of vaccination indicated that immunity may not be mediated by B cells (Else, 1974). There is some evidence that the antigenic determinant to which cellular immunity may be directed may be the nonvirion antigen present at the surface of lymphoblastoid cell lines derived from MD lymphomas which contain the viral genome (Witter *et al.*, 1975). Powell (1975) was able to immunize chickens against MD by glutaraldehyde-fixed lymphoma cells that contained nonvirion cell-surface antigen. Immunization of chickens with chicken kidney cells infected by MDV also protected against lymphoma development by MDV. The available evidence

(Powell, 1975) indicates that immunity to MDV may result in the restriction of infection, thus reducing the probability of malignant transformation of T lymphocytes, and that cellular immunity by T cells to nonvirion antigen at the surface of transformed lymphocytes may lead to the rejection of potentially transformed cells.

3. Epstein-Barr Virus

EBV is involved both in IM and BL, and patients suffering from both diseases respond immunologically to EBV-specified nonvirion (EBNA, EA) and virion (VCA, MA) antigens (W. Henle and G. Henle, 1973, 1974; Klein, 1973). Infection with EBV is widespread in the general population and is acquired in early childhood under lower socioeconomic conditions. The infected individuals acquire antibodies directed against EBV capsid antigens and also develop neutralizing antibodies. Individuals positive for EBV antibodies become immune to IM (Niederman et al., 1968). During the course of illness, antibodies to VCA, MA, and neutralizing antibodies develop which persist for long periods of time (G. Henle et al., 1968; Klein et al., 1968; Niederman et al., 1968; Miller et al., 1972). Antibodies to EA also develop during the acute phase of illness and decline rapidly after recovery (G. Henle et al., 1971). Antibodies to the D component of the EA complex are most prevalent in IM patients (G. Henle et al., 1971; W. Henle and G. Henle, 1974). Since healthy individuals contain antibodies to VCA and neutralizing antibodies but no antibody to EA, the demonstration of significant levels of EA antibodies in patients is indicative of current primary infection.

Antibodies to the nonvirion antigen (EBNA) appear much later in IM patients than the antibodies to VCA and EA, and persist for life (G. Henle et al., 1974). Antibodies to EBNA were also demonstrated in individuals with antibody to viral capsid antigens. Similar findings have also been reported with regard to antibodies to soluble antigen (Vonka et al., 1972).

During the course of infectious mononucleosis, atypical lymphocytes of T-cell origin are present in the circulation in large numbers. These T cells have now been shown to be the effector cells in cell-mediated immunity to membrane antigens associated with lymphoblastoid cell lines carrying EBV genome (Svedmyr and Jondal, 1975), indicating that the cell-mediated immunity may play an important role in limiting the proliferation of EBV-transformed lymphoid cells of B origin.

BL patients also develop an immune response to EBV-determined antigens. All patients have high antibody titers to VCA as compared to a control population (G. Henle et al., 1969). BL patients develop antibodies to EA, and they are directed predominantly to the R component (W. Henle et al., 1970, 1973). EA antibodies are present in higher titers in tumor-bearing patients than in tumor-free patients. Recurrence of the disease in remission patients is accompanied by a rise in anti-EA antibody titers. BL patients consistently develop antibodies to nonvirion nuclear antigen (EBNA). Antibodies to MA are also present in BL patients and they remain constant throughout the course of the disease. However, a decrease in anti-MA antibody titers at the time of recurrence, followed by a rise, has been observed (Klein *et al.,* 1969; Gunvén *et al.,* 1974). The decrease in anti-MA antibody titers is probably due to the absorption of antibody by the tumor cells. IgG eluted from the tumor cells has been shown to be directed to EBV-specified MA (Hewetson *et al.,* 1972). Whether the coating of BL cells *in vivo* with antibody leads to tumor enhancement is not known.

Convincing evidence exists which shows that an immune response plays a determining role in the regression of BL. Spontaneous regressions of the tumors in BL patients have been reported (Burkitt and Kyalwazi, 1967). Also, patients cured by chemotherapy survive for a long period of time (Clifford *et al.,* 1967), and delayed hypersensitivity reactions to autologous tumor-cell extracts have been observed in BL patients (Fass *et al.,* 1970). Recently, Jondal *et al.* (1975) have demonstrated the presence of T cells in a biopsy of BL, which were shown to be cytotoxic to autologous tumor cells and to the EBV-positive cell lines.

X. ROLE OF DNA-VIRUS-INDUCED ANTIGENS IN NEOPLASIA

Cells derived from tumors induced by viruses, chemical carcinogens, and physical agents, and from human tumors of unknown etiology, synthesize macromolecules that normal adult cells do not. Only those macromolecules that are antigenic in the autochthonous host and to which the host reacts by making either a humoral or a cellular immune response are involved in immunoregulation of tumor growth. Specific antigens in tumor cells, depending upon their location in the cells and upon the nature and magnitude of the immune response being elicited by the host against these antigens, will determine the tumor behavior *in vivo.*

The antigens that are located within the cells, such as T antigens in the nucleus of SV40θ and adenovirus-transformed cells, and EBNA in BL cells, do not play any role in the immunological modulation of the growth of DNA virus-induced tumors. EA antigen, an EBV-determined intracellular antigen, can also be ruled out because of its location in the transformed cells and its absence in the cells derived from biopsy of BL. However, as pointed out earlier, the magnitude of the immune response to intracellular antigens such as EA can be used to predict tumor growth *in vivo.*

Surface antigens, by virtue of their location at the surface of transformed or tumor cells, do play a very significant role in the progression and regression of DNA-virus-induced neoplasia. Surface antigens in DNA-virus-transformed cells may be a component of either virion or virus-specific nonvirion antigens. Additionally, tumor cells may express cross-reactive embryonic antigens at the cell surface. All of these classes of surface antigens may affect tumor growth in some manner.

Virion antigens have been demonstrated at the surface of cells transformed by viruses belonging to the herpesvirus group. Thus, cells derived from BL contain MA which are virion components, and a virion glycoprotein has been demonstrated at the surface of HSV-transformed cells. The virion antigens as a rule induce the synthesis of virus-neutralizing antibodies in the tumor-bearing host. The neutralizing antibodies may limit the spread of infectious virus in the permissive host in which the virus both replicates and transforms cells. Thus individuals with antibodies to EBV become immune to IM. The incidence of IM in Africans is significantly lower than elsewhere (Klein, 1973).

There are several lines of evidence that indicate that virion antigens at the cell surface do play an important role in the rejection of DNA-virus-induced tumors. In the case of Shope-fibroma-induced tumors, where regression of tumors in adult rabbits is common, the regressions may be mediated by the immune response to virion antigens at the cell surface (Tompkins et al., 1970a,b). The development of complement-dependent cytotoxic antibodies to antigens at the surface of fibroma-virus-infected cells has been demonstrated to correlate with tumor regression in vivo (Singh et al., 1973). The virion antigens at the surface of virus-transformed cells may also mediate the rejection of developing tumors induced by rabbit papilloma virus, human wart virus, simian herpesviruses, and EBV. The mechanism by which antibodies to the virion antigens may mediate the rejection of a tumor is not known at this time. It can, however, be speculated that either K or B cells may act as killer cells in the presence of antibodies. Antibody-dependent lymphocyte destruction of cells infected by herpesvirus saimiri has been demonstrated (Prevost et al., 1975); similar results with SV40-transformed hamster cells have been obtained in vitro (Lausch et al., 1975a). The virion antigens at the cell surface may also participate in T-cell-mediated cytotoxic killing of target cells (Svedmyr and Jondal, 1975).

The humoral immune response to virion antigens at the surface of tumor cells may also be involved in the protection of tumors from immune destruction by sensitized lymphocytes. Thus BL cells from biopsy are often coated with antibodies to EBV-determined membrane antigens (Klein, 1973).

It is not always the case that the virion antigens present at the surface of virus-transformed cells induce a rejection response in vivo. Both HSV- and CMV-transformed cells are not rejected by the HSV- or CMV-immunized syngeneic hamsters (Rapp and Duff, 1973; Murasko, 1975).

The nonvirion surface antigens associated with papovavirus- and adenovirus-transformed cells induce a rejection response in the host which leads to the inhibition of tumor growth. Animals receiving virus as newborns develop tumors after a long latent period; however, immunization during the latent period with either the virus or virus-transformed cells will prevent the appearance of tumors at the site of inoculation. The lack of tumor development in adult animals and tumor development in immunosuppressed adults upon virus administration indicates that an antigen (TrAg) is synthesized in the transformed and infected cells which induces a specific cellular immune response in the host. The appearance of TrAg *in vitro* at the surface of mouse cells abortively infected with SV40 has been demonstrated by specifically sensitizing normal lymphocytes *in vitro* by cultivating them on the SV40-infected cell monolayers. The sensitized lymphocytes inhibited the growth of SV40-transformed cells *in vivo*, indicating that the sequence of events observed *in vitro* actually takes place *in vivo* upon virus inoculation (Tevethia and Tevethia, 1976).

The immune response to TrAg may also affect the behavior of tumor cells *in vivo*. The tumor cells may develop immunoresistance. In this case tumor cells, although themselves immunogenic, are not rejected by the immunized host. When primary SV40 tumors are allowed to grow for prolonged time periods, the cells derived from these tumors and from metastases were claimed to have lost TrAg, since these cells were not rejected by the SV40-immunized hamsters (Deichman and Kluchareva, 1966). It was later demonstrated (Tevethia *et al.*, 1971) that such tumor cells possess TrAg and could immunize hamsters against a challenge of immunosensitive SV40 tumor cells but they could not be rejected by the immunized hamsters.

The TrAg release *in vivo* from the tumor cells may block the activity of sensitized lymphocytes, thus allowing the developing tumor to escape immune destruction (Thompson *et al.*, 1975). Although there is no direct evidence available which might indicate that the soluble TrAg from DNA-virus-transformed cells can block lymphocyte reactivity, indirect experimental evidence has indicated that the soluble antigen may play a role in the inhibition of lymphocyte reactivity. Sensitized lymphocytes can be demonstrated in animals either immunized by the virus or bearing small tumors induced by the SV40-transformed cells but cannot be detected in animals bearing large tumors (Blasecki and Tevethia, 1975b; Howell *et al.*, 1975). The lymphocytes capable of inhibiting syngeneic tumors can, however, be reactivated by extensive washing (Coggin *et al.*, 1974) or culturing *in vitro*, or by treatment of lymphocytes with low concentrations of proteolytic enzymes (Blasecki and Tevethia, 1975b), thus suggesting that the sensitized lymphocytes are present in the tumor-bearing animals but their activity is blocked, most probably by the soluble TrAg.

DNA-virus-transformed cells also possess cross-reacting embryonic antigens at the cell surface (for review, see Coggin and Anderson, 1974; Tevethia, 1975). Although experimental evidence does indicate that embryonic antigens might induce a weak resistance against tumor transplantation and tumor induction by SV40 (Coggin and Anderson, 1974), the resistance induced is not strong enough to prevent tumor induction and tumor transplantation *in vivo.* The cell-mediated immunity to embryonic antigens can, however, be demonstrated by the *in vitro* microcytotoxicity test (Hellström and Hellström, 1975*a,b*). No parallel experiments were carried out to determine whether the *in vitro* reactivity of lymphocytes sensitized to embryonic antigens correlated with *in vivo* rejection response. It is quite possible that immunity to embryonic antigens may play a minor role in regulating tumor growth.

XI. CONCLUSIONS

Virus-specific antigens associated with DNA-virus-transformed cells have several functions in studies of viral carcinogenesis. The presence of specific intracellular antigens in tumor cells, such as the intranuclear T antigen in papovavirus-transformed cells and EBNA in EBV-transformed cells, and the appearance of the identical antigen in the virus productive cycle indicate that the transformation, whether *in vitro* or *in vivo,* was caused by a particular oncogenic virus. The immune response to T antigen, EBNA, and EA in the tumor-bearing host is also helpful in following viral oncogenesis. The synthesis of T antigen and EBNA, whether in permissive or nonpermissive cells, has served as a marker for early viral functions.

Cells transformed by DNA tumor viruses also possess specific antigens at the cell surface. These antigen(s) can be detected by the classical transplantation-rejection test *in vivo* and by *in vitro* techniques which measure cellular immune reaction and by serological tests. Cell-surface antigens mediate the development of a cellular immune response in the host which leads to the rejection of developing tumors. The development of specific surface antigens in the virus cytolytic cycle indicates that the transformation of cells is not a prerequisite for their appearance. The existence of specific cell-surface antigens and cross-reactive embryonic antigens, which induce tumor immunity, offers an excellent opportunity for immunoregulation of virus-induced tumors. However, in order to exploit specific surface antigens for immunotherapeutic purposes, it is essential to understand their biochemical nature and the immune response of the host to these antigens.

ACKNOWLEDGMENTS

The studies reported here were supported in part by Research Grants CA 14939, CA 12924, and CA 18450 from the National Cancer Institute, National Institutes of Health, and by Contract No. N01 CP 53516 within The Virus

Cancer Program of the National Cancer Institute, National Institutes of Health, Bethesda, Maryland. The authors are grateful to Dr. Mary J. Tevethia for her suggestions and comments.

XII. REFERENCES

Abrahams, P. J., Mulder, C., Van der Voorde, A., Warnaar, S. O., and Van der Eb, A. J., 1975, Transformation of primary rat kidney cells by fragments of simian virus 40 DNA, *Virology* **16**:818–823.

Ahmed, M., and Schidlovsky, G., 1972, Detection of virus-associated antigen on membranes of cells productively infected with Marek's disease herpesvirus, *Cancer Res.* **32**: 187–192.

Albrecht, T., and Rapp, F., 1973, Malignant transformation of hamster embryo fibroblasts following exposure to ultraviolet-irradiated human cytomegalovirus, *Virology* **55**: 53–61.

Allison, A. C., and Law, L. W., 1968, Effects of antilymphocyte serum on virus oncogenesis, *Proc. Soc. Exp. Biol. Med.* **127**:207–212.

Allison, A. C., and Taylor, R. B., 1967, Observations on thymectomy and carcinogenesis, *Cancer Res.* **27**:703–707.

Allison, A. C., Chesterman, F. C., and Baron, S., 1967, Induction of tumors in adult hamsters with simian virus 40, *J. Natl. Cancer Inst.* **38**:567–572.

Allison, A. C., Monga, J. N., and Hammond, V., 1974, Increased susceptibility to virus oncogenesis of congenitally thymus-deprived nude mice, *Nature (London)* **252**: 746–747.

Altstein, A. D., Deichman, G. I., Sarycheva, O. F., Dodonova, N. N., Tsetlin, E. M., and Vassilieva, N. N., 1967a, Oncogenic and transforming activity of hydroxylamine-inactivated SV40 virus, *Virology* **33**:746–748.

Altstein, A. D., Sarycheva, O. F., and Dodonova, N. N., 1967b, Detection of defective (T-antigen inducing, but noninfectious) particles in preparations of SV40 virus, *Virology* **33**:744–746.

Ambrose, K. R., Anderson, N. G., and Coggin, J. H., 1971, Interruption of SV40 oncogenesis with human foetal cells, *Nature (London)* **233**:194.

Anderson, J. P., McCormick, K. J., Stenback, W. A., and Trentin, J. J., 1971, Induction of hepatomas by an avian adenovirus (CELO), *Proc. Soc. Exp. Biol. Med.* **137**:421–423.

Ankerst, J., and Sjögren, H. O., 1970, Demonstration of two group-specific TSTAs in adenovirus-induced tumors, *Int. J. Cancer* **6**:84–94.

Ankerst, J., Jonsson, N., Kjellén, L., Norrby, E., and Sjögren, H. O., 1974, Induction of mammary fibroadenomas in rats by adenovirus type 9, *Int. J. Cancer* **13**:286–290.

Aurelian, L., Strandberg, J. D., Melendez, L. V., and Johnson, L. A., 1971, Herpesvirus type 2 isolated from cervical tumor cells grown in tissue culture, *Science* **174**:704–707.

Baldwin, R. W., Embleton, M. J., Price, M. R., and Vose, B. M., 1974, Embryonic antigen expression on experimental rat tumors, *Transplant. Rev.* **20**:77–99.

Bansal, S. C. and Sjögren, H. O., 1971, "Unblocking" serum activity *in vitro* in the polyoma system may correlate with antitumor effects of antiserum *in vivo*, *Nature (London)* **233**:76–77.

Bansal, S. C., and Sjögren, H. O., 1972, Counteraction of the blocking of cell–mediated tumor immunity by inoculation of unblocking sera and splenectomy: immunotherapeutic effects on primary polyoma tumors in rats, *Int. J. Cancer,* 9:490–509.

Bansal, S. C., Hargreaves, R., and Sjögren, H. O., 1972, Facilitation of polyoma tumor growth in rats by blocking sera and tumor eluate, *Int. J. Cancer* 9:97–108.

Baranska, W., Koldovsky, P., and Koprowski, H., 1970, Antigenic study unfertilized mouse eggs: cross reactivity with SV40-induced antigens, *Proc. Natl. Acad. Sci. U.S.A.* 67:193–199.

Barski, G., and Youn, J. K., 1969, Evolution of cell-mediated immunity in mice bearing an antigenic tumor. Influence of tumor growth and surgical removal, *J. Natl. Cancer Inst.* 43:111–112.

Baum, S. G., Reich, P. R., Hybner, C. J., Rowe, W. P., and Weissman, S. M., 1966, Biophysical evidence for linkage of adenovirus and SV40 DNA's in adenovirus 7-SV40 hybrid particles, *Proc. Natl. Acad. Sci. U.S.A.* 56:1509–1515.

Berman, L. D., 1967, On the nature of transplantation immunity in the adenovirus tumor system, *J. Exp. Med.* 125:983–1000.

Biggs, P. M., 1973, Marek's disease, in: *The Herpesviruses* (A. Kaplan, ed.), pp. 557–594, Academic Press, New York.

Black, P. H., 1968, The oncogenic DNA viruses: A review of *in vitro* transformation studies, *Annu. Rev. Microbiol.* 22:391–426.

Black, P. H., Rowe, W.P., Turner, H. C., and Huebner, R. J., 1963, A specific complement-fixing antigen present in SV40 tumor and transformed cells, *Proc. Natl. Acad. Sci. U.S.A.* 50:1148–1156.

Blasecki, J. W., and Tevethia, S. S., 1973, *In vitro* assay of cellular immunity to tumor-specific antigen(s) of virus-induced tumors by macrophage migration inhibition, *J. Immunol.* 110:590–594.

Blasecki, J. W., and Tevethia, S. S., 1975a, *In vitro* studies on the cellular immune response of tumor-bearing mice to SV40-transformed cells, *J. Immunol.* 114:244–249.

Blasecki, J. W., and Tevethia, S. S., 1975b, Restoration of specific immunity against SV40 tumor-specific transplantation antigen to lymphoid cells from tumor-bearing mice, *Int. J. Cancer* 16:275–283.

Boiron, M., Lévy, J. P., and Thomas, M., 1965, Production de tumeurs chez le hamster par inoculation d'acide désoxyribonucléique extrait de cellules infectées par le virus SV40, *Ann. Inst. Pasteur Paris* 108:298–305.

Brugge, J. S., and Butel, J. S., 1975, Role of simian virus 40 gene A function in maintenance of transformation, *J. Virol.* 15:619–635.

Burkitt, D., and Kyalwazi, S. K., 1967, Spontaneous remission of African lymphoma. *Br. J. Cancer* 21:14–16.

Butel, J. S., Guentzel, M. J., and Rapp, F., 1969. Variants of defective simian papovavirus 40 (PARA) characterized by cytoplasmic localization of simian papovavirus 40 tumor antigen, *J. Virol.* 4:632–641.

Butel, J. S., Tevethia, S. S., and Nachtigal, M., 1971, Malignant transformation *in vitro* by "nononcogenic" variants of defective SV40 (PARA), *J. Immunol.* 106:969–974.

Butel, J. S., Tevethia, S. S., and Melnick, J. L., 1972, Oncogenicity and cell transformation by papovavirus SV40: The role of the viral genome, in: *Advances in Cancer Research,* Vol. 15 (G. Klein and S. Weinhouse, eds.), pp. 1–55, Academic Press, New York.

Carroll, R. B., Hager, L., and Dulbecco, R., 1974, Simian virus 40 T antigen binds to DNA, *Proc. Natl. Acad. Sci. U.S.A.* 71:3754–3757.

Casto, B. C., 1973, Biologic parameters of adenovirus transformation, *Prog. Exp. Tumor Res.* 18:166–198.

Cerottini, J. C., and Brunner, K. T., 1974, Cell mediated cytotoxicity: Allograft rejection and tumor immunity, *Adv. Immunol.* **18**:67–132.

Chen, J. H., and Purchase, H. G., 1970, Surface antigen on chick kidney cells infected with herpesvirus of Marek's disease, *Virology* **40**:410–412.

Chou, J. Y., and Martin, R. G., 1974, Complementation analysis of simian virus 40 mutants, *J. Virol.* **13**:1101–1109.

Chou, J. Y., and Martin, R. G., 1975, DNA infectivity and the induction of host DNA synthesis with temperature-sensitive mutants of simian virus 40, *J. Virol.* **15**: 145–150.

Clifford, P., Singh, S., Sternsward, J., and Klein, G., 1967, Long term survival of patients with Burkitt's lymphoma; an assessment of treatment and other factors which may relate to survival, *Cancer Res.* **27**:2578–2615.

Coggin, J. H., and Ambrose, K. R., 1969, A rapid *in vivo* assay for SV40 tumor immunity in hamsters, *Proc. Soc. Exp. Biol. Med.* **130**:246–252.

Coggin, J. H., and Anderson, N. G., 1974, Cancer, differentiation and embryonic antigens: some central problems, in: *Advances in Cancer Research*, Vol. 19 (G. Klein and S. Weinhouse, eds.), pp. 105–165, Academic Press, New York.

Coggin, J. H., Ambrose, K. R., and Anderson, N. G., 1970, Fetal antigen capable of inducing transplantation immunity against SV40 hamster tumor cells, *J. Immunol.* **105**:524–526.

Coggin, J. H., Ambrose, K. R., Bellomy, B. B., and Anderson, N. G., 1971, Tumor immunity in hamsters immunized with fetal tissue, *J. Immunol.* **107**:526–533.

Coggin, J. H., Ambrose, K. R., Dierlam, P. J., and Anderson, N. G., 1974, Proposed mechanism by which autochthonous neoplasms escape tumor rejection, *Cancer Res.* **34**:2092–2101.

Collard, W., Thornton, H., and Green, M., 1973, Cells transformed by human herpesvirus type 2 transcribe virus-specific RNA sequences shared by herpesvirus type 1 and 2, *Nature (London) New Biol.* **243**:264–266.

Collins, J. J., and Black, P. H., 1973*a*, Analysis of surface antigens on simian virus 40-transformed cells. I. Unique antigencity of simian virus 40-transformed outbred hamster kidney cell lines, *J. Natl. Cancer Inst.* **51**:95–114.

Collins, J. J., and Black, P. H., 1973*b*, Analysis of surface antigens on simian virus 40-transformed cells. II. Exposure of simian virus 40-induced antigens on transformed rabbit kidney and inbred hamster kidney cells by phospholipase C, *J. Natl. Cancer Inst.* **51**:115–134.

Collins, J. J., Black, P. H., Strosberg, A. D., Haber, E., and Bloch, K. J., 1974, Transformation by simian virus 40 of spleen cells from a hyperimmune-rabbit: evidence for synthesis of immunoglobulin by the transformed cells, *Proc. Natl. Acad. Sci. U.S.A.* **71**:260–262.

Datta, S. K., and Vandeputte, M., 1971, Studies on cellular and humoral immunity to tumor-specific antigens in polyoma virus-induced tumors of rats, *Cancer Res.* **31**:882–889.

Davoli, D., and Fareed, G. C., 1974, Formation of reiterated simian virus 40 DNA, *Cold Spring Harbor Symp. Quant. Biol.* **39**:137–146.

Defendi, V., 1963, Effects of SV40 virus immunization on growth of transplantable SV40 and polyoma virus tumors in hamsters, *Proc. Soc. Exp. Biol. Med.* **113**:12–16.

Defendi, V., and Jensen, F., 1967, Oncogenicity by DNA tumor viruses: Enhancement after ultraviolet and cobalt-60 radiation, *Science* **157**:703–705.

Deichman, G. I., 1969, Immunological aspects of carcinogenesis by deoxyribonucleic acid tumor viruses, in: *Advances in Cancer Research*, Vol. 12 (G. Klein and S. Weinhouse, eds.), pp. 101–136, Academic Press, New York.

Deichman, G. I., and Kluchareva, T. E., 1964, Immunological determinants of oncogenesis in hamsters infected with SV40 virus, *Virology* **24**:131–137.

Deichman, G. I., and Kluchareva, T. E., 1966, Loss of transplantation antigen in primary simian virus 40-induced tumors and their metastases, *J. Natl. Cancer Inst.* **36**:647–655.

Deinhardt, F. W., Falk, L. S., and Wolfe, L. G., 1974, Simian herpesviruses and neoplasia, in: *Advances in Cancer Research*, Vol. 19 (G. Klein and S. Weinhouse, eds.), pp. 167–205, Academic Press, New York.

Del Villano, B. C., and Defendi, V., 1973, Characterization of SV40 T antigen, *Virology* **51**:34–46.

Diamandopoulos, G. Th., 1973, Induction of lymphocytic leukemia, lymphosarcoma, reticulum cell sarcoma, and osteogenic sarcoma in the Syrian golden hamster by oncogenic DNA simian virus 40, *J. Natl. Cancer Inst.* **50**:1347–1365.

Diamandopoulos, G. Th., and McLane, M. F., 1974, Development of antibodies to viral and tumor antigens before tumor induction, *J. Immunol.* **13**:1450–1456.

Diamandopoulos, G. Th., Tevethia, S. S., Rapp, F., and Enders, J. F., 1968, Development of S and T antigens and oncogenicity in hamster embryonic cell lines exposed to SV40, *Virology* **34**:331–336.

Dierlam, P., Anderson, N. G., and Coggin, J. H., 1971, Immunization against tumors with fetal antigens: Detection of immunity by the colony inhibition test and by adoptive transfer, in: *Embryonic and Fetal Antigens in Cancer* (N. G. Anderson *et al.*, eds.), pp. 203–214, Proceedings of the First Conference and Workshop on Embryonic and Fetal Antigens in Cancer, Oak Ridge, Tenn., May 24–26, 1971.

Dougherty, R. M., and DiStefano, H. S., 1974, Isolation and characterization of a papovavirus from human urine, *Proc. Soc. Exp. Biol. Med.* **146**:481–487.

Drapkin, M. S., Apella, E., and Law, L. W., 1974, Immunogenic properties of a soluble tumor-specific transplantation antigen induced by simian virus 40, *J. Natl. Cancer Inst.* **52**:259–264.

Dubbs, D. R., Rachmeler, M., and Kit, S., 1974, Recombination between temperature-sensitive mutants of simian virus 40, *Virology* **57**:161–174.

Duff, R., and Rapp, F., 1970a, Reaction of serum from pregnant hamsters with surface of cells transformed by SV40, *J. Immunol.* **105**:521–523.

Duff, R., and Rapp, F., 1970b, Quantitative characteristics of the transformation of hamster cells by PARA (defective simian virus 40)–adenovirus 7, *J. Virol.* **5**:568–577.

Duff, R., and Rapp, R., 1971, Properties of hamster embryo fibroblasts transformed *in vitro* after exposure to ultraviolet-irradiated herpes simplex virus type 2, *J. Virol.* **8**:469–477.

Duff, R., and Rapp, F., 1973, Oncogenic transformation of hamster embryo cells after exposure to inactivated herpes simplex virus type 1, *J. Virol.* **12**:209–217.

Duff, R., Knight, P., and Rapp, F., 1972, Variation in oncogenic and transforming potential of PARA (defective simian virus 40)–adenovirus 7, *Virology* **47**:849–853.

Duff, R., Doller, E., and Rapp, F., 1973, Immunologic manipulation of metastases due to herpesvirus transformed cells, *Science* **180**:79–81.

Eddy, B., 1964, Simian virus 40 (SV40); an oncogenic virus, *Prog. Exp. Tumor Res.* **4**:1–26.

Else, R. W., 1974, Vaccinal immunity to Marek's disease in bursectomized chickens, *Vet. Rec.* **95**:182–187.

Epstein, M. A., 1970, Aspects of the EB virus, *Adv. Cancer Res.* **13**:383–411.

Epstein, M. A., Achong, B. G., and Barr, Y., 1964, Virus particles in cultured lymphoblasts from Burkitt's lymphoma, *Lancet* **1**:702–703.

Evans, C. A., and Ito, Y., 1966, Antitumor immunity in the Shope papilloma–carcinoma complex of rabbits. III. Response to reinfection with viral nucleic acid, *J. Natl. Cancer Inst.* **36**:1161–1166.

Evans, C. A., Weiser, R. S., and Ito, Y., 1962, Antiviral and antitumor immunologic mechanisms operative in the Shope papilloma–carcinoma system, *Cold Spring Harbor Symp. Quant. Biol.* 27:453–462.

Evans, R., and Grant, C. K., 1972, Role of macrophages in tumour immunity. III. Cooperation between macrophages and lymphoid factors in an *in vitro* allograft situation, *Immunology* 23:667–687.

Fass, L., Herberman, R. B., and Ziegler, J., 1970, Delayed cutaneous hypersensitivity reactions to autologous extracts of Burkitt-lymphoma cells. *N. Engl. J. Med.* 282: 776–780.

Feldman, L. A., Butel, J. S., and Rapp, F., 1966, Interaction of a simian papovavirus and adenoviruses. I. Induction of adenovirus tumor antigen during abortive infection of simian cells, *J. Bacteriol.* 91:813–818.

Finkelstein, J. Z., and McAllister, R. M., 1969, Ultraviolet inactivation of the cytocidal and transforming activities of human adenovirus type 1, *J. Virol.* 3:353–354.

Freeman, A. E., Black, P. H., Vanderpool, E. A., Henry, P. H., Austin, J. B., and Huebner, R. J., 1967, Transformation of primary rat embryo cells by adenovirus type 2, *Proc. Natl. Acad. Sci. U.S.A.* 58:1205–1212.

Frenkel, N., Roizman, B., Cassai, E., and Nahmias, A., 1972, A DNA fragment of herpes simplex 2 and its transcripts in human cervical cancer tissue, *Proc. Natl. Acad. Sci. U.S.A.* 69:3784–3789.

Frenkel, N., Locker, H., Roizman, B., and Rapp, F., 1975, Viral DNA sequences in hamster cell lines transformed by UV-irradiated HSV-2, Session W-33, *Third International Congress for Virology*, p. 120, Madrid, Spain.

Fujinaga, F., Sekikawa, K., Yamazaki, H., and Green, M., 1974, Analysis of multiple viral genome fragments in adenovirus 7-transformed hamster cells, *Cold Spring Harbor Symp. Quant. Biol.* 39:633–636.

Gallimore, P. H., 1972, Tumor production in immunosuppressed rats with cells transformed *in vitro* by adenovirus type 2, *J. Gen. Virol.* 16:99–102.

Gardner, S. D., Field, A. M., Coleman, D. V., and Hulme, B., 1971, New human papovavirus (B.K.) isolated from urine after renal transplantation, *Lancet* 1:1253–1257.

Gerber, P., and Hoyer, B. H., 1971, Induction of cellular DNA synthesis in human leukocytes by Epstein-Barr virus, *Nature (London)* 231:46–47.

Gerber, P., Whang-Peng, J., and Monroe, J. H., 1969, Transformation and chromosome changes induced by Epstein-Barr virus in normal human leukocyte cultures, *Proc. Natl. Acad. Sci. U.S.A.* 63:740–747.

Gerber, P., Nonoyama, M., Lucas, S., Perlin, E., and Goldstein, L. I., 1972, Oral excretion of Epstein-Barr virus by healthy subjects and patients with infectious mononucleosis, *Lancet* 2:988–989.

Gergely, L., Klein, G., and Ernberg, I., 1971*a*, Appearance of Epstein-Barr virus-associated antigens in infected Raji cells, *Virology* 45:10–21.

Gergely, L., Klein, G., and Ernberg, I., 1971*b*, The action of DNA antagonists on Epstein-Barr virus (EBV)-associated early antigen (EA) in Burkitt lymphoma lines, *Int. J. Cancer* 7:293–302.

Gilden, R. V., Kern, J., Heberling, R. L., and Huebner, R. J., 1968, Serological studies of the T and tumor antigens of the oncogenic simian adenoviruses, *Appl. Microbiol.* 16:1015–1018.

Gilead, Z., and Ginsberg, H. S., 1968, Characterization of the tumorlike (T) antigen induced by Type 12 adenovirus. II. Physical and chemical properties, *J. Virol.* 2:15–20.

Ginsberg, H. S., Ensinger, M. J., Kauffman, R. S., Mayer, A. J., and Lundholm, U., 1974, Cell transformation: A study of regulation with types 5 and 12 adenovirus temperature-sensitive mutants, *Cold Spring Harbor Symp. Quant. Biol.* 39:419–426.

Girardi, A. J., 1965, Prevention of SV40 virus oncogenesis in hamsters, I. Tumor resistance induced by human cells transformed by SV40, *Proc. Natl. Acad. Sci. U.S.A.* **54**: 445–451.

Girardi, A. J., 1967, Tumor resistance and tumor enhancement with SV40 virus-induced tumors, in: *Germinal Centers in Immune Responses* (H. Cottier, N. Odartchenko, R. Schindler, and C. C. Congdon, eds.), pp. 422–427, Springer-Verlag, New York.

Girardi, A. J., and Defendi, V., 1970, Induction of SV40 transplantation antigen (TrAg) during the lytic cycle, *Virology* **42**:688–698.

Girardi, A. J., and Roosa, R. A., 1967, Prevention of SV40 virus oncogenesis in hamsters. II. The effect of thymectomy on induction of tumor resistance by SV40-transformed human cells, *J. Immunol.* **99**:1217–1220.

Girardi, A. J., Reppucci, P., Dierlam, P., Rutala, W., and Coggin, J. H., 1973, Prevention of simian virus 40 tumors by hamster fetal tissue: Influence of parity status of donor females on immunogenicity of fetal tissue and on immune cell cytotoxicity, *Proc. Natl. Acad. Sci. U.S.A.* **70**:183–186.

Goldman, R. D., Chang, C., and Williams, J. F., 1974, Properties and behavior of hamster embryo cells transformed by human adenovirus type 5, *Cold Spring Harbor Symp. Quant. Biol.* **39**:601–614.

Goldner, H., Girardi, A. J., Larson, V. M., and Hilleman, M. R., 1964, Interruption of SV40 virus tumorigenesis using irradiated homologous tumor antigen, *Proc. Soc. Exp. Biol. Med.* **117**:851–857.

Graessmann, A., Graessmann, M., Hoffmann, H., Niebel, J., Brandner, G., and Mueller, N., 1974, Inhibition by interferon of SV40 tumor antigen formation in cells injected with SV40 cRNA transcribed *in vitro, FEBS Lett.* **39**:249–251.

Graham, F. L., Van der Eb, A. J., and Heijneker, H. L., 1974a, Size and location of the transforming region in human adenovirus type 5 DNA, *Nature (London)* **251**:687–691.

Graham, F. L., Abrahams, J., Mulder, C., Heijneker, H., Warnaar, S. O., deVries, F. A. J., and Van der Eb, A. J., 1974b, Studies on *in vitro* transformation by DNA and DNA fragments of human adenoviruses and simian virus 40, *Cold Spring Harbor Symp. Quant. Biol.* **39**:637–650.

Gunvén, P., Klein, G., Clifford, P., and Singh, S., 1974, Epstein-Barr virus-associated membrane-reactive antibodies during long term survival after Burkitt's lymphoma, *Proc. Natl. Acad. Sci. U.S.A.* **71**:1422–1426.

Habel, K., 1961, Resistance of polyoma virus immune animals to transplanted polyoma tumors, *Proc. Soc. Exp. Biol. Med.* **106**:722–725.

Habel, K., 1962, Immunological determinants of polyoma virus oncogenesis, *J. Exp. Med.* **115**:181–193.

Habel, K., and Eddy, B. E., 1963, Specificity of resistance to tumor challenge of polyoma and SV40 virus-immune hamsters, *Proc. Soc. Exp. Biol. Med.* **113**:1–4.

Hampar, B., Derge, J. G., Tanaka, A., and Nonoyama, M., 1974, Sequence of Epstein-Barr virus productive cycle in human lymphoblastoid cells, *Cold Spring Harbor Symp. Quant. Biol.* **39**:811–816.

Hargis, B. J., and Malkiel, S., 1975, Induction of sarcomas in mice by SV40 virus, *Fed. Proc.* **34**:973.

Hayry, P., and Defendi, V., 1968, Use of mixed hemagglutination technique in detection of virus-induced antigen(s) on SV40-transformed cell surface, *Virology* **36**:317–321.

Hayry, P., and Defendi, V., 1970, Surface antigen(s) of SV40-transformed tumor cells, *Virology* **41**:22–29.

Hellström, I., and Hellström, K. E., 1975a, Cytotoxic effect of lymphocytes from pregnant mice on cultivated tumor cells. I. Specificity, nature of effector cells and blocking by serum, *Int. J. Cancer* **15**:1–16.

Hellström, I., and Hellström, K. E., 1975b, Cytotoxic effect of lymphocytes from pregnant mice on cultivated tumor cells. II. Blocking and unblocking of cytotoxicity, *Int. J. Cancer* 15:30–38.

Hellström, I., and Sjögren, H. O., 1965, Demonstration of H-2 isoantigens and polyoma specific tumor antigens by measuring colony formation *in vitro, Exp. Cell Res.* 40:212–215.

Hellström, I., and Sjögren, H. O., 1967, *In vitro* demonstration of humoral and cell-bound immunity against common specific transplantation antigen(s) of adenovirus 12-induced mouse and hamster tumors, *J. Exp. Med.* 125:1105–1118.

Hellström, I., Evans, C. A., and Hellström, K. E., 1969, Cellular immunity and its serum-mediated inhibition in Shope-virus-induced rabbit papillomas, *Int. J. Cancer* 4: 601–607.

Hellström, K. E., and Hellström, I., 1969, Cellular immunity against tumor antigens, in: *Advances in Cancer Research,* Vol. 12 (G. Klein and W. Weinhouse, eds.), pp. 167–223, Academic Press, New York.

Hellström, K. E., and Hellström, I., 1974, Lymphocyte-mediated cytotoxicity and blocking serum activity to tumor antigens, *Adv. Immunol.* 18:209–277.

Henle, G., and Henle, W., 1966, Immunofluorescence in cells derived from Burkitt's lymphoma, *J. Bacteriol.* 91:1248–1256.

Henle, G., Henle, W., and Diehl, V., 1968, Relation of Burkitt's tumor associated herpes type virus to infectious mononucleosis, *Proc. Natl. Acad. Sci. U.S.A.* 59:94–101.

Henle, G., Henle, W., Clifford, P., Diehl, V., Kafuko, G. W., Kirya, B. B., Klein, G., Morrow, R. H., Munube, G. M. R., Pite, P., Tukei, P. M., and Ziegler, J. L., 1969, Antibodies to Epstein-Barr virus in Burkitt's lymphoma and control groups, *J. Natl. Cancer Inst.* 43:1147–1157.

Henle, G., Henle, W., and Klein, G., 1971, Demonstration of two distinct components in the early antigen complex of Epstein-Barr virus-infected cells, *Int. J. Cancer* 8:272–282.

Henle, G., Henle, W., and Horwitz, C. A., 1974, Antibodies to Epstein-Barr virus associated nuclear antigen in infectious mononucleosis, *J. Infect. Dis.* 130:231–239.

Henle, W., and Henle, G., 1973, Epstein-Barr virus, and infectious mononucleosis, *N. Engl. J. Med.* 288:263–264.

Henle, W., and Henle, G., 1974, Epstein-Barr virus and human malignancies, *Cancer* 34:1368–1374.

Henle, W., Diehl, V., Kohn, G., Zur Hausen, H., and Henle, G., 1967, Herpes-type virus and chromosome marker in normal leukocytes after growth with irradiated Burkitt cells, *Science* 157:1064–1065.

Henle, W., Henle, G., Zajac, B., Pearson, G., Waubke, R., and Scriba, M., 1970, Differential reactivity of human sera with early antigens induced by Epstein-Barr virus, *Science* 169:188–190.

Henle, W., Henle, G., Gunvén, P., Klein, G., Clifford, P., and Singh, S., 1973, Patterns of antibodies to Epstein-Barr virus induced early antigens in fatal cases of Burkitt's lymphoma and long term survivors, *J. Natl. Cancer Inst.* 50:1163–1173.

Hewetson, J., Gothoskar, B., Klein, G., and Singh, S., 1972, Radioiodine labeled antibody test for the detection of membrane antigens associated with Epstein-Barr virus, *J. Natl. Cancer Inst.* 48:87–94.

Hinuma, Y., and Grace, J. T., 1967, Cloning of immunoglobulin-producing human leukemic and lymphoma cells in long-term cultures, *Proc. Soc. Exp. Biol. Med.* 124:107–111.

Hinze, H. C., 1971, Induction of lymphoid hyperplasia and lymphoma-like disease in rabbits by Herpesvirus sylvilagus, *Int. J. Cancer* 8:514–522.

Howell, S. B., Dean, J. H., Esber, E. C., and Law, L. W., 1974, Cell interactions in adoptive immune rejection of a syngeneic tumor, *Int. J. Cancer* 14:662–674.

Howell, S. B., Dean, J. H., and Law, L. W., 1975, Defects in cell-mediated immunity during growth of a syngeneic simian virus-induced tumor, *Int. J. Cancer* **15**:152–169.

Hudson, L., and Payne, L. N., 1973, An analysis of the T and B cells in Marek's disease lymphoma of the chicken, *Nature (London)* **241**:52–53.

Huebner, R. J., Rowe, W. P., Turner, H. C., and Lane, W. T., 1963, Specific adenovirus complement-fixing antigens in virus-free hamster and rat tumors, *Proc. Natl. Acad. Sci. U.S.A.* **50**:379–389.

Huebner, R. J., Chanock, R. M., Rubin, B. A., and Casey, M. J., 1964a, Induction by adenovirus type 7 of tumors in hamsters having the antigenic characteristics of SV40 virus, *Proc. Natl. Acad. Sci. U.S.A.* **52**:1333–1340.

Huebner, R. J., Pereira, H. G., Allison, A. C., Hollinshead, A. C., and Turner, H. C., 1964b, Production of type specific C antigen in virus-free hamster tumor cells induced by adenovirus type 12, *Proc. Natl. Acad. Sci. U.S.A.* **51**:432–439.

Huebner, R. J., Casey, M. J., Chanock, R. M., and Schell, K., 1965, Tumors induced in hamsters by a strain of adenovirus type 3: Sharing of tumor antigens and "neoantigens" with those produced by adenovirus type 7 tumors, *Proc. Natl. Acad. Sci. U.S.A.* **54**:381–388.

Inbar, M., Rabinowitz, Z., and Sachs, L., 1969, The formation of variants with a reversion of properties of transformed cells. III. Reversion of the structure of the cell surface membrane, *Int. J. Cancer* **4**:690–696.

Irlin, I. S., 1967, Immunofluorescent demonstration of a specific surface antigen in cells infected or transformed by polyoma virus, *Virology* **32**:725–728.

Jaenisch, R., and Mintz, B., 1974, Simian virus 40 DNA sequences in DNA of healthy adult mice derived from preimplantation blastocysts injected with viral DNA, *Proc. Natl. Acad. Sci. U.S.A.* **71**:1250–1254.

Jensen, F., and Defendi, V., 1968, Transformation of African green monkey kidney cells by irradiated adenovirus 7–simian virus 40 hybrid, *J. Virol.* **2**:173–177.

Jessel, D., Hudson, J., Landau, T., Tenen, D., and Livingston, D. M., 1975, Interaction of partially purified simian virus 40 T antigen with circular viral DNA molecules, *Proc. Natl. Acad. Sci. U.S.A.* **72**:1960–1969.

Jondal, M., Svedmyr, E., Klein, E., and Klein, G., 1975, Epstein-Barr virus (EBV) specific T and K cell cytotoxicity *in vitro*, *Proc. VIIth Int. Symp. Comp. Leuk. Res.* (in press).

Kaplan, P. M., Melnick, J. L., and Tevethia, S. S., 1971, Development of nononcogenic SA 7-adenovirus 2 populations that immunize against SA 7-transformed cells, *J. Natl. Cancer Inst.* **46**:565–576.

Kelly, F., and Sambrook, J., 1974, Variants of simian virus 40-transformed mouse cells resistant to cytochalasin B, *Cold Spring Harbor Symp. Quant. Biol.* **39**:345–353.

Kelly, T. J., Jr., and Rose, J. A., 1971, Simian virus 40 integration site in an adenovirus 7-simian virus 40 hybrid DNA molecule, *Proc. Natl. Acad. Sci. U.S.A.*, **68**:1037–1041.

Kelly, T. J., Lewis, A. M., Levine, A. S., and Siegel, S., 1974, Structural studies on two adenovirus 2-SV40 hybrids containing the entire SV40 genome, *Cold Spring Harbor Symp. Quant. Biol.* **39**:409–417.

Khera, K. S., Ashkenazi, A., Rapp, F., and Melnick, J. L., 1963, Immunity in hamsters to cells transformed *in vitro* and *in vivo* by SV40. Tests for antigenic relationship among papovaviruses, *J. Immunol.* **91**:604–613.

Khoury, G., Howley, P., Garon, C., Mullarkey, M. F., Takemoto, K. K., and Martin, M. A., 1975, Homology and relationship between the genomes of papovaviruses, BK virus and simian virus 40, *Proc. Natl. Acad. Sci. U.S.A.* **72**:2563–2567.

Kimura, G., and Itagaki, A., 1975, Initiation and maintenance of cell transformation by simian virus 40: A viral genetic property, *Proc. Natl. Acad. Sci. U.S.A.* **72**:673–677.

Kimura, S., Esparza, J., Benyesh-Melnick, M., and Schaffer, P. A., 1974, Enhanced replication of temperature-sensitive mutants of herpes simplex virus type 2 (HSV-2) at the nonpermissive temperature in cells transformed by HSV-2, *Intervirology* 3:162–169.

Kimura, S., Flannery, V. L., Levy, B., and Schaffer, P., 1975, Oncogenic transformation of primary hamster cells by herpes simplex virus type 2 (HSV-2) and an HSV-2 temperature-sensitive mutant, *Int. J. Cancer* 15:786–798.

Kirschstein, R. L., and Gerber, P., 1962, Ependymomas produced after intracerebral inoculation of SV40 into newborn hamsters, *Nature (London)* 195:299–300.

Kit, S., Kurimura, T., and Dubbs, D. R., 1969, Transplantable mouse tumor line induced by injection of SV40-transformed mouse kidney cells, *Int. J. Cancer* 4:384–392.

Klein, G., 1966, Tumor antigens, *Annu. Rev. Microbiol.* 20:223–252.

Klein, G., 1969, Experimental studies in tumor immunology, *Fed. Proc.* 28:1739–1753.

Klein, G., 1973, The Epstein-Barr virus, in: *The Herpesviruses* (A. S. Kaplan, ed.), pp. 521–555, Academic Press, New York.

Klein, G., 1974, Studies on the Epstein-Barr virus genome and the EBV-determined nuclear antigen in human malignant disease, *Cold Spring Harbor Symp. Quant. Biol.* 39: 783–790.

Klein, G., and Vonka, V., 1974, Relationship between the Epstein-Barr virus-determined complement-fixing antigen and the nuclear antigen detected by anticomplement fluorescence, *J. Natl. Cancer Inst.* 53:1645–1646.

Klein, G., Clifford, P., Klein, E., and Stjernswärd, J., 1966, Search for tumor specific immune reactions in Burkitt lymphoma patients by the membrane immunofluorescence reaction, *Proc. Natl. Acad. Sci. U.S.A.* 55:1628–1635.

Klein, G., Clifford, P., Klein, E., Smith, R. T., Minowada, J., Kourilsky, F. M., and Burchenal, J. H., 1967, Membrane immunofluorescence reactions of Burkitt lymphoma cells from biopsy specimens and tissue cultures, *J. Natl. Cancer Inst.* 39:1027–1044.

Klein, G., Pearson, G., Henle, W., Diehl, V., and Niederman, J. C., 1968, Relation between Epstein-Barr viral and cell membrane immunofluorescence in Burkitt tumor cells, *J. Exp. Med.* 128:1021–1030.

Klein, G., Clifford, P., Henle, G., Henle, W., Geering, G., and Old, L. J., 1969, EBV-associated serological patterns in a Burkitt lymphoma patient during regression and recurrence, *Int. J. Cancer* 4:416–421.

Klein, G., Gergely, L., and Goldstein, G., 1971, Two-color immunofluorescence studies on EBV-determined antigens, *Clin. Exp. Immunol.* 8:593–602.

Klein, G., Giovanella, B. C., Lindahl, T., Fialkow, P. J., Singh, S., and Stehlin, J. S., 1974, Direct evidence for the presence of EBV DNA and nuclear antigen in malignant epithelial cells from patients with poorly differentiated carcinoma of the nasopharynx, *Proc. Natl. Acad. Sci. U.S.A.* 71:4737–4741.

Kluchareva, T. E., Shachanina, K. L., Belova, S., Chibisova, V., and Deichman, G. I., 1967, Use of immunofluorescence for detection of specific membrane antigen in simian virus 40-infected nontransformed cells, *J. Natl. Cancer Inst.* 39:825–832.

Koprowski, H., Sawicki, W., and Koldovsky, P., 1971, Immunological cross-reactivity between antigen of unfertilized mouse eggs and mouse cells transformed by simian virus 40, *J. Natl. Cancer Inst.* 46:1317–1323.

Kutinová, L., Vonka, V., and Brouček, J., 1973, Increased oncogenicity and synthesis of herpesvirus antigens in hamster cells exposed to herpes simplex type 2 virus, *J. Natl. Cancer Inst.* 50:759–766.

Lai, C., and Nathans, D., 1974, Mapping of temperature-sensitive mutants of simian virus 40: Rescue of mutants by fragments of viral DNA, *Virology* 60:466–475.

Larson, V. M., Girardi, A. J., Hilleman, M. R., and Zwickey, R. E., 1965, Studies of oncogenicity of adenovirus type 7 viruses in hamsters, *Proc. Soc. Exp. Biol. Med.* **118**:15–24.

Lausch, R. N., and Rapp, F., 1971, Concomitant immunity in hamsters bearing syngeneic transplants of tumors induced by PARA-adenovirus 7, simian adenovirus 7 and 9, 10 dimethylbenzanthracene, *Int. J. Cancer* **7**:322–330.

Lausch, R. N., Tevethia, S. S., and Rapp, F., 1968. Evidence of SV40-specific transplantation and surface antigens in cells transformed by PARA-adenovirus 12, *J. Immunol.* **101**:645–649.

Lausch, R. N., Tevethia, S. S., and Rapp, F., 1970, Evidence for tolerance to SV40 tumor antigen in hamsters bearing PARA-adenovirus 12 tumor transplants, *J. Immunol.* **104**:305–311.

Lausch, R. N., Sofranko, J., and Prather, S. O., 1975a, Analysis of sera from SV40 immunized and tumor bearing hosts for blocking activity and antibody dependent cellular cytotoxicity, *J. Immunol.* **115**:682–687.

Lausch, R. N., Jones, C., Christie, D., Hay, K. A., and Rapp, F., 1975b, Spleen cell mediated cytotoxicity of hamster cells transformed by herpes simplex virus: Evidence for virus specific membrane antigen, *J. Immunol.* **114**:459–465.

Laux, D., and Lausch, R. N., 1974, Reversal of tumor-mediated suppression of immune reactivity by *in vitro* incubation of spleen cells, *J. Immunol.* **112**:1900–1908.

Lavi, S., and Winocour, E., 1972, Acquisition of sequences homologous to host deoxyribonucleic acid by closed circular simian virus 40 deoxyribonucleic acid, *J. Virol.* **9**: 309–316.

Law, L. W., 1966, Immunologic responsiveness and the induction of experimental neoplasms, *Cancer Res.* **26**:1121–1132.

Law, L. W., and Ting, R. C., 1965, Immunologic competence and induction of neoplasms by polyoma virus, *Proc. Soc. Exp. Biol. Med.* **119**:823–829.

Law, L. W., Ting, R. C., and Leckband, E., 1967, Prevention of virus induced neoplasms in mice through passive transfer of immunity by sensitized syngeneic lymphoid cells, *Proc. Natl. Acad. Sci. U.S.A.* **57**:1068–1075.

Levin, M. J., Oxman, M. N., Diamandopoulos, G. Th., Levine, A. S., Henry, P. H., and Enders, J. F., 1969, Virus-specific nucleic acids in SV40 exposed hamster embryo cell lines: Correlation with S and T antigens, *Proc. Natl. Acad. Sci. U.S.A.* **62**:589–596.

Levine, A. S., Oxman, M. N., Henry, P. H., Levin, M. J., Diamandopoulos, G. Th., and Enders, J. F., 1970, Virus-specific deoxyribonucleic acid in simian virus 40-exposed hamster cells: Correlation with S and T antigens, *J. Virol.* **6**:199–207.

Levy, M. H., and Wheelock, E. F., 1974, The role of macrophages in defense against neoplastic disease, *Adv. Cancer Res.* **20**:131–163.

Lewis, A. M., Jr., and Rowe, W. P., 1970, Isolation of two plaque variants from the adenovirus type 2-simian virus 40 hybrid population which differ in their efficiency in yielding simian virus 40, *J. Virol.* **5**:413–420.

Lewis, A. M., Jr., and Rowe, W. P., 1971, Studies on nondefective adenovirus-simian virus hybrid viruses. I. A newly characterized simian virus 40 antigen induced by the Ad2+ND$_1$ virus. *J. Virol.* **7**:189–197.

Lewis, A. M., Jr., and Rowe, W. P., 1973, Studies of nondefective adenovirus 2-simian virus 40 hybrid viruses. VIII. Association of simian virus 40 transplantation antigen with a specific region of the early viral genome, *J. Virol.* **12**:836–840.

Lewis, A. M., Jr., Levin, M. J., Weise, W. H., Crumpacker, C. S., and Henry, P. H., 1969, A nondefective (competent) adenovirus-SV40 hybrid isolated from the Ad2-SV40 hybrid population, *Proc. Natl. Acad. Sci. U.S.A.* **63**:1128–1135.

Lewis, A. M., Jr., Levine, A. S., Crumpacker, C. S., Levin, M. J., Samaha, R. J., and Henry,

P. H., 1973, Studies of nondefective adenovirus 2-simian virus 40 hybrid viruses. V. Isolation of additional hybrids which differ in their simian virus 40-specific biological properties, *J. Virol.* **11**:655–664.

Lewis, A. M., Rabson, A. S., and Levine, A. S., 1974*a*, Studies of nondefective adenovirus 2-simian virus 40 hybrid viruses. Transformation of hamster kidney cells by adenovirus 2 and nondefective hybrid viruses, *J. Virol.* **13**:1291–1301.

Lewis, A. M., Breeden, J. H., Wewerka, Y. L., Schnipper, L. E., and Levine, A. S. 1974*b*, Studies of hamster cells transformed by adenovirus 2 and the nondefective Ad2-SV40 hybrids, *Cold Spring Harbor Symp. Quant. Biol.* **39**:651–656.

Lherisson, A. M., Meyer, G., and Bonneau, H., 1967, Détection d'un antigène de membrane dans le système tumoral polyome-hamster, *Bull. Cancer* **54**:419–422.

Mackaness, G. B., 1971, Delayed hypersensitivity and the mechanism of cellular resistance to infection, *Prog. Immunol.* **1**:413–424.

Macnab, J. C. M., 1974, Transformation of rat embryo cells by temperature-sensitive mutants of herpes simplex virus, *J. Gen. Virol.* **24**:143–153.

Major, E. O., and Di Mayorca, G., 1973, Malignant transformation of BHK_{21} clone 13 cells by BK virus—A human papovavirus, *Proc. Natl. Acad. Sci. U.S.A.* **70**:3210–3212.

Malmgren, R. A., Takemoto, K. K., and Carney, P. G., 1968, Immunofluorescent studies of mouse and hamster cell surface antigens induced by polyoma virus, *J. Natl. Cancer Inst.* **40**:263–268.

Marek, J. 1908, Multiple Nerventzündung (polyneuritis) bei Hühnern, *Dtsch. Tieraerztl. Wochenschr.* **15**:417–421.

Martin, R. G., and Chou, J. Y., 1975, Simian virus 40 functions required for the establishment and maintenance of malignant transformation, *J. Virol.* **15**:599–612.

McAllister, R. M., Nicholson, M. O., Reed, G., Kern, J., Gilden, R. V., and Huebner, R. J., 1969, Transformation of rodent cells by adenovirus 19 and other group D adenoviruses, *J. Natl. Cancer Inst.* **43**:917–923.

McDougall, J. K., Dunn, A. R., and Gallimore, P. H., 1974, Recent studies on the characteristics of adenovirus-infected and -transformed cells, *Cold Spring Harbor Symp. Quant. Biol.* **39**:591–600.

Melendez, L. V., Daniel, M. D., Hunt, R. D., and Garcia, F. G., 1968, An apparently new herpesvirus from primary kidney culture of the squirrel monkey *(Saimiri sciureus)*, *Lab. Anim. Care* **18**:374–381.

Melendez, L. V., Hunt, R. D., King, N. W., Barahona, H. H., Daniel, M. D., Fraser, C. E. O., and Garcia, F. G., 1972, Herpesvirus ateles, a new lymphoma of monkeys, *Nature (London) New Biol.* **235**:182–184.

Mertz, J. E., Carbon, J., Herzberg, M., Davis, R. W., and Berg, P., 1974, Isolation and characterization of individual clones of simian virus 40 mutants containing deletions, duplications and insertions in their DNA, *Cold Spring Harbor Symp. Quant. Biol.* **39**:69–84.

Metzgar, R. S., and Oleinick, S. R., 1968, The study of normal and malignant cell antigens by mixed agglutination, *Cancer Res.* **28**:1366–1371.

Meyer, G., and Birg, F., 1970, Sensitivity to inactivation by ultraviolet light of certain functions of polyoma virus: Cell surface antigen, *J. Gen. Virol.* **9**:127–131.

Mikulska, Z. B., Smith, C., and Alexander, P., 1966, Evidence for an immunological reaction of the host directed against its own actively growing primary tumor, *J. Natl. Cancer Inst.* **36**:29–35.

Miller, G., Niederman, J. C., and Stitt, D. A., 1972, Infectious mononucleosis: Appearance of neutralizing antibody to Epstein-Barr virus measured by inhibition of formation of lymphoblastoid cell lines, *J. Infect. Dis.* **125**:403–406.

Miller, G., Niederman, J. C., and Andrews, L. L., 1973, Prolonged oropharyngeal excretion of Epstein-Barr virus after infectious mononucleosis, *N. Engl. J. Med.* 288:229–232.

Miller, G., Robinson, J., Heston, L., and Lipman, M., 1974, Differences between laboratory strains of Epstein-Barr virus based on immortalization, abortive infection and interference, *Proc. Natl. Acad. Sci. U.S.A.* 71:4006–4010.

Murasko, D. M., 1975, Demonstration of virus associated antigens on hamster cells transformed by cytomegalovirus, Ph.D. thesis, Pennsylvania State University.

Murasko, D. M., and Lausch, R. N., 1974, Cellular immune response to virus specific antigen in hamsters bearing isografts of cytomegalovirus-transformed cells, *Int. J. Cancer* 14:451–460.

Nadkarni, J. S., Nadkarni, J. J., Klein, G., Henle, W., Henle, G., and Clifford, P., 1970, EB viral antigens in Burkitt tumor biopsies and early cultures, *Int. J. Cancer* 6:10–17.

Nahmias, A. J., Josey, W. E., Naib, Z. M., Luce, C., and Guest, B., 1970a, Antibodies to herpesvirus hominis types 1 and 2 in humans. II. Women with cervical cancer, *Am. J. Epidemiol.* 91:547–552.

Nahmias, A. J., Naib, Z. M., Josey, W. E., Murphy, F. A., and Luce, C. F., 1970b, Sarcomas after inoculation of newborn hamsters with herpesvirus hominis type 2 strains, *Proc. Soc. Exp. Biol. Med.* 134:1065–1069.

Nazerian, K., 1973, Marek's disease: a neoplastic disease of chickens caused by a herpesvirus, in: *Advances in Cancer Research*, Vol. 17 (G. Klein and S. Weinhouse, eds.), pp. 279–315, Academic Press, New York.

Nazerian, K., and Chen, J. H., 1973, Immunoferritin studies of Marek's disease virus directed intracellular and membrane antigens, *Arch. Gesamte Virusforsch.* 41:59–65.

Nazerian, K., Lindahl, T., Klein, G., and Lee, L. F., 1973, Deoxyribonucleic acid of Marek's disease virus in virus-induced tumors, *J. Virol.* 12:841–846.

Nelson, D. S., 1974, Immunity to infection, allograft immunity and tumour immunity: Parallels and contrasts, *Transplant. Rev.* 19:226–254.

Niederman, J. C., McCollum, R. W., Henle, G., and Henle, W., 1968, Infectious mononucleosis: Clinical manifestations in relation to EB virus antibodies, *J. Amer. Med. Assoc.* 203:205–209.

Nilsson, K., Klein, G., Henle, W., and Henle, G., 1971, The establishment of lymphoblastoid lines from adult and fetal human lymphoid tissue and its dependence on EBV, *Int. J. Cancer* 8:443–450.

Nonoyama, M., Huang, C. H., Pagano, J. S., Klein, G., and Singh, S., 1973, DNA of Epstein-Barr virus detected in tissue of Burkitt's lymphoma and nasopharyngeal carcinoma, *Proc. Natl. Acad. Sci. U.S.A.* 70:3265–3268.

Okazaki, W., Purchase, H. G., and Burmester, B. R., 1970, Protection against Marek's disease by vaccination with a herpesvirus of turkeys (HVT), *Avian Dis.* 14:413–429.

Osborn, M., and Weber, K., 1975, Simian virus 40 gene A function and maintenance of transformation, *J. Virol.* 15:636–644.

Oxman, M. N., and Black, P. H., 1966, Inhibition of SV40 T antigen formation by interferon, *Proc. Natl. Acad. Sci. U.S.A.* 55:1133–1140.

Oxman, M. N., Takemoto, K. K., and Eckhart, W., 1972, Polyoma T antigen synthesis by temperature-sensitive mutants of polyoma virus, *Virology* 49:675–682.

Padgett, B. L., Walker, D. L., ZuRhein, G. M., Eckroade, R. J., and Dessel, B. H., 1971, Cultivation of papova-like virus from human brain with progressive multifocal leukoencephalopathy, *Lancet* 1:1257–1260.

Pattengale, P. K., Smith, R. W., and Gerber, P., 1974, B-Cell characteristics of human peripheral and cord blood lymphocytes transformed by Epstein-Barr virus, *J. Natl. Cancer Inst.* 52:1081–1086.

Paulin, D., and Cuzin, F., 1975, Polyoma virus T antigen. I. Synthesis of modified heat-labile T antigen in cells transformed with a *ts-a* mutant, *J. Virol.* 15:393–397.

Pauluzzi, S., and Rapp, F., 1969, Antigenic and oncogenic properties of a cell line derived from a hamster brain tumor induced by simian adenovirus 7, *J. Natl. Cancer Inst.* 43:1165–1173.

Payne, L. N., and Biggs, P. M., 1967, Studies on Marek's disease. II. Pathogenesis, *J. Natl. Cancer Inst.* 39:281–302.

Payne, L. N., and Rennie, M., 1970, Lack of effect of bursectomy on Marek's disease, *J. Natl. Cancer Inst.* 45:387–397.

Penny, J. B., and Narayan, O., 1973, Studies of the antigenic relationships of the new human papovaviruses by electron microscopy agglutination, *Infect. Immun.* 8: 299–300.

Pollack, R. E., Green, H., and Todaro, G. J., 1968, Growth control in cultured cells: Selection of sublines with increased sensitivity to contact inhibition and decreased tumor-producing ability, *Proc. Natl. Acad. Sci. U.S.A.* 60:126–133.

Pope, J. H., and Rowe, W. P., 1964, Detection of specific antigen in SV40-transformed cells by immunofluorescence, *J. Exp. Med.* 120:121–127.

Pope, J. H., Horne, M. K., and Scott, W., 1969, Identification of the filterable leukocyte-transforming factor of QIMR-WIL cells as herpes-like virus, *Int. J. Cancer* 4:255–260.

Powell, P. C., 1975, Immunity to Marek's disease induced by glutaraldehyde treated cells of Marek's disease lymphoblastoid cell lines, *Nature (London)* 257:684–685.

Powell, P. C., Payne, L. N., Frazier, J. A., and Rennie, M., 1974, Lymphoblastoid cell lines from Marek's disease lymphomas, *Nature (London)* 251:79–80.

Prevost, J. M., Orr, T. W., and Pearson, G. R., 1975, Augmentation of lymphocyte cytotoxicity by antibody to Herpesvirus saimiri associated antigens, *Proc. Natl. Acad. Sci. U.S.A.* 72:1671–1675.

Purchase, H. G., 1974, Marek's disease virus and the herpesvirus of turkeys, in: *Progress in Medical Virology*, Vol. 18 (J. L. Melnick, ed.), pp. 178–197, S. Karger, Basel.

Purchase, H. G., and Biggs, P. M., 1967, Characterization of five isolates of Marek's disease, *Res. Vet. Sci.* 8:440–449.

Purchase, H. G., and Okazaki, W., 1971, Effect of vaccination with herpesvirus of turkeys (HVT) on horizontal spread of Marek's disease (herpesvirus), *Avian Dis.* 15:391–397.

Purchase, H. G., and Sharma, J. M., 1975, Amelioration of Marek's disease and absence of vaccine protection in immunologically deficient chickens, *Nature* 248:419–421.

Pyrhönen, S., and Johansson, E., 1975, Regression of warts, an immunological study, *Lancet* 1:1–10.

Rabinowitz, Z., and Sachs, L., 1968, Reversion of properties in cells transformed by polyoma virus, *Nature (London)* 220:1203–1206.

Rabinowitz, Z., and Sachs, L., 1969, The formation of variants with a reversion of properties of transformed cells. I. Variants from polyoma-transformed cells grown *in vivo*, *Virology* 38:336–342.

Rabinowitz, Z., and Sachs, L. 1970, The formation of variants with reversion of properties of transformed cells. IV. Loss of detectable polyoma transplantation antigen, *Virology* 40:193–198.

Rapp, F., 1974, Herpesviruses and cancer, in: *Advances in Cancer Research*, Vol. 19 (G. Klein and S. Weinhouse, eds.), pp. 265–302, Academic Press, New York.

Rapp, F., and Duff, R., 1971, Quantitative aspects of virus-induced transformation of mammalian cells, in: *From Molecules to Man: The Gustav Stern Symposium on Perspectives in Virology VII*, pp. 37–53, Academic Press, New York.

Rapp, F., and Duff, R. G., 1973, Transformation of hamster embryo fibroblasts by herpes simplex viruses type 1 and type 2, *Cancer Res.* 33:1527–1534.

Rapp, F., and Li, J. L. H., 1974, Demonstration of the oncogenic potential of herpes simplex viruses and human cytomegalovirus, *Cold Spring Harbor Symp. Quant. Biol.* 39:747–763.

Rapp, F., and Westmoreland, D., 1976, Cell transformation by DNA-containing viruses, *Biochim. Biophys. Acta* 458:167–211.

Rapp, F., Butel, J. S., and Melnick, J. L., 1964a, Virus induced intranuclear antigen in cells transformed by papovavirus SV40, *Proc. Soc. Exp. Biol. Med.* 116:1131–1135.

Rapp, F., Kitahara, T., Butel, J. S., and Melnick, J. L., 1964b, Synthesis of SV40 tumor antigen during replication of simian papovavirus (SV40), *Proc. Natl. Acad. Sci. U.S.A.* 52:1138–1142.

Rapp, F., Melnick, J. L., Butel, J. S., and Kitahara, T., 1964c, The incorporation of SV40 genetic material into adenovirus 7 as measured by intranuclear synthesis of SV40 tumor antigen, *Proc. Natl. Acad. Sci. U.S.A.* 52:1348–1352.

Rapp, F., Butel, J. S., Feldman, L. A., Kitahara, T., and Melnick, J. L., 1965, Differential effects of inhibitors on the steps leading to the formation of SV40 tumor and virus antigens, *J. Exp. Med.* 121:935–944.

Rapp, F., Tevethia, S. S., and Melnick, J. L., 1966, Papovavirus SV40 transplantation immunity conferred by an adenovirus-SV40 hybrid, *J. Natl. Cancer Inst.* 36:707–708.

Rapp, F., Tevethia, S. S., Rawls, W. E., and Melnick, J. L., 1967, Production of antibodies to papovavirus SV40 tumor antigen in African green monkeys, *Proc. Soc. Exp. Biol. Med.* 125:794–798.

Rapp, F., Jerkofsky, M., Melnick, J., and Levy, B., 1968, Variation in the oncogenic potential of human adenoviruses carrying a defective SV40 genome (PARA), *J. Exp. Med.* 127:77–90.

Rapp, F., Pauluzzi, S., and Butel, J. S., 1969, Variation in properties of plaque progeny of PARA (defective simian papovavirus 40)–adenovirus 7, *J. Virol.* 4:626–631.

Rapp, F., Li, J. L. H., and Jerkofsky, M., 1973, Transformation of mammalian cells by DNA-containing viruses following photodynamic inactivation, *Virology* 55:339–346.

Rapp, F., Geder, L., Murasko, D., Lausch, R., Ladda, R., Huang, E.-S., and Webber, M. M., 1975, Long-term persistence of cytomegalovirus genome in cultured human cells of prostatic origin, *J. Virol.* 16:982–990.

Rawls, W. E., Tompkins, W. A. F., and Melnick, J. L., 1969, The association of herpes-virus type 2 and carcinoma of the uterine cervix, *Am. J. Epidemiol.* 89:547–554.

Reed, C. L., Cohen, G. H., and Rapp, F., 1975, Detection of a virus-specific antigen on the surface of herpes simplex virus-transformed cells, *J. Virol.* 15:668–670.

Reed, S. I., Ferguson, J., Davis, R., and Stark, G. R., 1975, T antigen binds to Simian virus 40 DNA at the origin of replication, *Proc. Natl. Acad. Sci. U.S.A.* 72:1605–1609.

Reedman, B. M., and Klein, G., 1973, Cellular localization of an Epstein-Barr virus (EBV)-associated complement-fixing antigen in producer and non-producer lymphoblastoid cell lines, *Int. J. Cancer* 11:499–502.

Riggs, J. L., Takemori, N., and Lennette, E. H., 1968, Cross-reactivity between T antigens of adenoviral immunotypes of proved and currently unproved oncogenic potential, *J. Immunol.* 100:348–354.

Risser, R., Rifkin, D., and Pollack, R., 1974, The stable classes of transformed cells induced by SV40 infection of established 3T3 cells and primary rat embryonic cells, *Cold Spring Harbor Symp. Quant. Biol.* 39:317–324.

Robb, J. A., and Martin, R. G., 1972, Genetic analysis of simian virus 40. III. Characterization of a temperature sensitive mutant blocked at an early stage of productive infection in monkey cells, *J. Virol.* 9:956–968.

Robb, J. A., Tegtmeyer, P., Ishikawa, A., Stark, G. R., and Ozer, H. L., 1974, Antigenic phenotypes and complementation groups of temperature-sensitive mutants of simian virus 40, *J. Virol.* 13:662–665.

Robinson, J., and Miller, G., 1975, Assay for Epstein-Barr virus based on stimulation of DNA synthesis in mixed leukocytes from human umbilical cord blood, *J. Virol.* 15:1065–1072.

Roizman, B., and Kieff, D., 1975, Herpes simplex and Epstein-Barr viruses in human cells and tissues: A study in contrasts, in: *Cancer: A Comprehensive Treatise,* Vol. 2 (F. Becker, ed.), pp. 241–322, Plenum Press, New York.

Röllinghoff, M., and Warner, N. L., 1973, Specificity of *in vivo* tumor rejection assessed by mixing immune spleen cells with target and unrelated tumor cells, *Proc. Soc. Exp. Biol. Med.* 144:813–818.

Rowe, W. P., and Baum, S. G., 1964, Evidence for a possible genetic hybrid between adenovirus type 7 and SV40 viruses, *Proc. Natl. Acad. Sci. U.S.A.* 52:1340–1347.

Royston, I., and Aurelian, L., 1970, Immunofluorescent detection of herpesvirus antigens in exfoliated cells from human cervical carcinoma, *Proc. Natl. Acad. Sci. U.S.A.* 67: 204–212.

Sadowski, J. M., and Rapp, F., 1975, Inhibition by levamisole of metastases by cells transformed by herpes simplex virus type 1, *Proc. Soc. Exp. Biol. Med.* 149:219–222.

Sambrook, J., 1973, Transformation by polyoma virus and simian virus 40, in: *Advances in Cancer Research,* Vol. 16 (G. Klein and S. Weinhouse, eds.), pp. 141–180, Academic Press, New York.

Sambrook, J., Botchan, M., Gallimore, P. M., Ozanne, B., Pettersson, U., Williams, J., and Sharp, P., 1974, Viral DNA sequences in cells transformed by simian virus 40, adenovirus type 2 and adenovirus type 5, *Cold Spring Harbor Symp. Quant. Biol.* 39:615–632.

Sambrook, J., Williams, J., Sharp, P. A., and Grodzicker, T., 1975, Physical mapping of temperature-sensitive mutations of adenoviruses, *J. Mol. Biol.* 97:369–390.

Sauer, G., Koprowski, H., and Defendi, V., 1967. The genetic heterogeneity of simian virus 40, *Proc. Natl. Acad. Sci. U.S.A.* 58:599–606.

Schaller, J. P., and Yohn, D. S., 1974, Transformation potential of the noninfectious (defective) component in pools of adenoviruses type 12 and simian adenovirus 7, *J. Virol.* 14:392–401.

Seemayer, N. H., Hirai, K., and Defendi, V., 1973, Analysis of minimal functions of simian virus 40. I. Oncogenic transformation of Syrian hamster kidney cells *in vitro* by photodynamically inactivated SV40, *Int. J. Cancer* 12:524–531.

Sharma, J. M., 1975, The role of T cells in herpesvirus induced Marek's disease lymphoma, in: *VIIth International Symposium on Comparative Leukemia Research,* in press.

Shin, S. I., Freedman, V. H., Risser, R., and Pollack, R., 1975, Tumorigenicity of virus-transformed cells in nude mice is correlated specifically with anchorage independent growth *in vitro, Proc. Natl. Acad. Sci. U.S.A.* 72:4435–4439.

Shope, T., Dechairo, D., and Miller, G., 1973, Malignant lymphoma in cottontop marmosets following inoculation with Epstein-Barr virus, *Proc. Natl. Acad. Sci. U.S.A.* 70: 2487–2491.

Silvestre, D., Kourilsky, F., Klein, G., Yata, Y., Neauport-Sautes, C., and Levy, J., 1971, Relationship between EBV-associated membrane antigen on Burkitt lymphoma cells and the viral envelope, demonstrated by immunoferritin labelling, *Int. J. Cancer* 8:222–233.

Singh, S. B., Smith, J. W., Rawls, W. E., and Tevethia, S. S., 1973, Demonstration of cytotoxic antibodies in rabbits bearing tumors induced by Shope fibroma virus, *Infect. Immun.* 5:352–358.

Sjögren, H. O., 1964, Studies on specific transplantation resistance to polyoma-virus-induced tumors. II. Mechanism of resistance induced by polyoma virus infection, *J. Natl. Cancer Inst.* 32:375–393.

Sjögren, H. O., 1965, Transplantation methods as a tool for detection of tumor-specific antigens, *Prog. Exp. Tumor Res.* 6:289–322.

Sjögren, H. O., and Bansal, S. C., 1971, Antigens in virally induced tumors, in: *Progress in Immunology*, (B. Amos, ed.), pp. 921–938, Academic Press, New York.

Sjögren, H. O., and Borum, K., 1971, Tumor-specific immunity in the course of primary polyoma and Rous tumor development in intact and immunosuppressed rats, *Cancer Res.* 31:890–900.

Sjögren, H. O., Hellstrom, I., and Klein, G., 1961, Resistance of polyoma virus immunized mice against transplantation of established polyoma tumors, *Exp. Cell Res.* 23: 204–208.

Sjögren, H. O., Minowada, M. D., and Ankerst, J., 1967, Specific transplantation antigens of mouse sarcomas induced by adenovirus type 12, *J. Exp. Med.* 125:689–701.

Smith, H. S., Scher, C. D., and Todaro, G. J., 1971, Induction of cell division in medium lacking serum growth factor by SV40, *Virology* 44:359–370.

Smith, H. S., Gelb, L. D., and Martin, M. A., 1972, Detection and quantitation of simian virus 40 genetic material in abortively transformed BALB/3T3 clones, *Proc. Natl. Acad. Sci. U.S.A.* 69:152–156.

Smith, R. W., Morganroth, J., and Mora, P. T., 1970, SV40 virus-induced tumor specific transplantation antigen in cultured mouse cells, *Nature (London)* 227:141–145.

Stutman, O., 1975, Tumor development after polyoma infection in athymic nude mice, *J. Immunol.* 114:1213–1217.

Svedmyr, E., Demissie, A., Klein, G., and Clifford, P., 1970, Antibody patterns in different human sera against intracellular and membrane antigen complexes associated with Epstein-Barr virus, *J. Natl. Cancer Inst.* 44:595–610.

Svedmyr, E., and Jondal, M., 1975, Cytotoxic effector cells for B cell lines transformed by Epstein-Barr virus present in patients with infectious mononucleosis, *Proc. Natl. Acad. Sci. U.S.A.* 72:1622–1626.

Syverton, J. T., Dascomb, H. E., Wells, E. B., Koomen, J., and Berry, G. P., 1950, The virus-induced papilloma-to-carcinoma sequence. II. Carcinomas in the natural host, the cottontail rabbit, *Cancer Res.* 10:440.

Tai, H. T., Smith, C. A., Sharp, P. A., and Vinograd, J., 1972, Sequence heterogeneity in closed simian virus 40 deoxyribonucleic acid, *J. Virol.* 9:317–325.

Takemoto, K. K., and Mullarkey, M. F., 1973, Human papovavirus, BK strain: Biological studies including antigenic relationship to simian virus 40, *J. Virol.* 12:625–631.

Takemoto, K. K., Ting, R. C. Y., Ozer, H. L., and Fabisch, P., 1968, Establishment of a cell line from an inbred mouse strain for viral transformation studies: simian virus 40 transformation and tumor production, *J. Natl. Cancer Inst.* 41:1401–1409.

Tegtmeyer, P., 1972, Simian virus 40 deoxyribonucleic acid synthesis: The viral replicon, *Virology* 10:591–598.

Tegtmeyer, P., 1975, Function of simian virus 40 gene *A* in transforming infection, *J. Virol.* 15:613–618.

Tegtmeyer, P., and Ozer, H. L., 1971, Temperature-sensitive mutants of simian virus 40: Infection of permissive cells, *J. Virol.* 8:516–524.

Tegtmeyer, P., and Ozer, H. L., 1972, Synthesis and assembly of simian virus 40 II.

Synthesis of the major capsid protein and its incorporation into viral particles, *J. Virol.* 9:52–60.

Tegtmeyer, P., Schwartz, M., Collins, J. K., and Rundell, K., 1975, Regulation of tumor antigen synthesis by simian virus 40 gene *A, J. Virol.* 16:168–178.

Tenser, R. B., and Hsiung, G. D., 1973, Infection of thymus cells *in vivo* and *in vitro* with a guinea pig herpes-like virus and the effect of antibody on virus replication in organ culture, *J. Immunol.* 110:552–560.

Tevethia, M. J., and Tevethia, S. S., 1976, Biology of SV40 transplantation antigen (TrAg). I. Demonstration of SV40 TrAg on gluteraldehyde-fixed SV40-infected African green monkey kidney cells, *Virology* 69:474–489.

Tevethia, S. S., 1967, Characterization of hamster antibody reacting with papovavirus SV40 tumor antigen, *J. Immunol.* 98:1257–1264.

Tevethia, S. S., 1970, Immune response of rabbits to purified papovavirus SV40, *J. Immunol.* 104:72–78.

Tevethia, S. S., 1974, Evidence for virus-specific transplantation antigen in cells of lymphoid neoplasms induced by papovavirus SV40, *Int. J. Cancer* 13:494–499.

Tevethia, S. S., 1975, Immunofluorescence staining of DNA tumor virus-induced antigens, *Ann. N.Y. Acad. Sci.* 254:541–550.

Tevethia, S. S., and McMillan, V. L., 1974, Acquisition of malignant properties by SV40-transformed mouse cells: relationship to type-C viral antigen expression, *Intervirology* 3:269–276.

Tevethia, S. S., and Tevethia, M. J., 1975*a*, DNA virus (SV40) induced antigens, in: *Cancer, A Comprehensive Treatise*, Vol. 4 (F. Becker, ed.), 185–207, Plenum Press, New York.

Tevethia, S. S., and Tevethia, M. J. 1975*b*, Cell surface antigens of DNA virus (SV40) infected and transformed cells, in: *Cellular Membranes and Tumor Cell Behavior*, pp. 447–467, Williams and Wilkins, Baltimore.

Tevethia, S. S., and Tevethia, M. J., 1976, Cell-mediated immunity to virus-induced tumors: Generation of lymphocytes sensitized to specific transplantation antigen in mouse cells infected with papovavirus SV40, in: *Progress in Medical Virology*, Vol. 21 (F. Rapp, ed.), pp. 103–117, S. Karger, Basel.

Tevethia, S. S., and Zarling, J. M., 1972, Participation of macrophages in tumor immunity, *Natl. Cancer Inst. Monogr.* 35:279–282.

Tevethia, S. S., Katz, M., and Rapp, F., 1965, New surface antigen in cells transformed by simian papovavirus SV40, *Proc. Soc. Exp. Biol. Med.* 119:896–901.

Tevethia, S. S., Couvillon, L. A., and Rapp, F., 1968*a*, Development in hamsters of antibodies against surface antigens present in cells transformed by papovavirus SV40, *J. Immunol.* 100:358–362.

Tevethia, S. S., Diamandopoulos, G. Th., Rapp, F., and Enders, J. F., 1968*b*, Lack of relationship between virus-specific and transplantation antigens in hamster cells transformed by simian papovavirus SV40, *J. Immunol.* 101:1192–1198.

Tevethia, S. S., Dreesman, G. R., Lausch, R. N., and Rapp, F., 1968*c*, Effect of anti-hamster thymocyte serum on papovavirus SV40-induced transplantation immunity, *J. Immunol.* 101:1105–1110.

Tevethia, S. S., Crouch, N. A., Melnick, J. L., and Rapp, F., 1970, Detection of specific surface antigens by colony inhibition in cells transformed by papovavirus SV40, *Int. J. Cancer* 5:176–184.

Tevethia, S. S., McMillan, V. L., Kaplan, P. M., and Bushong, S. C., 1971, Variation in immunosensitivity of SV40 transformed hamster cells, *J. Immunol.* 106:1295–1300.

Tevethia, S. S., Blasecki, J. W., Waneck, G., and Goldstein, A., 1974, Requirement of thymus-derived θ positive lymphocytes for rejection of DNA virus (SV40) tumors in mice, *J. Immunol.* 113:1417–1423.

Tevethia, S. S., Zarling, J. M., and Flax, M., 1976, Macrophages and the destruction of syngeneic virus-induced tumors, in: *Immunology of Macrophage* (D. S. Nelson, ed.), Academic Press, New York, in press.

Thompson, D. M. P., 1975, Soluble tumor-specific antigen and its relationship to tumor growth, *Int. J. Cancer* 15:1016–1029.

Ting, C. C., and Herberman, R. B., 1971, Detection of tumor-specific antigen of simian virus 40-induced tumors by the isotopic antiglobulin technique, *Int. J. Cancer* 7:499–506.

Ting, C. C., Larvin, D. H., Shiv, G., and Herberman, R. B., 1972, Expression of fetal antigens in tumor cells, *Proc. Natl. Acad. Sci. U.S.A.* 69:1664–1668.

Ting, C. C., Rodrigues, D., and Herberman, R. B., 1973, Expression of fetal antigens and tumor-specific antigens in SV40-transformed cells. II. Tumor transplantation studies, *Int. J. Cancer* 12:519–523.

Tockstein, G., Polasa, H., Piña, M., and Green, M., 1968, A simple purification procedure for adenovirus type 12 T and tumor antigens and some of their properties, *Virology* 36:377–386.

Tompkins, W. A. F., Adams, C., and Rawls, W. E., 1970a, An *in vitro* measure of cellular immunity to fibroma virus, *J. Immunol.* 104:502–510.

Tompkins, W. A. F., Crouch, N. A., Tevethia, S. S., and Rawls, W. E., 1970b, Characterization of surface antigen on cells infected by fibroma virus, *J. Immunol.* 105:1181–1189.

Tooze, J. (ed), 1973, The molecular biology of tumor viruses, *Cold Spring Harbor Laboratory*, New York.

Trentin, J. J., and Bryan, E., 1966, Virus induced transplantation immunity to human adenovirus type 12 tumors of the hamster and mouse, *Proc. Soc. Exp. Biol. Med.* 121:1216–1219.

Trentin, J. J., Yabe, Y., and Taylor, G., 1962, The quest for human cancer viruses, *Science* 137:835–841.

Trentin, J. J., Van Hoosier, G. L., Jr., and Samper, L., 1968, The oncogenicity of human adenoviruses in hamsters, *Proc. Soc. Exp. Biol. Med.* 127:683–689.

Tubergen, D. G., and Feldman, J. D., 1971, The role of thymus and bone marrow cells in delayed hypersensitivity, *J. Exp. Med.* 134:1144–1154.

Uchida, S., and Watanabe, S., 1969. Tumorigenicity of the antigen-forming defective virions of simian virus 40, *Virology* 35:166–168.

Uchida, S., Yoshiike, K., Watanabe, S., and Furino, A., 1968, Antigen forming defective virions of simian virus 40, *Virology* 34:1–8.

Vandeputte, M., 1969, Antilymphocyte serum and polyoma virus oncogenesis in rats, *Transplant. Proc.* 1:100–105.

Vandeputte, M., Denys, P., Leyten, R., and De Somer, P., 1963, The oncogenic activity of the polyoma virus in thymectomized rats, *Life Sci.* 2:475–478.

Vandeputte, M., Eyssen, H., Sobis, H., and De Somer, P., 1974, Induction of polyoma virus tumors in athymic nude mice, *Int. J. Cancer* 14:445–450.

Van Der Noordaa, J., 1968, Transformation of rat cells by adenovirus types 1, 2, and 3, *J. Gen. Virol.* 3:303–304.

Volkers, S., and Pitts, J., 1973, Virus specific surface antigens in cells productively infected with polyoma virus, *Nature (London) New Biol.* 244:274–275.

Volkman, A., and Collins, F. M., 1971, The restorative effect of peritoneal macrophages on delayed hypersensitivity following ionizing radiation, *Cell Immunol.* 2:552–566.

Vonka, V., Zavadova, H. Kutinova, L., and Rezacova, D., 1967, Development of antibodies against viral and tumor antigens of papovavirus SV40 in monkeys, *Proc. Soc. Exp. Biol. Med.* **125**:790–793.

Vonka, V., Benyesh-Melnick, M., and McCombs, R., 1970, Antibodies in human sera to soluble and viral antigens found in Burkitt lymphoma and other lymphoblastoid cell lines, *J. Natl. Cancer Inst.* **44**:865–872.

Vonka, V., Vlckova, I., Zonadova, H., Kouba, K., Lazovska, J., and Duber, J., 1972, Antibodies to EBV virus capsid antigen and to soluble antigen of lymphoblastoid cells in infectious mononucleosis patients, *Int. J. Cancer* **9**:529–535.

Walker, D. L., Padgett, B. L., ZuRhein, G. M., Albert, A. E., and Marsh, R. F., 1973, Human papovavirus (JC): Induction of brain tumors in hamsters, *Science* **181**:674–676.

Weiner, L. P., Herndon, R. M., Narayan, O., and Johnson, R. T., 1972, Further studies of a simian virus 40 like virus isolated from human brain, *J. Virol.* **10**:147–152.

Weiss, A. F., Portmann, R., Fischer, H., Simon, J., and Zang, K. D., 1975, Simian virus 40-related antigens in three human meningiomas with defined chromosome loss, *Proc. Natl. Acad. Sci. U.S.A.* **72**:609–613.

Wesslen, T., 1970. SV40 tumorigenesis in mouse, *Acta Pathol. Microbiol. Scan.* **78**: 479–487.

Wilkie, N. M., Ustacelebi, S., and Williams, J. F., 1973, Characterization of temperature-sensitive mutants of adenovirus type 5: nucleic acid synthesis, *Virology* **51**:499–503.

Williams, J. F., Young, C. S. H., and Austin, P. E., 1974, Genetic analysis of human adenovirus type 5 in permissive and nonpermissive cells, *Cold Spring Harbor Symp. Quant. Biol.* **39**:427–437.

Witter, R. L., 1972, Turkey herpesvirus: Lack of oncogenicity for turkeys, *Avian Dis.* **16**:660–670.

Witter, R. L., Solomon, J. J., Champion, L. R., and Nazerian, K., 1971, Long term studies of Marek's disease infection in individual chickens, *Avian Dis.* **15**:346–365.

Witter, R. L., Stephens, E. A., Sharma, J. M., and Nazerian, K., 1975, Demonstration of a tumor-associated surface antigen in Marek's disease, *J. Immunol.* **115**:177–183.

Wolf, H., zur Hausen, H., and Becker, V., 1973, EB viral genomes in epithelial nasopharyngeal carcinoma cells, *Nature (London) New Biol.* **244**:245–247.

Wright, P. W., and Law, L. W., 1971, Quantitative *in vitro* measurement of simian virus 40 tumor-specific antigens, *Proc. Natl. Acad. Sci. U.S.A.* **69**:973–976.

Wright, P. W., Smith, H. S., and McCoy, J., 1973, Tumorigenicity and antigenicity of mouse cells infected with simian virus 40. I. Relationship of growth *in vitro* and *in vivo* in immunosuppressed and immunocompetent recipients, *J. Natl. Cancer Inst.* **51**: 951–959.

Yohn, D. S., 1973, Sex related resistance in hamsters to adenovirus oncogenesis, *Prog. Exp. Tumor Res.* **18**:138–165.

Yoshiike, K., 1968, Studies on DNA from low-density particles of SV40. II. Noninfectious virions associated with a large-plaque variant, *Virology* **34**:402–409.

Zarling, J. M., and Tevethia, S. S., 1973*a*, Transplantation immunity to simian virus 40-transformed cells in tumor-bearing mice. I. Development of cellular immunity to simian virus 40 tumor-specific transplantation antigens during tumorigenesis by transformed cells, *J. Natl. Cancer Inst.* **50**:137–147.

Zarling, J. M., and Tevethia, S. S., 1973*b*, Transplantation immunity to simian virus 40-transformed cells in tumor bearing mice. II. Evidence for macrophage participation at the effector level of tumor cell rejection, *J. Natl. Cancer Inst.* **50**:149–157.

Zbar, B., Wepsic, H. T., Rapp, H. J., Stewart, L. C., and Borsos, T., 1970, Two-step mechanism of tumor graft rejection in syngeneic guinea pigs. II. Initiation of reaction by a cell fraction containing lymphocytes and neutrophils, *J. Natl. Cancer Inst.* **44**:701–717.

Zembala, M., Ptak, W., and Hanczakowska, M., 1973, The role of macrophages in the cytotoxic killing of tumor cells *in vitro*. I. Primary immunization of the lymphocytes *in vitro* for target cell killing and the mechanism of lymphocyte macrophage cooperation, *Immunology* **25**:631–644.

zur Hausen, H., Henle, W., Hummeler, K., Diehl, V., and Henle, G., 1967, Comparative study of cultured Burkitt tumor cells by immunofluorescence, autoradiography and electron microscopy, *J. Virol.* **1**:830–837.

zur Hausen, H., Schulte-Holthausen, H., Klein, G., Henle, W., Henle, G., Clifford, P., and Santesson, L., 1970, EB-virus DNA in biopsies of Burkitt tumors and anaplastic carcinomas of the nasopharynx, *Nature (London)* **228**:1056–1058.

Chapter 2

Immunity to Leukemia, Lymphoma, and Fibrosarcoma in Cats: A Case for Immunosurveillance

M. Essex

Department of Microbiology
Harvard University School of Public Health
Boston, Massachusetts 02115

I. INTRODUCTION

Central to the discipline of tumor immunology is the hypothesis of immu-nosurveillance. Does the immune response act to eliminate developing clones of cancer cells in the same manner that it eliminates injurious microorganisms or grafted tissues from unrelated individuals? A great amount of work has been done in response to this question using either virus-induced tumors or transplant-able tumors in inbred mice, but very few studies have been done with sponta-neous tumors of outbred animals. Evidence that immunosuppressed people have a greater risk of developing certain types of tumors (Gatti and Good, 1971; Penn, 1974, 1975; Wilson and Penn, 1975) is compatible with, but not conclu-sive proof of, the immunosurveillance hypothesis. Further proof requires not only the demonstration of a depressed immune response to specific tumor cell membrane antigens in outbred individuals prior to tumor development but also the reciprocal—evidence of an enhanced immune response in individuals who remain free of tumors following exposure to the same oncogenic agents. Our general lack of information concerning either the etiological agents of sponta-neous tumors or the existence of tumor cell membrane antigens on such tumors probably represents the major roadblock against the design of such experiments for application to outbred individuals with spontaneous tumors.

Knowledge of the etiology and natural history of leukemia and lymphoma of outbred cats has expanded significantly in the last 5 years, thus making the feline system an appropriate model for the testing of the immunosurveillance hypothesis. Much of the information concerning the virology and pathology of feline leukemia, lymphoma, and fibrosarcoma has been recently reviewed elsewhere (Essex *et al.*, 1973*a*, 1976*a*; W. Jarrett, 1975; Deinhardt, 1975; Essex, 1975*a,b;* Hardy *et al.*, 1976*a*). Thus, both in keeping with the theme of this volume and in concentrating on information that has not been reviewed in detail before, the emphasis for this chapter will be on the apparent role of tumor immunity in the pathogenesis of spontaneous neoplasia.

II. IMMUNOSURVEILLANCE HYPOTHESIS

Individuals with either inherited immune deficiency disease or drug-induced immunosuppression have a greatly increased risk of development of neoplastic diseases, especially the lymphomas and leukemias (Gatti and Good, 1971; Penn, 1974, 1975). Patients with ataxia-telangiectasia, the Wiskott-Aldrich syndrome, and certain agammaglobulinemias, for example, have up to a 10,000-fold increase in risk for the development of certain types of tumors. This increased risk is apparently not due to an increased susceptibility for transformation to occur at the cellular level (Kersey *et al.*, 1972). Under experimental conditions in laboratory animals, the administration of immunosuppressive agents, such as antilymphocyte serum, greatly increases risk for development of both primary tumors and subsequent metastasis (Allison and Law, 1968; Hellmann *et al.*, 1968; Hirsch and Murphy, 1968).

Such observations led Burnet (1970) to propose the hypothesis of immunological surveillance. The hypothesis postulated that tumor cells possessed cell-surface antigens that would be recognized as "foreign" by adult immunologically competent animals, and that under normal circumstances this recognition would result in elimination of developing clones of malignant cells. Burnet, like Thomas (1959) before him, subscribed to the concept that tumor immunity would be analogous in principle to homograft rejection, and possibly even the evolutionary explanation for the development of homograft rejection responses. As homograft rejection had been quite conclusively shown to be a function of thymus-derived (T) lymphocytes, participation by the bone marrow-derived (B) population of lymphocytes or humoral antibody was considered to have either an insignificant or a deleterious effect (Hellström and Hellström, 1970).

With this background, observations that neither thymusless (nude) mice (Rygaard and Povlsen, 1974; Stutman, 1974) nor neonatally thymectomized mice (Sanford *et al.*, 1973) had a significant increase in incidence of most spontaneous or induced tumors were considered contradictory to the hypothesis (Prehn, 1974; Schwartz, 1974). An alternative explanation for these observations would be that the B-cell immune compartment might be a mediator of immune surveillance in some tumor systems. Although certain herpesvirus-associated tumors such as Burkitt's lymphoma of man (Jondal *et al.*, 1975) and Marek's disease of chickens (Sharma *et al.*, 1975) do seem to have operative T-cell-mediated immunosurveillance mechanisms, there is equally convincing evidence that either antibodies or non-T lymphocyte populations play important roles in certain oncornavirus systems (Lamon *et al.*, 1973; G. Pearson *et al.*, 1973; Thompson and Linna, 1973; Senik *et al.*, 1974).

Immunoglobulin, complement receptor, and thymocyte markers have been used extensively for identification of cell populations in various lymphoid malignancies. Burkitt's lymphoma and chronic lymphocytic leukemia, for example, appear to be tumors of B lymphocytes, while acute lymphoblastic leukemia of children appears to be a tumor of T lymphocytes (Jondal and Klein, 1973; Kersey *et al.*, 1973; Belpomme *et al.*, 1974; Brown *et al.*, 1974). It is logical that T-cell-mediated immunity should be developed to control malignancies involving B-type target cells. In the case of malignancies involving T-type target cells, however, the possibility that B-lymphocyte mechanisms would mediate immunosurveillance must be considered. In this regard, early evidence suggests that most lymphomas and lymphoid leukemias of cats appear to involve transformed T lymphoid cells (Mackey *et al.*, 1975a; Cockerell *et al.*, 1976; Cerny and Essex, unpublished observations).

III. FELINE ONCORNAVIRUSES

Two distinctly different groups of oncornaviruses have been found in domestic cats. The first group, comprised of the feline leukemia (FeLV) and sarcoma viruses (FeSV), was discovered in tumor tissue or blood plasma from field cases of spontaneous lymphoma (W. Jarrett *et al.*, 1964a,b; Kawakami *et al.*, 1967; Theilen *et al.*, 1968; Rickard *et al.*, 1969) or fibrosarcoma (Snyder and Theilen, 1969; Gardner *et al.*, 1970; Snyder, 1971; McDonough *et al.*, 1971). The second group, the endogenous oncornaviruses designated RD-114, was isolated from cultured or fresh tissues from normal healthy cats (Fischinger *et al.*, 1973; Livingston and Todaro, 1973; Sarma *et al.*, 1973; Noronha *et al.*, 1974). Studies to characterize the RD-114 class of agents (Baluda and Roy-Burman, 1973; Gillespie *et al.*, 1973; McAllister *et al.*, 1973; Neiman, 1973; Okabe *et al.*, 1973; Ruprecht *et al.*, 1973) revealed that the group had been discovered earlier by McAllister *et al.* (1972) in their attempts to isolate human oncornaviruses. All the endogenous RD-114-type oncornaviruses isolated thus far from domestic cats appear similar or identical. Yet the RD-114 agents show only a distant relationship to the FeLV-FeSV group by either serological (McAllister *et al.*, 1973; Schafer *et al.*, 1973; Gilden *et al.*, 1974) or nucleic acid hybridization techniques (Baluda and Roy-Burman, 1973; Gillespie *et al.*, 1973; Ruprecht *et al.*, 1973; Quintrell *et al.*, 1974; Gillespie and Gallo, 1975). The FeLV-FeSV group appears to have no greater relatedness to the RD-114 group, for example, than either group has to the murine leukemia-sarcoma oncornavirus group or the simian leukemia-sarcoma group.

A close relationship does occur between the endogenous feline group and an endogenous group of oncornaviruses isolated from normal healthy baboons, designated the M7 group (Benveniste *et al.*, 1974; Sherr *et al.*, 1974; Todaro *et al.*, 1974). In apparent analogy with the FeLV-FeSV and RD-114 agents of cats, however, the simian sarcoma and gibbon lymphoma agents of primates appear to be unrelated to the endogenous primate M7 group (Sherr *et al.*, 1974; Gillespie and Gallo, 1975). This is different from the situation in inbred mice and chickens, however, where the endogenous and exogenous viruses are much more closely related within each species (Essex, 1975*a*).

The major antigens of the RD-114 viruses and cells infected by them have been identified (Gilden *et al.*, 1974; Riggs *et al.*, 1974; Sarma *et al.*, 1974*a*), but very few studies have been done to determine the *in vivo* immune response to them in cats. Additionally, since no successful attempts to demonstrate oncogenicity have been reported for either the RD-114 group or endogenous oncornaviruses of other species, the significance of such information would be difficult to interpret.

Several excellent reviews are available on oncornavirus structure (Bauer, 1974; Bolognesi, 1974; Schäfer and Bolognesi, 1976). They should be consulted if detailed information on the structural nature of FeLV-FeSV antigens is desired. Operationally, the viral structural proteins that appear important for interpretation of the immune response are those designated p15, p30, and gp70 (August *et al.*, 1974). These proteins also appear in infected producer cells, in both cytoplasmic and membrane sites (Ubertini *et al.*, 1971; Hilgers *et al.*, 1972; Hardy *et al.*, 1973*a,b;* Friedman *et al.*, 1974; Strand *et al.*, 1974; Yoshiki *et al.*, 1974; Del Villano *et al.*, 1975; Kurth, 1975). Like other oncornaviruses, the FeLV-FeSV group buds from cell membranes, is type C in morphology, is about 100 nm in diameter, and is of buoyant density 1.14–1.17 g/cm^3 in sucrose (Essex, 1975*a*). Unlike the RD-114 group, which grows productively only in cells from nonfeline species (Fischinger *et al.*, 1973; Livingston and Todaro, 1973), the FeLV-FeSV group replicates from most feline cells either *in vitro* or *in vivo* (O. Jarrett *et al.*, 1968; Dougherty *et al.*, 1969; Hardy *et al.*, 1969; Rickard *et al.*, 1969; Theilen *et al.*, 1969; W. Jarrett *et al.*, 1973*b*). The FeLV-FeSV group will also grow in and/or transform cells from numerous other species, such as dog, man, ox, and dolphin (O. Jarrett *et al.*, 1969, 1970; Chang *et al.*, 1970; Deinhardt *et al.*, 1970; Hampar *et al.*, 1970; Sarma *et al.*, 1970; O. Jarrett, 1971; Lee, 1971; Essex *et al.*, 1972*a,b;* Monti-Bragadin and Ulrich, 1972; McDonald *et al.*, 1972; McAllister *et al.*, 1973; Chan *et al.*, 1974*a,b*).

Three distinct subgroups of the FeLV-FeSV group have been identified on the functional basis of serum antibody neutralization or host-cell surface attachment site interference (Sarma and Log, 1971, 1973). These functions are presumed to be specified by the virus envelope gp70. The subgroups, designated A, B, and C, have somewhat different infectivity patterns, at least for cells from nonfeline species (O. Jarrett et al., 1973, Sarma et al., 1975).

FeLVs induce only minor physiological changes in fibroblastic or epithelial cells (Bardell and Essex, 1974), and induce formation of syncitia in lymphoid lines of human or canine origin (Hampar et al., 1973; Noronha, personal communication). The Epstein-Barr herpesvirus and the Abelson murine leukemia virus will convert normal lymphoid cells from their respective species to permanently established lines (Pope et al., 1969; Nilsson et al., 1971; Sklar et al., 1974). Similar experiments with leukemogenic oncornavirus isolates from cats or other outbred species have not been reported. FeSVs are among the most efficient transforming viruses available for susceptible fibroblastic or epithelial cells. Transformation of primary or early passage secondary tissues from fetal or neonatal cats is most efficient (Sarma et al., 1971a,b, 1972; McDonald et al., 1972), but comparable tissues of canine, bovine, monkey, or human origin can also be transformed (Chang et al., 1970; Deinhardt et al., 1970; Sarma et al., 1970, 1971a,b; McAllister et al., 1971; McDonald et al., 1972; Melnick et al., 1973; Chan et al., 1974a,b; Theilen et al., 1974). All isolates of FeSV thus far tested contain a hundred- to a thousandfold excess of nontransforming particles in the virus pools (Sarma et al., 1971a,b, 1972). Sarcomagenic oncornaviruses of mice are defective in that an excess of associated "helper" nonsarcomagenic virus is necessary for completion of the replication cycle and release of progeny virus particles (Hartley and Rowe, 1966). This property has been used to establish murine sarcoma virus positive, helper leukemia virus negative cultures by infection with end-point dilutions (Aaronson and Rowe, 1970; Bassin et al., 1970). Such cultures are then valuable for titration of leukemia virus stocks, because infection with leukemia virus results in rescue and release of the sarcoma virus, with the development of foci.

A feline cell line that contains defective murine sarcoma virus was developed by Fischinger et al. (1974) for assay of the FeLVs and the xenotrophic murine oncornaviruses. The sensitivity of the line for focus formation by either field strains or purified subgroups of FeLV has made the line very valuable for isolation and titration of FeLV, and for detection and titration of virus neutralizing antibody.

The viral structural proteins can be detected in the cytoplasm of infected producer cells with antisera made to these antigens in heterologous species, such as rabbits or goats. The indirect immunofluorescence procedure for the detection of cytoplasmic FeLV antigens has been adopted for use on blood films by Hardy et al. (1973a,b). This modification was extremely valuable because it was shown that the presence or absence of FeLV antigens detected in this manner was an accurate reflection of the presence of circulating infectious FeLV, or viremia (Hardy *et al.*, 1973*b*; Hardy, 1974; Deinhardt, 1975; Hardy and McClelland, 1975; O. Jarrett, personal communication). Thus since only a drop of blood is needed from each cat and the air-dried films can be stored for long periods before examination, this test is ideal for the seroepidemiological screening of large numbers of cats. On a more limited scale, complement fixation (Sarma *et al.*, 1971*c*; Gardner *et al.*, 1974), immunodiffusion (Hardy *et al.*, 1969), electron microscopy (Laird *et al.*, 1968), and radioimmunoassay (Scolnick *et al.*, 1972) have also been used for the detection of FeLV in tissues. For the detection of nonneutralizing antibody to virus proteins complement-fixation inhibition (Olsen and Yohn, 1972; Olsen *et al.*, 1975), the paired radioactive iodine labeling test (Yohn and Olsen, 1973), or radioimmunoprecipitation have been used (Aaronson, personal communication; Charman *et al.*, 1976).

IV. FELINE ONCORNAVIRUS-ASSOCIATED CELL MEMBRANE ANTIGEN

We originally suggested the term "feline oncornavirus-associated cell membrane antigen" (FOCMA) for the cell-surface reactivity observed on a feline lymphoma cell line when serum from cats that were resistant to tumor growth was used (Essex *et al.*, 1971*a,b*, 1972*b*). The target cell that was used in the original studies, designated Fl 74, was derived from a cat with a laboratory-induced lymphoma (Theilen *et al.*, 1969). The same cell line is still used as the reference positive target for FOCMA. This cell line actively produces feline leukemia virus (FeLV) of all three subgroups (Sarma and Log, 1973). Similar or identical FOCMA activity has been detected on other feline lymphoma cell lines, such as the F422, which produces subgroup A virus only, and leukemic lymphoblasts taken by biopsy or at autopsy from neoplastic cats (Essex, unpublished observations).

Antibody activity to FOCMA developed only following exposure to live FeLV or feline sarcoma virus (FeSV), and high titers occurred only when cats resisted the development of progressive tumors (Essex *et al.*, 1971*a,b*, 1973*a,b*). Specificity of the antigen was determined by observations that (1) antibody activity developed only under either laboratory or natural conditions following exposure to FeLV or FeSV, (2) antibody activity was present in all infected cats that resisted tumor development, regardless of genetic background of the cat, (3) buffy coat lymphocytes from unexposed cats were always negative for the antigen, regardless of genetic background, and (4) the FOCMA antigen showed no cross-reactivity with analogous cell membrane antigens induced by other agents, such as the avian, simian, or murine oncornaviruses, or the Epstein-Barr herpesvirus (Essex, 1974, 1975*a*; Boone *et al.*, 1973; Oshiro *et al.*, 1974). The infection of human or canine lymphoid cells with FeLV resulted in the specific induction of a membrane antigen which was detectable with monkey or canine serum from FeLV- or FeSV-infected animals (Essex *et al.*, 1972*b*, 1973*b*).

Most serological studies for detection of FOCMA and titration of FOCMA antibody have used indirect membrane immunofluorescence. We have recently found that the antibody-mediated cytotoxicity test gives comparable results (Mathes *et al.*, 1976). Mackey *et al.* (1975*b*) have adapted the mixed-cell hemadsorption test for titrating FOCMA antibody (Mackey *et al.*, 1975*b*; Rogerson *et al.*, 1975).

When considering the nature of FOCMA, several classes of antigens can be considered on the basis of studies done with the murine and avian oncornavirus systems. Representative publications for the various antigen classes are given in Table I. In murine systems, numerous oncornavirus-associated cell membrane antigens have been described (Aoki, 1974). Some of the antigens appear specific for certain virus strains (Cerny and Essex, 1974; Ting *et al.*, 1974) while others appear to have wide-ranging subgroup or group specificity (Klein and Klein, 1964; Yoshiki *et al.*, 1974). Few, if any, have been characterized for both specificity according to virus strain or group and biological class of antigen, i.e., derepressed embryonic, virus structural, or tumor specific. The identification and characterization of true "tumor-specific" antigens seem most important, but this issue becomes solely academic if it can be shown that derepressed embryonic antigens or viral structural proteins can function in the same capacity.

Table I. Tumor Cell Membrane Antigens Found on Cells Transformed by Murine and Avian Oncornaviruses

Species	Class	References
Murine	Embryonic	Ishimoto *et al.* (1974)
	Virus structural proteins	
	1. p30	Yoshiki *et al.* (1974)
	2. p15	Friedman *et al.* (1974), Strand *et al.* (1974), Ihle *et al.* (1974)
	3. gp70	Aaronson and Stephenson (1974), Ihle *et al.* (1974), Hanna *et al.* (1975)
	Tumor specific	Moroni *et al.* (1974), Chang *et al.* (1975)
Avian	Embryonic	Kurth and Bauer (1973)
	Virus structural proteins	
	1. gp70	Chen and Hanafusa (1974), Phillips and Perdue (1974)
	Tumor specific	Kurth (1975), Rohrschneider *et al.* (1975), Bauer *et al.* (1976)

In the avian system, a cell membrane antigen that appears to be tumor specific has been identified (Kurth, 1975; Rohrschneider et al., 1975; Bauer et al., 1976). It is group specific, unlike the virus envelope glycoproteins, and expressed only on transformed cells, regardless of whether or not they produce progeny virus. The antigen is a glycoprotein of approximately 100,000 daltons.

As yet, relatively little is known about the nature of FOCMA, but several observations suggest that it is not one of the major viral structural proteins, gp70, p30, or p15. The gp70 antigen is the main target for virus neutralization, and numerous studies indicate that FOCMA antibody titers and virus-neutralizing antibody titers for given animals or groups of animals are not necessarily related (Schaller et al., 1975; Hardy et al., 1976a). Cats can be viremic, for example, in the presence of high FOCMA antibody titers (Aldrich and Pederson, 1974; Essex et al., 1975c), but such cats do not have detectable virus-neutralizing antibody (Hardy et al., 1976a). Inactivated virus can also induce virus-neutralizing antibody in adult cats, but FOCMA antibody is never induced unless viable virus is given (Olsen et al., 1976b).

Similar evidence suggests that cell-surface FOCMA is not the viral structural protein p30. First, serological studies indicate that titers of antibody to p30 in individual cats by radioimmunoprecipitation do not correspond to antibody titers to FOCMA by membrane immunofluorescence (Charman et al., 1976; Aaronson and Essex, unpublished observations). Second, vaccination of adult cats with inactivated FeLV or pure p30 may result in the production of high titers of antibody to p30, but such cats have no FOCMA antibody (Olsen et al., 1975; Charman and Essex, unpublished observations).

Using goat or rabbit antisera to the pure FeLV structural components, gp70, p30, and p15, we have recently shown that the FOCMA-positive target cell, Fl 74, contains these antigens on the cell surface in amounts sufficient for detection by membrane immunofluorescence (Essex, Oroszlan, Noronha, and Hardy, unpublished observations). Using either disrupted whole FeLV or pure virus fractions, we could adsorb antibody activity in the antisera of goat or rabbit origin that was directed to these components. Such membrane-reactive FOCMA antibody activity in cat sera could not be removed by adsorption with either whole disrupted FeLV or pure gp70, p30, or p15.

The question of virus group versus subgroup specificity for FOCMA has been more difficult to address. All sera from cats with either laboratory or natural exposure to FeLV or FeSV had evidence of FOCMA antibody production if they resisted tumor development. All "transformed" lymphoid or fibroblastic cultures of feline origin contain subgroup A virus, however, as do all the standard strains used for tumor induction and all field isolates thus far described. It is therefore not yet possible to say if FOCMA is specific only for subgroup A virus, or common for all subgroups as is the TSTA (tumor-specific transplantation antigen) described in avian oncornavirus systems. Nontransformed fibroblasts of human or canine lymphoid lines are available which are infected with only subgroup B or C virus. These cultures do contain cell-surface reactivity as determined by membrane immunofluorescence, but whether this activity is adsorbable with virus fractions p30, gp70, and p15 has not been determined.

Olsen *et al.* (1976*a*) have studied the expression of FOCMA in the Fl 74 target cell under varying culture conditions. They found that FOCMA expression is cell cycle dependent, and that the rate at which the cells passed through the cycle determined both the pattern and intensity of expression. Cells grown in static suspension were most highly positive, but cells grown in spinner cultures could be induced to express as much FOCMA by synchronization using either exposure to cold or amino acid deprivation. Similar studies with murine oncornavirus-associated cell membrane antigens indicated that the greatest expression occurred during G_1 (Cikes, 1970).

V. LABORATORY-INDUCED AND NATURALLY OCCURRING TUMORS OF CATS

Very extensive evidence now exists that oncornaviruses cause leukemia, lymphoma, and fibrosarcoma in outbred cats under natural conditions. The evidence that the causative agents of leukemia and lymphoma are primarily transmitted in a horizontal fashion, as truly contagious viruses, is almost as extensive. The evidence for horizontal transmission will be reviewed briefly because the method of acquisition of the causative agent is obviously an important factor in determining immunogenicity for both the causative agent and the transformed cell.

The lymphoproliferative and myeloproliferative tumors of cats have recently been classified by W. Jarrett and Mackey (1974). The FeLV-induced lymphoid malignancies occur as both true leukemias and lymphomas, with subclassification of the lymphomas into thymic, multicentric, alimentary, and atypical forms. The relative frequency of the different forms varies considerably. The alimentary form of lymphoma, for example, accounts for more than half of the lymphoid tumors in Glasgow, with fewer than 5% of the cases being true lymphoid leukemia, while in Boston the reverse is seen (Essex *et al.,* 1975*d*). If FeLV strain differences rather than a genetically determined response of the host determines the pathological response, then this presumably reflects geographic differences in the relative frequency of virus strains or subgroups. Analogous geographic differences are seen in the relative ratio of myeloproliferative tumors to lymphoproliferative tumors (Ott, personal communication). These observations suggest that data collected in one locality on either the total incidence of feline leukemia-lymphoma or the relative incidence according to age, sex, breed, or pathological form are probably not valid for other geographic areas or possibly even different time periods for the same geographic areas. There is general agreement, however, that leukemias and lymphomas represent the most common malignancies of cats.

In our study of one large breeding household containing cats of Western, African, and Oriental origin with the same exposure to FeLV, no apparent differences were observed in infection rates. More than 97% of the cats in each group had evidence of infection based on either persistent viremia or development of antibody to FOCMA or both (Essex *et al.*, 1975c). The lymphoproliferative diseases of cats are common at an early age. More than half of the 106 cases we collected at a large Boston hospital during a 2-year period were in cats less than 4 years of age and more than 25% were in cats less than 2 years of age (Essex *et al.*, 1975d).

Numerous virus isolates from spontaneous cases of lymphoma-leukemia (W. Jarrett *et al.*, 1964b; Kawakami *et al.*, 1967; Rickard *et al.*, 1969; Theilen *et al.*, 1970) and fibrosarcoma (Snyder and Theilen, 1969; Gardner *et al.*, 1970; McDonough *et al.*, 1971; Snyder, 1971) have been used to induce tumors in neonatal cats. In the case of leukemia-lymphoma, the incubation period for experimental induction varies with FeLV strain and dose, host age at time of inoculation, inoculation route, and probably genetic susceptibility of the host (Essex, 1975a,b). The incidence of tumor induction is 90% or higher when the Rickard strain is parenterally inoculated into neonatal kittens, but much lower when the same virus is given to cats 3 months of age or older, or given by intranasal instillation to neonates (Hoover *et al.*, 1972, 1976). In newborn kittens inoculated with another strain of FeLV, the incidence of leukemia-lymphoma was much lower and the incubation period several months to several years in length (Mackey *et al.*, 1972). Since lower incidences of neoplasia and longer incubation periods are seen following induced horizontal contact, they probably more accurately reflect natural conditions (W. Jarrett, 1972; Essex *et al.*, 1973a; W. Jarrett *et al.*, 1973b). Many kittens inoculated with FeLV die with either nonregenerative anemia or thymic atrophy with various associated secondary infections before the development of neoplasms (Anderson *et al.*, 1971; Mackey *et al.*, 1972; Hoover *et al.*, 1973, 1974, 1976). Spontaneous isolates of FeLV have all consisted of either subgroup A alone, subgroup A plus B, or subgroup A plus B plus C (Sarma and Log, 1973; Sarma *et al.*, 1974b). As for the strains most commonly employed for experimental purposes, the Rickard strain is subgroup A, the Jarrett FeLV-5 is subgroup AB, and the Theilen strain is subgroup ABC. Subgroup B or C viruses have not been isolated without the presence of A subgroup. The Rickard strain of FeLV-A has also been used to induce lymphoma in dogs (Rickard *et al.*, 1973).

Spontaneous fibrosarcomas are relatively uncommon in cats as compared to lymphoproliferative tumors, but FeSVs can be isolated from most of the tumors in young cats (Snyder, 1971). In apparent contrast, many of the fibrosarcomas of older cats appear to be free of FeSV. All fibrosarcoma viruses thus far characterized have been subgroup AB (Sarma and Log, 1973). The isolates from spontaneous cases have varying degrees of oncogenicity (Snyder, 1971; Essex and Snyder, 1973; Snyder and Dungworth, 1973). The Snyder-Theilen isolate, for example, will induce tumors in neonates with a latent period of only 1–2 weeks and most animals die from a large tumor load with 3–4 weeks. Incubation and survival periods are considerably longer with the Gardner isolate (Essex and Snyder, 1973). Most induced fibrosarcomas are highly undifferentiated, and widespread metastasis in various body organs is common. The pathology of the induced tumors has been described in detail by Snyder et al. (1970). Incubation periods and survival periods are greatly prolonged when cats older than 3 months of age are inoculated or when low virus doses are employed (Snyder et al., 1970; Essex et al., 1971a,b, 1973b). Tumor regression is common when older animals or lower doses are used. The FeSVs have also been used to induce fibrosarcomas in numerous nonfeline species, such as dogs, monkeys, pigs, and sheep (Snyder and Theilen, 1969; Deinhardt et al., 1970; Gardner et al., 1970; Essex et al., 1972b; Rabin et al., 1972; Wolfe et al., 1972; L. Pearson et al., 1973; Theilen et al., 1974; Slauson et al., 1975).

A. Horizontal Transmission

Various experimental observations made under both laboratory and field conditions have provided indisputable evidence that FeLVs are rapidly and effeciently transmitted in a horizontal fashion when cats are in close contact. The first suggestions that FeLV was a contagious virus were made when clusters of spontaneous leukemia were observed (Schneider et al., 1967; Brodey, 1971). Defendants of the oncogene hypothesis (Huebner and Todaro, 1969; Todaro and Huebner, 1972) deemphasized the significance of such observations as evidence for horizontal transmission, and instead chose to interpret them as being due to genetic relatedness of cats in the same household (and thus vertical virus transmission), or being due to chance alone (Schneider, 1971). We became convinced that such clusters could not be due to chance alone when we observed a continuing high incidence of spontaneous leukemia, occurring in a prospective sense, in several households that had previously been designated as "high-risk" environments (Cotter et al., 1973, 1974, 1975; Essex et al., 1975c). One household with a population at risk of 35, for example, came to our attention after three cases of leukemia had occurred within a 1-year period. We then undertook a concentrated serological, virological, and pathological study of the household, and observed the spontaneous development of nine more cases of leukemia in the same population within the ensuing 3-year period (Cotter et al.,

1973, 1974). Since the cases of leukemia in this house were not in related individuals, the vertical transmission hypothesis did not appear to be a tenable explanation for the findings (Cotter *et al.*, 1974).

The second major line of evidence for horizontal transmission was the observation of a higher-than-expected number of cases of lymphoproliferative disease in cats known to be exposed to FeLV-infected cats. This observation was originally made under laboratory conditions by Rickard (1969), who observed five cases of leukemia among 26 contact-control kittens, and Snyder (personal communication), who observed a few cases of fibrosarcoma in uninoculated kittens maintained under similar conditions. Such observations were appreciated only after experiments designed specifically to address this question proved successful. When uninoculated control "tracers" were deliberately exposed to FeLV-inoculated or naturally infected cagemates under either laboratory or field conditions, a higher-than-expected incidence of leukemia was observed (Essex *et al.*, 1973a; W. Jarrett *et al.*, 1973b; Hardy *et al.*, 1973b).

Serological studies were then undertaken using various test procedures on both healthy "tracer" cats that were deliberately exposed to virus-inoculated or naturally infected cagemates, and healthy pet cats residing in private households where one or more cases of spontaneous feline leukemia had been recently documented. The tests used were for FOCMA antibody, virus-neutralizing antibody, antibody to virus core p30 antigen, detection of virus core antigens in peripheral blood cells by the "Hardy test," and the isolation of infectious FeLV.

Our studies on detection of FOCMA antibody in FeLV-exposed and unexposed cats are summarized in Table II. More than three-fourths of the cats that were contact-exposed to FeLV in either laboratory or field environments had evidence of an antibody response to FOCMA (Essex and Snyder, 1973; W. Jarrett *et al.*, 1973b; Essex *et al.*, 1975c,d,e, 1976a). In contrast, cats of comparable genetic backgrounds that were deliberately housed away from known infected cats had very low frequencies of detectable FOCMA antibody and much lower geometric mean titers (Essex *et al.*, 1975a). Pet cats living in suburban or urban private household environments were less frequently positive for detectable FOCMA antibody when compared to cats in laboratory or private environments known to be exposed to FeLV, but more frequently positive than colony cats that were kept away from known infected cats (Essex *et al.*, 1973a, 1975a). Similar results were obtained when cats were tested for the presence of virus-neutralizing antibody (Hardy *et al.*, 1976a). Forty-four percent of the cats known to be exposed to FeLV under natural circumstances had detectable, neutralizing antibody. Only 5% of the pet or stray cats of unknown exposure status and none of 34 cats assumed to be isolated from exposure to FeLV had such antibody. We observed antibody to pure FeLV p30 in 20 of 33 healthy cats from similar environments using radioimmunoprecipitation. None of 11 cats from environments where FeLV exposure was unlikely had antibody against anti-p30 by radioimmunoprecipitation (Charman *et al.*, 1976).

Table II. Detection and Titration of FOCMA Antibody in Healthy Cats from Various Environments

Population	Number positive/ total	Titer range	Geometric mean titer	References
FeLV exposed (natural)				Essex et al.
Exposure group No. 1	100/121 (83)[a]	0–256	5.87	(1975b,c, 1976a,b)
Exposure group No. 2	13/17 (77)	0–64	4.65	
Exposure group No. 3	10/14 (71)	0–32	2.60	
Exposure group No. 4	8/10 (80)	0–64	4.23	
Exposure group No. 5	4/8 (50)	0–32	3.87	
FeLV exposed (laboratory)				Essex and Snyder
Experiment 1	9/10 (90)	0–32	6.12	(1973), W. Jarrett
Experiment 2	11/13 (85)	0–64	6.72	et al. (1973b),
Totals	20/23 (87)	0–64	6.45	Essex et al.
				(1975a,c)
Unexposed laboratory cats[b]				Essex et al.
Colony No. 1	1/70 (2)	0–1	0.01	(1975b)
Colony No. 2	0/50 (0)	–	0	
Colony No. 3	3/70 (4)	0–16	0.07	
Colony No. 4	2/31 (7)	0–4	0.01	
Totals	6/221 (3)	0–16	0.04	
Street cats of unknown exposure status[c]				Essex et al. (1973b, 1975a)
Group No. 1	102/163 (63)	0–256	1.18	
Group No. 2	1/33 (3)	0–1	0.02	
Group No. 3	15/32 (47)	0–32	0.66	
Group No. 4	11/28 (40)	0–8	0.59	
Totals	129/256 (50)	0–256	0.85	

[a]Percent positive.
[b]Cats maintained under pathogen-free or disease-free conditions and never knowingly exposed to FeLV.
[c]Except for group No. 2, which represents pet cats from single-cat households.

The same groups of cats were examined for the presence of FeLV in peripheral blood leukocytes and platelets, as an index of persistent viremia (Hardy et al., 1973a, 1976a; W. Jarrett et al., 1973b; Essex et al., 1973a, 1975b,c,e; Cotter et al., 1974, 1975; Hoover et al., 1976). About half of the healthy cats that were known to be exposed to an FeLV-infected cat under either private household or laboratory conditions were virus positive. This should be compared to an incidence of FeLV detection of 1% or less for either stray cats, those from "clean" laboratory environments, or those from "single-cat" private pet households (see Table III). The significance of these results is further emphasized by observations that FeLV-exposed cats with detectable

Table III. Detection of FeLV Antigens in Healthy Cats from Different Environments

Environment	Number of cats tested	Number positive	Percent positive	References
1. Private households with known presence of an FeLV-infected cat				Essex *et al.* (1975*b,c*)
House No. 1	125	64	51.2	
House No. 2	17	5	29.4	
House No. 3	14	8	57.1	
House No. 4	10	6	60.0	
Totals	166	83	50.0	
2. Private households with a previous history of feline leukemia or a related disease[a]	543	177	32.6	Hardy *et al.* (1973*a,b*; 1976*a*)
3. Experimental cats with deliberate contact exposure to FeLV-infected cagemates				W. Jarrett *et al.* (1973*b*), Essex *et al.* (1976*b*)
Experimental series 1	39	19	48.7	
Experimental series 2	9	6	66.7	
Totals	48	25	52.1	
4. Suburban and urban stray and pet cats of unknown exposure	752	4	0.5	Hardy *et al.* (1973*a,b*; 1976*a*), Cotter *et al.* (1975), Essex *et al.* (1975*a*)
5. Pet cats from single cat households	497	0	0	Hardy *et al.* (1973*a,b*, 1976*a*)
6. Unexposed laboratory colony cats	228	0	0	Hardy *et al.* (1973*a,b*; 1976*a*) Essex *et al.* (1975*a*)

[a]Leukemia, lymphoma, fibrosarcoma, nonregenerative anemia, thymic atrophy syndrome, granulomatous disease, and infectious peritonitis.

virus-neutralizing or anti-FOCMA antibody are less likely to be virus-infected than antibody negative cats living in the same house (Essex *et al.*, 1975*c*). Thus 90% or more of the cats in such contact environments have evidence of present or prior infection by FeLV when several serological tests are used, while cats of comparable genetic backgrounds that are housed in isolated environments rarely show evidence of infection.

The results listed in Tables II and III for experimental or laboratory contact FeLV-exposed cats were based on cats that had been serologically tested and found negative prior to exposure. They therefore provide confirmation by prospective seroconversion for the earlier observations based on single samples from cats in cluster households. These observations have also been confirmed and extended by Hoover *et al.* (1976). Almost all of the cats horizontally exposed to FeLV in the first month or 2 of age appear to develop persistent viremia. At weaning age, the incidence of development of persistent viremia decreases to 50–75%. As for cats first exposed as immunocompetent adults, observations on both laboratory and field populations suggest that the conversion rate is probably quite low.

If the above observations do not seem sufficiently convincing by themselves, then the recent experiments by Hardy *et al.* (1976*a*) on control of spontaneous leukemia by elimination of FeLV-excretor cats provides virtual proof for the hypothesis. The procedure of "test and eliminate" was used, a principle which has long been applied to problems with infectious diseases in preventive veterinary medicine. In a large serological survey based on healthy cats known to be residing in FeLV-exposure households, the blood smear immunofluorescence test was used to test before and after a 3-month interval. During this period, 32 of the 268 (11.9%) uninfected cats that were allowed to remain in contact with infected cats converted to positive. In otherwise comparable households where all infected cats were removed at the start of the 3-month examination period, only 3 of 564 (0.5%) converted to become FeLV positive (Hardy *et al.*, 1976*b*).

FeLV replicates efficiently in salivary gland tissue and oral and nasal epithelium (Gardner *et al.*, 1971; W. Jarrett *et al.*, 1973*b*; Hardy *et al.*, 1976*a*). Since cats frequently groom each other, this could probably be an easy way for FeLV transmission to occur.

FeLV can be readily detected in most cases of either induced or naturally occurring leukemia or lymphoma (Laird *et al.*, 1968; Hardy *et al.*, 1969, 1973*a,b*, 1976*a*; W. Jarrett *et al.*, 1973*a*; Gardner *et al.*, 1974; Essex *et al.*, 1975*d*). The incidence of virus positivity appears to vary with age, tumor type, and/or geographic location (Hardy *et al.*, 1973*b*; W. Jarrett *et al.*, 1973*a*; Essex *et al.*, 1975*d*; Gardner *et al.*, 1974). Old cats with either lymphoproliferative neoplasia, nonregenerative anemia, infectious peritonitis, or other bacterial or viral diseases were less likely to have circulating FeLV than young cats with the same diseases. Certain types of lymphoproliferative neoplasms, such as the alimentary form which is the most common in Glasgow, were found to be less frequently FeLV-positive than the other forms.

B. Immunosuppressive Potential of FeLV

Numerous reports have documented that oncornaviruses of mice, at least the Friend, Rauscher, and Moloney strains, are immunosuppressive (Notkins *et al.*, 1970; Dent, 1972). Since Friend and Rauscher viruses cause erythroblastic rather than lymphoblastic leukemia, it appears likely that the virus-associated immunosuppressive functions are expressed independently from the functions responsible for malignant transformation. Such oncornaviruses could presumably then regulate oncogenesis in two ways: first by actively transforming cells, and second by interfering with whatever immunosurveillance mechanism the host might mount toward the developing tumor. By extension of this reasoning, one can postulate that oncornaviruses which have lost their transforming potential could still render the infected host more sensitive to infectious disease processes in general, or even tumors caused by unrelated agents. It seemed logical to determine if the observations reported for the rather artificially selected viruses of inbred mice were also true for an outbred species, such as the cat, with oncornavirus infections that were naturally acquired.

Early experiments on the induction of leukemia, lymphoma, or fibrosarcoma by inoculation of neonatal or young cats were characterized by a higher-than-expected incidence of fatalities due to concurrent infections by various cytopathic viruses and bacteria (Rickard et al., 1969; Theilen et al., 1970; Anderson et al., 1971; Essex and Snyder, 1973). The true incidence of the development of such diseases was probably greatly underestimated, because the experimental design often excluded such "nonspecific" early deaths from the data analysis. Another relevant observation was the recognition of premature atrophy of the thymus as a routine pathological lesion in young cats with both induced and spontaneous leukemia (Anderson et al., 1971; Gilmore and Holzworth, 1971; Hoover et al., 1973; W. Jarrett et al., 1973c).

With this background, we decided to test for FeLV infection cats that were presented to a large veterinary hospital with infectious processes other than the neoplastic diseases and nonregenerative anemias which were already known to be associated with FeLV (Cotter et al., 1975; Essex et al., 1975b,d, 1976a). From one-half to two-thirds of the cats with such diseases were found to be viremic with FeLV, as compared to 2% or less of the cats with physical trauma, urolithiasis, or normal health (see Table IV). Since many of these diseases occur more frequently than leukemia, especially in certain geographic areas (Table V), it seemed possible that FeLV might be even more important as an immuno-suppressive agent than as a cause of neoplasia.

Our next approach was to prospectively examine cats that were naturally infected with FeLV for subsequent development of these infectious diseases, as well as leukemia. We found that FeLV-infected healthy cats were about fivefold more likely to subsequently develop various nonneoplastic diseases than uninfected cats living in the same households (Essex et al., 1975b). Complete hemograms were done on both the FeLV-infected and uninfected healthy cats. Although there was no evidence of either subclinical anemia or altered total white blood cell counts in the infected cats, the total peripheral lymphocyte count for the same FeLV-infected healthy cats was substantially reduced as compared to the uninfected housemates (Essex et al., 1975b).

Very little work has been done to evaluate specific immune functions in cats with either experimentally induced or naturally acquired infections. Two studies

Table IV. Detection of Feline Leukemia Virus in Cats
with Nonneoplastic Infectious Diseases

Diagnosis	Number of cats tested	Number positive	Percent Positive	References
Hemobartonellosis	23	13	57	Essex et al.
Infectious peritonitis				(1975b,d)
and granulomatous disease	59	34	58	Cotter et al.
Bacterial infections	95	47	50	(1974, 1975)
Abortion and fetal				
resorption	26	13	50	
Glomerulonephritis	7	3	43	
Total	210	110	52	
Physical (trauma and				
urethral obstruction)	27	1	4	

Table V. Relative Frequency of Detectable Circulating FeLV in Cats
According to Age, Disease Form, and Geographic Location

Variable	Class	Number tested	Number positive	Percent positive	References
Geographic	Boston	144	97	67	Essex (1975a,b),
location	New York	33	28	85	Essex et al. (1975b,d),
(leukemia-	Glasgow	56	28	50	Hardy et al. (1973b),
lymphoma only)					W. Jarrett et al.
					(1973a)
Disease form	Lymphatic leukemia	66	46	70	Essex (1975a,b),
	Thymic lymphoma	33	24	73	Essex et al. (1975b,d)
	Multicentric				
	lymphoma	20	14	70	
	Alimentary				
	lymphoma	10	5	50	
	Other forms of				
	lymphoma[a]	15	8	53	
	Nonregenerative				
	anemia	128	89	70	
Age (both	Less than 5				Essex (1975a,b),
leukemia–	years	207	148	72	Essex et al.
lymphoma	5 years or				(1975b,d)
and other	over	83	45	54	
diseases)					

[a]For example, skin, central nervous system.

have reported on the immunosuppressive potential of R-FeLV during the preleu-kemic state following virus inoculation. The first study (Perryman *et al.*, 1972) indicated a substantial defect in the cell-mediated immune homograft rejection mechanism during the incubation period before leukemia development. Sixteen of 18 FeLV-infected cats had significantly prolonged allograft survival times as compared to their controls. In the second study, Cockerell *et al.* (1976) found that FeLV-inoculated kittens had depressed blast transformation responses to both conconavalin A and pokeweed mitogen as early as 4 weeks after virus inoculation. This time period was at least 2 months before clinical leukemia had appeared.

VI. IMMUNE RESPONSE TO LABORATORY-INDUCED TUMORS

Our first attempts to detect antibody to a tumor cell membrane antigen involved cats of different ages inoculated with oncogenic ST-FeSV. Most cats that were first given the virus at 1 month of age or older developed no detectable tumors, or had only temporary tumor growth with subsequent regression (Essex *et al.*, 1971*b*). These cats were examined for the presence of humoral antibody to the FeLV producer line established from an experimental case of lymphoma (Theilen *et al.*, 1969). All such "regressor" or "tumor-free" cats were found to have detectable antibody to the FOCMA antigen by indirect membrane immuno-fluorescence. Most newborn kittens and a lower percentage of older cats that were inoculated with the same virus died with rapidly progressing, metastasizing tumors (Snyder and Theilen, 1969; Snyder *et al.*, 1970; Snyder, 1971; Essex *et al.*, 1971*a,b*; Snyder and Dungworth, 1973). Such "progressor" animals did not have high titers of antibody to FOCMA, as did the regressors.

Figure 1 summarizes our experience with the detection of FOCMA antibody in susceptible cats inoculated with several strains of viable FeSV (Essex *et al.*, 1971*b*, 1973*b*, 1976*a*; Essex and Snyder, 1973; Essex, 1974, 1975*a,b*). It is apparent that "progressor" animals have either no detectable antibody or very low levels, when compared to "regressor" or "no-tumor" animals. Fifty-six of 57 (98%) of the "progressor" cats we studied failed to develop FOCMA antibody titers as high as 8. About half had no detectable antibody at all. The geometric mean for all 57 was less than 1.0. All of 30 "regressor" cats developed FOCMA antibody titers of 4 or higher, and all of 11 cats that failed to develop tumors had titers of 8 or higher. The geometric mean anti-FOCMA titer for "regressor" cats was more than twentyfold higher than for "progressor" cats, and the geometric mean titer for those that developed no tumors was about thirtyfold higher than for the progressors.

Similar studies with tumors induced by the Gardner-Arnstein (GA) strain of FeSV confirmed the association of efficient antibody production against

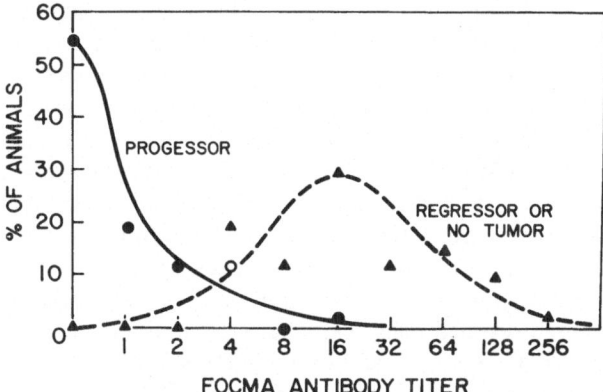

Fig. 1. Comparison of FOCMA antibody titers for cats with experimentally induced progressive fibrosarcomas to titers for cats that developed only "regressor" tumors or no tumors at all following inoculation with FeSV.

FOCMA with tumor resistance (Schaller *et al.*, 1975). Since the GA strain of FeSV is associated with longer inoculation periods before tumor development and with slower-growing tumors, additional questions about the correlation between tumor growth and FOCMA antibody were asked. It was determined that cats with either slowly progressing tumors or temporary regression had FOCMA antibody titers that were intermediate between the values for cats in the "rapid-progressor" and "no-tumor" or "permanent-regressor" categories. It was also determined that "regressor" cats had a much more rapid anti-FOCMA response than "progressor" cats. "Regressor" cats generally had high antibody titers by 6–10 weeks after exposure to FeSV, while "progressor" cats usually did not develop significant levels of FOCMA antibody until 18–20 weeks after virus injection (Schaller *et al.*, 1975).

In early experiments where varying doses of ST-FeSV were given to neonates it was noted that some kittens had detectable levels of FOCMA antibody within a few days of birth, and that this was associated with protection from the effects of ST-FeSV oncogenesis (Essex *et al.*, 1971*a*, 1973*b*). It was later apparent that the antibody had been passively acquired from the nursing mothers, who themselves had become horizontally infected with suboncogenic doses of FeLV or FeSV while nursing previous litters of inoculated kittens.

Several observations suggested that FOCMA antibody and virus-neutralizing antibody are independent entities. First, we found no correlation between the presence of FOCMA antibody and virus-neutralizing antibody in the same animals (W. Jarrett *et al.*, 1973*b*; Schaller *et al.*, 1975). Progressor animals actually developed detectable virus-neutralizing antibody before regressor animals, but neither group appeared to have high enough titers to have much effect.

Second, Aldrich and Pederson (1974) found that animals still had high levels of circulating ST-FeSV after regression had occurred. Such cats had high levels of anti-FOCMA. Since they were simultaneously viremic with FeSV, it is apparent that they did not have operationally effective virus-neutralizing antibody. Third, cats that remained healthy following natural exposure to FeLV had both a higher frequency of anti-FOCMA and virus-neutralizing antibody (see next section), but only the nonviremic cats had detectable virus-neutralizing antibody (Hardy *et al.*, 1976*a*). In apparent agreement with these observations, we failed to adsorb anti-FOCMA antibody with intact FeLV (Oroszlan and Essex, unpublished observations). Finally, radioimmunoprecipitation tests for antibody in cat sera to pure FeLV gp70 revealed many cats that were positive for anti-FOCMA but negative for anti-gp70 (Aaronson and Essex, unpublished).

Cats inoculated with FeLV have a similar anti-FOCMA response (W. Jarrett *et al.*, 1973*b*; Essex, 1974; Hoover *et al.*, 1976). Regression or reversal of growth is apparent in the case of small FeSV-induced fibrosarcomas because the initial tumor response occurs at the readily palpable inoculation site. Such reversal of growth for a comparable number of malignant lymphoid cells in the bone marrow or visceral lymphoid organs would obviously not be as apparent, so no such "regressor" category is available for study. Of seven cats we studied that developed leukemia or lymphoma following virus inoculation, none developed significant titers of FOCMA antibody prior to death at 12–20 weeks post inoculation (Essex, 1974). Those that resisted leukemia development had developed titers of 8–256 by the same time period.

Similar results were obtained by Hoover *et al.* (1976). They found that all newborn cats inoculated with moderate doses of R-FeLV developed persistent viremia and died with lymphoma or nonregenerative anemia. None developed significant titers of either anti-FOCMA or virus-neutralizing antibody. Only 15% of the cats inoculated with the same virus preparation at 3 months of age or older developed either persistent viremia or disease. The cats in this group that remained free of persistent viremia developed significant titers of anti-FOCMA and virus-neutralizing antibody. None developed either lymphoma or other FeLV-related diseases within a 40-week observation period.

Thus it appears that cats which develop experimental leukemia are serologically analogous to those that develop progressive fibrosarcomas, while those that resist leukemia development are comparable to the FeSV-inoculated "regressor" or "no-tumor" group.

Encouraged by these results, vaccination of cats was attempted using either whole cells, cell membrane preparations, attenuated live virus, or killed virus (W. Jarrett *et al.*, 1974; Hardy *et al.*, 1976*b*; Olsen *et al.*, 1976*b*; Yohn *et al.*, 1976). The immunization of young kittens with either UV- or formalin-inactivated FeLV or FeSV was unsuccessful. Cats vaccinated in this manner developed low titers of virus-neutralizing antibody and antibody to virus core antigens, but they were completely unable to resist challenge with oncogenic virus (Hardy *et al.*,

1976*b*; Olsen *et al.*, 1975, 1976*b*; Yohn *et al.*, 1976). Some success was obtained by vaccinating pregnant mothers with killed FeSV, and allowing them to passively transmit neutralizing antibody to suckling neonates (Olsen *et al.*, 1976*b*; Yohn *et al.*, 1976). Such procedures would provide only very transient protection, however, for periods of only 6–8 weeks after birth (Essex *et al.*, 1973b).

Vaccination with attenuated live FeLV or FeSV resulted in successful induction of high neutralizing antibody titers (Hardy *et al.*, 1976*b*), but this procedure seemed impractical, since the seeding of viable virus into the environment and the possible redevelopment of oncogenic potential cannot be ruled out.

Vaccines containing either whole cells or cell fractions have thus far been the most successful, both in the sense of inducing high FOCMA antibody titers and in protecting from challenge with oncogenic FeSV or FeLV (W. Jarrett *et al.*, 1974; Olsen *et al.*, 1976*b*; Yohn *et al.*, 1976). W. Jarrett *et al.* (1974) were able to completely protect kittens from oncogenic challenge by vaccinating with viable F1 74 cells, the standard FOCMA-positive target line. This procedure is also not feasible for field conditions, however. In addition to the risk for introducing live FeLV as mentioned above, the administration of unpurified cell membrane material in moderate or large doses could cause such diseases as immune complex glomerulonephritis. Olsen *et al.* (1976*b*) and Yohn *et al.* (1976) have found, however, that FOCMA-containing cells can be equally protective after inactivation by heat or irradiation, suggesting that fractionation and purification of FOCMA antigen for preparation of an immunogen is probably a logical approach.

The ability of anti-FOCMA antibody to exert a cytotoxic effect on the target cell has been studied by Mathes *et al.* (1976). It was found that most FeLV-inoculated cats that developed FOCMA antibody as assayed by indirect membrane immunofluorescence also had significant titers of cytotoxic antibody. The same target cell, F1 74, was used, but rabbit complement was found to be much more efficient than cat or guinea pig complement. When serum from FeLV-inoculated cats was used up to 6–8 weeks post inoculation, an almost perfect correlation existed between cytotoxic effect and reactivity by membrane immunofluorescence. Serum either from the same cats at later periods following FeLV inoculation or from healthy field cats that had been chronically exposed to FeLV for long periods showed a less perfect correlation between the two tests.

VII. IMMUNE RESPONSE TO NATURALLY OCCURRING LEUKEMIA AND LYMPHOMA

Cats with naturally occurring leukemia, lymphoma, and nonregenerative anemia were examined for antibody to FOCMA (Essex, 1974; Essex *et al.*,

1975*d*, 1976*a*). As a group, they had the same general picture for FOCMA antibody as did cats with FeSV-induced progressive fibrosarcoma, or cats with FeLV-induced leukemia or lymphoma. Less than 5% of the cats with the diseases had antibody titers of 8 or more. Only about 10% had antibody titers of 4 or more, and less than half had any detectable FOCMA antibody at all. The geometric mean titer for all cats with FeLV-associated diseases was 0.58 (see Table VI).

Cats with naturally occurring lymphoproliferative neoplasms had low titers to FOCMA antibody regardless of pathological form of the disease, whether they were FeLV positive or negative by the Hardy test, geographic origin, sex, or age at the time of diagnosis (Essex *et al.*, 1975*d*).

For a control group that would be comparable to the cats injected with FeLV or FeSV that resist progressive tumors and remain healthy, we chose cats that were healthy despite being exposed to FeLV under natural conditions for a year or more in leukemia "cluster" households (Essex *et al.*, 1975*c*, 1976*a*). Although viremic healthy cats from such environments had a geometric mean antibody titer that was somewhat lower than for uninfected cats in the same environments, the mean titer for all the healthy cats was about tenfold higher than for cats with leukemia or lymphoma. About two-thirds of the healthy exposed cats had titers of 4 or higher and half had titers of 8 or higher. Figure 2 compares the distribution of anti-FOCMA titers for cats with leukemia, lymphoma, and nonregenerative anemia to the figures for cats that remained healthy following natural exposure to FeLV.

When healthy cats from the same cluster households were examined for antibody to FeLV by radioimmunoprecipitation, a partial correlation was seen between anti-FOCMA and anti-p30 activities (Charman *et al.*, 1976). While titers

Table VI. FOCMA Antibody Titers for Cats with Naturally Occurring Leukemia, Lymphoma, and Anemia

Health status	Number of cats with FOCMA antibody titers of							Total	Geometric mean titer
	0	1	2	4	8	16	32		
Lymphoid leukemia[a]	23	9	7	6	1			46	0.75
Lymphoma[a]	30	9	3	2				44	0.34
Anemia[a]	46	17	10	5	1	1	1	81	0.63
Totals	99	35	20	13	2	1	1	171	0.58

[a]Collected at the Angell Memorial Animal Hospital in Boston.

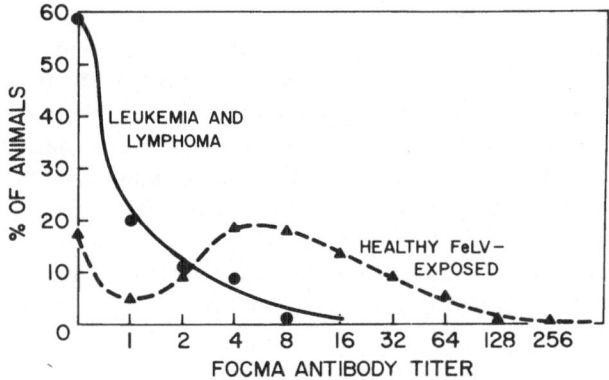

Fig. 2. Comparison of FOCMA antibody titers for cats with naturally occurring leukemia or lymphoma to titers for healthy, naturally FeLV-exposed cats.

of antibody of 200 or greater to p30 were seen only in cats with high titers of antibody to FOCMA (32 or greater), many cats with high titers of anti-FOCMA did not have significant levels of antibody to FeLV p30.

In the case of spontaneous leukemia or lymphoma, although the anti-FOCMA titers were obviously low when a cat with disease had been seen at a veterinary hospital, no information on the immunological status of such cats prior to the development of neoplasia was available. In the case of experimentally induced neoplasia, it had been possible to check the cats at several intervals before development of tumors. Since the cats with experimentally induced leukemia had never shown significant levels of humoral antibody to FOCMA during the incubation period for disease development, it seemed unlikely that the low titers were due to either (1) a "soaking-up" of preexisting humoral antibody or (2) suppression of the immunological system in general by the debilitation or cachexia of advanced neoplasia.

To consider the same issues for naturally occurring leukemia or lymphoma, we undertook a prospective seroepidemiological study of about 100 cats in a single high-risk leukemia cluster household (Essex *et al.*, 1975*f*). We had previously conducted a single spot-check of all of the cats for anti-FOCMA antibody and demonstrated that most had significant levels (Essex *et al.*, 1975*c*). Each cat was then examined for the presence of FeLV and FOCMA antibody at intervals of 3–5 months for up to 2½ years.

Eight cats subsequently developed new cases of leukemia and lymphoma, and 36 developed other lethal nonneoplastic diseases during the examination period. As expected, all eight leukemic cats had either no detectable FOCMA antibody or low titers after clinical leukemia was present. More important, however, was the observation that all eight also had very low or negative titers throughout the study period, long before disease development, while they were still healthy (see Table VII). The geometric mean anti-FOCMA titer for the eight leukemic cats was 1.36 at the time of last sampling, 3–5 months before signs of clinical leukemia, and 1.97 when the first sample was taken from each cat at the time the study started. The geometric mean titer for uninfected cats in the same household was about tenfold higher, and the mean for all cats in the house that remained healthy was five- to tenfold higher. Cats living in the same house that developed nonneoplastic diseases had antibody titers that were lower than for cats that remained healthy, but not nearly as low as for cats that subsequently developed leukemia.

VIII. SUMMARY AND CONCLUSIONS

Leukemias and lymphomas of outbred cats are caused by horizontally transmitted oncornaviruses. This system represents the best evidence currently

Table VII. FOCMA Antibody Titers According to Health Status for Cats from a Single Household Exposure Environment

Health status	Number and percent of cats with FOCMA antibody titers of				Geometric mean titer
	<4	4–16	>16	Total	
Subsequently developed leukemia (all FeLV positive)					
a. Last sample during health[a]	8 (100)	0 (0)	0 (0)	8	1.36
b. First sample[b]	5 (63)	3 (38)	0 (0)	8	1.97
Subsequently developed other diseases[c]					
a. FeLV positive	16 (53)	11 (37)	3 (10)	30	3.34
b. FeLV negative	1 (17)	4 (67)	1 (17)	6	9.90
Total	17 (47)	15 (42)	4 (11)	36	4.05
Remained healthy[d]					
a. FeLV positive	4 (27)	10 (67)	1 (7)	15	5.36
b. FeLV negative	2 (7)	18 (64)	8 (29)	28	15.90
Total	6 (14)	28 (65)	9 (21)	43	11.01

[a] 3–5 months before first signs of clinical illness.
[b] Taken at the start of the study.
[c] Last sample 3–5 months before disease development.
[d] Last sample at end of study.

available that naturally occurring malignant tumors of outbred mammals may be caused by viruses, although equally convincing evidence is available for the Marek's disease tumor of birds (Nazerian, 1973).

Studies with cats inoculated with feline sarcoma virus (FeSV) or feline leukemia virus (FeLV) have clearly demonstrated that an efficient humoral immune response to the feline oncornavirus-associated cell membrane antigen (FOCMA) is associated with protection from development of lethal tumors. Cats that develop no tumors, or tumors that subsequently regress, develop high titers of antibody to FOCMA. Cats with laboratory-induced progressive tumors or spontaneous leukemia or lymphoma have either no detectable FOCMA antibody or very low titers.

With this background, we attempted to test the general concept of immunosurveillance as it applies to FOCMA immunity in outbred cats that develop spontaneous leukemia under natural conditions. By concentrating the study on a single large feline leukemia-cluster household, it was possible to follow 43 contact-exposed healthy cats and eight that subsequently developed leukemia. The results clearly indicate that leukemic animals have poor antibody responses to FOCMA, the tumor cell membrane antigen, several months or years before any clinical signs of leukemia are apparent. In contrast, cats that remain healthy while living in the same exposure environment have humoral antibody titers to FOCMA that are much higher. Although the study concentrated on B-cell rather than T-cell immune effector mechanisms, the results clearly support the concept of immunosurveillance. Indirect evidence was also found that FeLV can act as an immunosuppressive agent. Such a mechanism might provide an explanation for the large number of cats with nonneoplastic diseases that are also coincidentally viremic with FeLV.

Several conclusions emerge from these studies:

1. Oncogenic C-type viruses exist under natural circumstances in at least one outbred mammalian species, the cat.
2. In the same species, these oncogenic viruses are primarily transmitted in a horizontal manner.
3. Most cats that are naturally exposed to FeLV mount an efficient immunosurveillance response that is directed to FOCMA.
4. Humoral antibody appears to contribute in a beneficial way to the immunosurveillance mechanism.

For researchers whose primary experience has been with the oncornavirus-induced tumors of inbred mice, these conclusions probably seem heretical. Yet, studies with oncornaviruses recently isolated from tumors of outbred monkeys are compatible with a major role for both horizontal virus transmission and antibody-associated immunosurveillance (Kawakami and Buckley, 1974; Gillespie and Gallo, 1975).

ACKNOWLEDGMENTS

This work was supported by grants from the National Cancer Institute (CA-13885), the Anna Fuller Fund, the Jane Coffin Childs Fund for Medical Research, and the National (DT-32) and Massachusetts Branches of the American Cancer Society. M. E. is a Scholar of the Leukemia Society of America.

IX. REFERENCES

Aaronson, S. A., and Rowe, W. P., 1970, Non-producer clones of murine sarcoma virus transformed Balb/3T3 cells, *Virology* **42**:9.

Aaronson, S. A., and Stephenson, J. R., 1974, Wide-spread natural occurrence of high titers of neuralizing antibody to a specific class of endogenous mouse-type C-virus, *Proc. Natl. Acad. Sci. U.S.A.* **71**:1957.

Aldrich, C. D., and Pederson, N. C., 1974, Persistent viremia after regression of primary virus-induced feline fibrosarcomas, *Am. J. Vet. Res.* **35**:1383.

Allison, A. C., and Law, L. W., 1968, Effects of antilymphocyte serum on virus oncogenesis, *Proc. Soc. Exp. Biol. Med.* **127**:207.

Anderson, L. J., Jarrett, W. F. H., Jarrett, O., and Laird, H. M., 1971, Feline leukemia-virus infection of kittens: Mortality associated with atrophy of the thymus and lymphoid depletion, *J. Natl. Cancer Inst.* **47**:807.

Aoki, T., 1974, Murine type-C RNA viruses: A proposed reclassification, other possible pathogenicities, and a new immunologic function, *J. Natl. Cancer Inst.* **52**:1029.

August, J. T., Bolognesi, D. P., Fleissner, E., Gilden, R. V., and Nowinski, R. C., 1974, A proposed nomenclature for the virion proteins of oncogenic RNA viruses, *Virology* **60**:595.

Baluda, M. A., and Roy-Burman, P., 1973, Partial characterization of RD 114 virus by DNA-RNA hybridization studies, *Nature (London) New Biol.* **244**:59.

Bardell, D., and Essex, M., 1974, Glycolysis during early infection of feline and human cells with feline leukemia virus, *Infect. Immun.* **9**:824.

Bassin, R. H., Tuttle, N., and Fischinger, P. J., 1970, Isolation of murine sarcoma virus-transformed mouse cells which are negative for leukemia virus from agar suspension cultures, *Int. J. Cancer* **6**:95.

Bauer, H., 1974, Virion and tumor cell antigens of C-type RNA tumor viruses, *Adv. Cancer Res.* **20**:275.

Bauer, H., Kurth, R., Gelderblom, H., and Rohrschneider, L., 1976, The immune response to oncornaviruses and tumor associated antigens in the chicken, *Cancer Res.* **36**:598.

Belpomme, D., Dantchev, D., Du Rusquec, E., Grandjon, D., Huchet, R., Pouillart, P., Schwarzenberg, L., Amiel, J. L., and Mathé, G., 1974, T and B lymphocyte markers on the neoplastic cell of 20 patients with acute and 10 patients with chronic lymphoid leukemia, *Biomedicine* **20**:109.

Benveniste, R. E., Lieber, M., Livingston, D., Sherr, C., and Todaro, G., 1974, Infectious C-type virus isolated from a baboon placenta, *Nature (London)* **248**:17.

Bolognesi, D. P., 1974, Structural components of RNA tumor viruses, *Adv. Virus Res.* **19**:315.

Boone, C. W., Church, E. C., and McAllister, R., 1973, Testing by the "paired-label" antibody binding technique for feline leukemia virus-induced cell surface antigens (FeLV-CSA) on the surface of human rhabdomyosarcoma cells releasing RD-114 virus, *Virology* **55**:157.

Brodey, R. S., 1971, Comments on epidemiologic aspects of feline leukemia virus, *J. Am. Vet. Med. Assoc.* **158**:1123.

Brown, G., Greaves, M. F., Lister, T. A., Rapson, N., and Papamichael, M., 1974, Expression of human T and B lymphocyte cell surface markers on leukemic cells, *Lancet* **2**:753.

Burnet, F. M., 1970, The concept of immunological surveillance, *Prog. Exp. Tumor Res.* **13**:1.

Cerny, J., and Essex, M., 1974, Membrane antigens of murine leukemia cells, *Nature (London)* **251**:742.

Chan, E. W., Schiop-Stansky, P. E., and O'Connor, T. E., 1974*a*, Mammalian sarcoma-leukemia viruses. I. Infection of feline, bovine, and human cell cultures with Snyder-Theilen feline sarcoma virus, *J. Natl. Cancer Inst.* **52**:473.

Chan, E. W., Schiop-Stansky, P. E., and O'Connor, T. E., 1974*b*, Rescue of cell-transforming virus from a non-virus-producing bovine cell culture transformed by feline sarcoma virus, *J. Natl. Cancer Inst.* **52**:469.

Chang, K. S. S., Law, L. W., and Appella, E., 1975, Distinction between tumor-specific transplantation antigen and virion antigens in solubilized products from membranes of virus-induced leukemic cells, Int. J. Cancer **15**:483.

Chang, R. S., Golden, H. D., and Harrold, B., 1970, Propagation in human cells of a filterable agent from the ST feline sarcoma, *J. Virol.* **6**:599.

Charman, H. P., Kim, N., Gilden, R. V., Hardy, W. D., Jr., and Essex, M., 1976, Humoral immune responses of cats to feline leukemia virus: Comparison of responses to the major structural protein, p30, and to a virus specific cell membrane antigen (FOCMA), *J. Natl. Cancer Inst.* **56**:859.

Chen, J. H., and Hanafusa, H., 1974, Detection of a protein of avian leukoviruses in uninfected chick cells by radioimmunoassay, *J. Virol.* **13**:340.

Cikes, M., 1970, Relationship between growth rate, cell volume, cell cycle kinetics, and antigenic properties of cultured murine lymphoma cells, *J. Natl. Cancer Inst.* **45**:979.

Cockerell, G. L., Krakowka, S. G., Hoover, E. A., Olsen, R. G., and Yohn, D. S., 1976, Lymphocyte mitogen reactivity in feline leukemia virus infected cats and identification of feline T and B lymphocytes, in: *Comparative Leukemia Research 1975* (J. Clemmensen and D. S. Yohn, eds.), pp. 81–83, Karger, Basel.

Cotter, S. M., Gilmore, C. E., and Rollins, C., 1973, Multiple cases of feline leukemia and feline infectious peritonitis in a household, *J. Am. Vet. Med. Assoc.* **162**:1054.

Cotter, S. M., Essex, M., and Hardy, W. D., Jr., 1974, Serological studies of normal and leukemic cats in a multiple-case leukemia cluster, *Cancer Res.* **34**:1061.

Cotter, S. M., Hardy, W. D., Jr., and Essex, M., 1975, Association of feline leukemia virus with lymphosarcoma and other disorders in the cat, *J. Am. Vet. Med. Assoc.* **166**:449.

Deinhardt, F., 1975, Cat leukemia virus and immunology, *Blood* **46**:143.

Deinhardt, F., Wolfe, L. G., Theilen, G. H., and Snyder, S. P., 1970, ST-feline fibrosarcoma virus: Induction of tumors in marmoset monkeys, *Science* **167**:881.

Del Villano, B. C., Nave, B., Croker, B. P., Lerner, R. A., and Dixon, F. J., 1975, The oncornavirus glycoprotein gp69/71: A constituent of the surface of normal and malignant thymocytes, *J. Exp. Med.* **141**:172.

Dent, P. B., 1972, Immunodepression by oncogenic viruses, *Prog. Med. Virol.* **14**:1.

Dougherty, E., Post, J. E., and Richard, C. G., 1969, Distribution of C-type viral particles in a spontaneous case of lymphatic leukemia in a cat, *Can. Vet. J.* **10**:291.

Essex, M., 1974, The immune response to oncornavirus infections, in: *Viruses, Evolution and Cancer,* (E. Kurstak and K. Maramorosch, eds.), pp. 513–548, Academic Press, New York.

Essex, M., 1975*a,* Horizontally and vertically transmitted oncornaviruses of cats, *Adv. Cancer Res.* **21**:175.

Essex, M., 1975*b,* Tumors induced by oncornaviruses in cats, *Pathobiol. Annu.* **5**:169.

Essex, M., and Snyder, S. P., 1973, Feline oncornavirus associated cell membrane antigen. I. Serological studies with kittens exposed to cell-free materials from various feline fibrosarcomas, *J. Natl. Cancer Inst.* **51**:1007.

Essex, M., Klein, G., Snyder, S. P., and Harrold, J. B., 1971*a,* Antibody to feline oncornavirus-associated cell membrane antigen in neonatal cats, *Int. J. Cancer* **8**:384.

Essex, M., Klein, G., Snyder, S. P., and Harrold, J. B., 1971*b,* Feline sarcoma virus (FSV) induced tumors: Correlation between humoral antibody and tumor regression, *Nature (London)* **233**:195.

Essex, M., Kawakami, T. G., and Kurata, K., 1972*a,* Continuous long-term replication of feline leukemia virus (FeLV) in an established canine cell culture (MDCK), *Proc. Soc. Exp. Biol. Med.* **139**:295.

Essex, M., Klein, G., Deinhardt, F., Wolfe, L., Hardy, W. D., Jr., Theilen, G., and Pearson, L., 1972*b,* Induction of the feline oncornavirus-associated cell membrane antigen in human cells, *Nature (London) New Biol.* **238**:187.

Essex, M., Cotter, S. M., and Carpenter, J. L., 1973*a,* Role of the immune response in the development and progression of virus-induced tumors of cats, *Am. J. Vet. Res.* **34**:809.

Essex, M., Snyder, S. P., and Klein, G., 1973*b,* Relationship between humoral antibodies and the failure to develop progressive tumors in cats injected with feline sarcoma virus, in: *Unifying Concepts of Leukemia* (R. M. Dutcher and L. Chieco-Bianchi, eds.), pp. 777–791, Karger, New York.

Essex, M., Cotter, S. M., Carpenter, J. L., Hardy, W. D., Jr., Hess, P., Jarrett, W., and Yohn, D. S., 1975*a,* Feline oncornavirus-associated cell membrane antigen. II. Antibody titers in healthy cats from pet household and laboratory colony environments, *J. Natl. Cancer Inst.* **54**:631.

Essex, M., Hardy, W. D., Jr., Cotter, S. M., Jakowski, R. M., and Sliski, A., 1975*b,* Naturally occurring persistent feline oncornavirus infections in the absence of disease, *Infect. Immun.* **11**:470.

Essex, M., Jakowski, R. M., Hardy, W. D., Jr., Cotter, S. M., Hess, P., and Sliski, A., 1975*c,* Feline oncornavirus-associated cell membrane antigen. III. Antibody titers in cats from leukemia cluster households, *J. Natl. Cancer Inst.* **54**:637.

Essex, M., Cotter, S. M., Hardy, W. D., Jr., Hess, P., Jarrett, W., Jarrett, O., Mackey, L., Laird, H., Perryman, L., Olsen, R. G., and Yohn, D. S., 1975*d,* Feline oncornavirus-associated cell membrane antigen. IV. Antibody titers in cats with naturally occurring leukemia, lymphoma, and other disease, *J. Natl. Cancer Inst.* **55**:463.

Essex, M., Hardy, W. D., Jr., Cotter, S. M., and Jakowski, R. M., 1975*e,* Immune response of healthy and leukemic cats to the feline oncornavirus-associated cell membrane antigen (FOCMA), in: *Comparative Leukemia Research, 1973* (Y. Ito and R. M. Dutcher, eds.), pp. 483–488, Karger, University of Tokyo Press, Tokyo.

Essex, M., Sliski, A., Cotter, S. M., Jakowski, R. M., and Hardy, W. D., Jr., 1975*f,* Immunosurveillance of naturally occurring feline leukemia, *Science* **190**:790.

Essex, M., Sliski, A., Hardy, W. D., Jr., and Cotter, S. M., 1976*a,* The immune response to leukemia virus and tumor associated antigens in cats, *Cancer Res.* **36**:640.

Essex, M., Cotter, S. M., Sliski, A., Hardy, W. D. Jr., Stephenson, J. R., Aaronson, S. A., and

Jarrett, O., 1976b, Horizontal transmission of feline leukemia virus under natural conditions in a feline, leukemia cluster household, *Int. J. Cancer*, in press.

Fischinger, P. J., Peebles, P. T., Nomura, S., and Haapala, D. K., 1973, Isolation of an RD-114-like oncornavirus from a cat cell line, *J. Virol.* 11:978.

Fischinger, P. J., Blevins, C. S., and Nomura, S., 1974, Simple quantitative assay for both xenotropic murine leukemia and ecotropic feline leukemia viruses, *J. Virol.* 14:177.

Friedman, M., Lilly, F., and Nathenson, S. G., 1974, Cell surface antigen induced by Friend murine leukemia virus is also in the virion, *J. Virol.* 14:1126.

Gallagher, R. E., and Gallo, R. C., 1975, Type C RNA tumor virus isolated from cultured human acute myelogenous leukemia cells, *Science* 187:350.

Gardner, M. B., Arnstein, P., Rongey, R. W., Estes, J. D., Sarma, P. S., Rickard, C. F., and Huebner, R. J., 1970, Experimental transmission of feline fibrosarcoma to cats and dogs, *Nature (London) New Biol.* 226:807.

Gardner, M. B., Rongey, R. W., Johnson, E. Y., DeJournett, R., and Huebner, R. J., 1971, C-type tumor virus particles in salivary tissue of domestic cats, *J. Natl. Cancer Inst.* 47:561.

Gardner, M. B., Rasheed, S., Rongey, R. W., Charman, H. P., Alena, B., Gilden, R. V., and Huebner, R. J., 1974, Natural expression of feline type C virus genomes, *Int. J. Cancer* 14:97.

Gatti, R. A., and Good, R. A., 1971, Occurrence of malignancy in immunodeficiency diseases, *Cancer* 28:89.

Gilden, R. V., Oroszlan, S., and Hatanaka, M., 1974, Comparison and evolution of RNA tumor virus components, in: *Viruses, Evolution and Cancer* (E. Kurstak and K. Maramorosch, eds.), pp. 235–258, Academic Press, New York.

Gillespie, D., and Gallo, R. C., 1975, RNA processing and RNA tumor virus origin and evolution, *Science* 188:802.

Gillespie, D., Gillespie, S., Gallo, R. C., East, J. L., and Dmochowski, L., 1973, Genetic origin of RD-114 and other RNA tumor viruses assayed by molecular hybridization, *Nature (London) New Biol.* 244:51.

Gilmore, C. E., and Holzworth, J., 1971, Naturally occurring feline leukemia: Clinical, pathologic, and differential diagnostic features, *J. Am. Vet. Med. Assoc.* 158:1013.

Hampar, B., Kelloff, G. J., Martos, L. M., Oroszlan, S., Gilden, R. V., and Walker, J. L., 1970, Replication of murine and feline RNA-containing C-type viruses in human lymphoblastoid cells, *Nature (London)* 228:857.

Hampar, B., Rand, K. H., Lerner, R. A., del Villano, B. C., Jr., McAllister, R. M., Maftos, L. M., Derge, J. G., Long, C. W., and Gilden, R. V., 1973, Formation of syncytia in human lymphoblastoid cells infected with type C viruses, *Virology* 55:453.

Hanna, M. G., Ihle, J. N., Batzing, B. L., Tennant, R. W., and Schenley, C. K., 1975, Assessment of reactivities of natural antibodies to endogenous RNA tumor virus envelope antigens and virus induced cell surface antigens, *Cancer Res.* 35:164.

Hardy, W. D., Jr., 1974, Immunology of oncornavirus, *Vet. Clin. North Am.* 4:133.

Hardy, W. D., Jr., and McClelland, A. J., 1975, Infectious spread and control of feline leukemia virus, *Transplant. Proc.* 7:265.

Hardy, W. D., Jr., Geering, G., Old, L. J., de Harven, E., Brodey, R. B., and McDonough, S., 1969, Feline leukemia virus: Occurrence of viral antigen in the tissues of cats with lymphosarcoma and other diseases, *Science* 166:1019.

Hardy, W. D., Jr., Hirshaut, Y., and Hess, P., 1973a, Detection of the feline leukemia virus and other mammalian oncornaviruses by immunofluorescence, in: *Unifying Concepts of Leukemia* (R. M. Dutcher and L. Chieco-Bianchi, eds.), pp. 778–799, Karger, New York.

Hardy, W. D., Jr., Old, L. J., Hess, P. W., Essex, M., and Cotter, S. M., 1973*b*, Horizontal transmission of feline leukemia virus, *Nature (London)* 244:266.

Hardy, W. D., Jr., Hess, P. W., MacEwen, E. G., McClelland, A. J., Zuckerman, E. E., Essex, M., and Cotter, S. M., 1976*a*, The biology of feline leukemia virus in the natural environment, *Cancer Res.* 36:582.

Hardy, W. D., Jr., Zuckerman, E. E., McClelland, A. J., Hess, P. W., MacEwen, E. G., Essex, M., and Cotter, S. M., 1976*b*, Feline leukemia virus control and vaccination, in: *Comparative Leukemia Research 1975* (J. Clemmensen and D. S. Yohn, eds.), pp. 511–514, Karger, Basel.

Hartley, J. W., and Rowe, W. P., 1966, Production of altered cell foci in tissue culture by defective Moloney sarcoma virus particles, *Proc. Natl. Acad. Sci. U.S.A.* 55:780.

Hellmann, K., Hawkins, R. I., and Whitecross, S., 1968, Antilymphocytic serum and tumour dissemination, *Brit. Med. J.* 2:533.

Hellström, K. E., and Hellström, I., 1970, Immunological enhancement as studied by cell culture techniques, *Annu. Rev. Microbiol.* 24:373.

Hilgers, J., Nowinski, R. C., Geering, G., and Hardy, W. D., Jr., 1972, Detection of avian and mammalian oncogenic RNA viruses (oncornaviruses) by immunofluorescence, *Cancer Res.* 32:98.

Hirsch, M. S., and Murphy, F. A., 1968, Effects of anti-thymocyte serum on Rauscher virus infection of mice, *Nature (London)* 218:478.

Hoover, E. A., McCullough, C. B., and Griesmer, R. A., 1972, Intranasal transmission of feline leukemia, *J. Natl. Cancer Inst.* 48:973.

Hoover, E. A., Perryman, L. E., and Kociba, G. J., 1973, Early lesions in cats inoculated with feline leukemia virus, *Cancer Res.* 33:145.

Hoover, E. A., Kociba, G. J., Hardy, W. D., Jr., and Yohn, D. S., 1974, Erythroid hypoplasia in cats inoculated with feline leukemia virus, *J. Natl. Cancer Inst.* 53:1271.

Hoover, E. A., Olsen, R. G., Hardy, W. D., Jr., Schaller, J. P., Mathes, L. E., and Cockerell, G. L., 1976, Biologic and immunologic response of cats to experimental infection with feline leukemia virus, in: *Comparative Leukemia Research 1975* (J. Clemmensen and D. S. Yohn, eds.), pp. 180–183, Karger, Basel.

Huebner, R. J., and Todaro, G. J., 1969. Oncogenes of RNA tumor viruses as determinants of cancer, *Proc. Natl. Acad. Sci. U.S.A.* 64:1087.

Ihle, J. N., Hanna, M. G., Jr., Roberson, L. E., and Kenney, F. T., 1974, Autogenous immunity to endogenous RNA tumor virus: Identification of antibody reactivity to select viral antigens, *J. Exp. Med.* 139:1568.

Ishimoto, A., Suzuki, Y., Yoshida, T., and Ito, Y., 1974, Further studies on mouse fetal antigen cross-reactive with Rauscher leukemia, *Cancer Res.* 34:2338.

Jarrett, O., 1971, Virology and host range of feline leukemia virus, *J. Am. Vet. Med. Assoc.* 158:1032.

Jarrett, O., 1973, Antigenic determinants shared by polypeptides of feline leukemia virus, in: *Unifying Concepts of Leukemia* (R. M. Dutcher and L. Chieco-Bianchi, eds.), pp. 810–812, Karger, New York.

Jarrett, O., Laird, H. M., Hay, D., and Crighton, G. W., 1968, Replication of cat leukemia virus in cell cultures, *Nature (London)* 219:521.

Jarrett, O., Laird, H. M., and Hay, D., 1969, Growth of feline leukemia virus in human cells, *Nature (London)* 224:1208.

Jarrett, O., Laird, H. M., and Hay, D., 1970, Growth of feline leukemia virus in human, canine, and porcine cells, in: *Comparative Leukemia Research 1969* (R. M. Dutcher, ed.), pp. 387–392, Karger, Basel and New York.

Jarrett, O., Laird, H. M., and Hay, D., 1972, Leukemia virus: restricted host range of a feline leukemia virus, *Nature (London)* **238**:220.

Jarrett, O., Laird, H. M., and Hay, D., 1973, Determinants of the host range of feline leukemia virus, *J. Gen. Virol.* **20**:169.

Jarrett, W. F. H., 1972. Feline leukemia, *J. Clin. Pathol.* **25**:43.

Jarrett, W. F. H., 1975, The relation of immune response to pathogenesis, vaccination, and epidemiology in virus-induced leukemia, *Br. J. Cancer*, **31**:147.

Jarrett, W. F. H., and Mackey, L. J., 1974, Neoplastic diseases of the haematopoietic and lymphoid tissues, *Bull. WHO* **50**:21.

Jarrett, W. F. H., Crawford, E., Martin, W. B., and Davie, F., 1964*a*, Leukemia in the cat: A virus-like particle associated with leukemia (lymphosarcoma), *Nature (London)* **202**: 567.

Jarrett, W. F. H., Martin, W. B., Crighton, G. W., Dalton, R. G., and Stewart, M. F., 1964*b*, Transmission experiments with leukemia lymphosarcoma, *Nature (London)* **202**:566.

Jarrett, W. F. H., Essex, M., Mackey, L. J., Jarrett, O., and Laird, H., 1973*a*, Antibodies in normal and leukemia cats to feline oncornavirus-associated cell membrane antigens, *J. Natl. Cancer Inst.* **51**:261.

Jarrett, W. F. H., Jarrett, O., Mackey, L., Laird, H., Hardy, W. D., Jr., and Essex, M., 1973*b*, Horizontal transmission of leukemia virus and leukemia in the cat, *J. Natl. Cancer Inst.* **51**:833.

Jarrett, W. F. H., Mackey, L. J., Jarrett, O., and Laird, H. M., 1973*c*, Feline leukemia virus induced infection–the spectrum of associated disease and its relevance to the pathogenesis and immunology of leukemia, in: *Unifying Concepts of Leukemia* (R. M. Dutcher and L. Chieco-Bianchi, eds.), pp. 93–101, Karger, New York.

Jarrett, W. F. H., Mackey, L., Jarrett, O., Laird, H., and Hood, C., 1974, Antibody response and virus survival in cats vaccinated against feline leukaemia, *Nature (London)* **248**: 230.

Jondal, M., and Klein, G., 1973, Surface markers on human B and T lymphocytes. II. Presence of Epstein-Barr virus receptors on B lymphocytes. *J. Exp. Med.* **138**:1365.

Jondal, M., Svedmya, E., Klein, E., and Singh, S., 1975, Killer T cells in Burkitt's lymphoma biopsy, *Nature (London)* **225**:405.

Kawakami, T. G., and Buckley, P. M., 1974, Antigenic studies on gibbon type-C viruses, *Transplant. Proc.* **6**:193.

Kawakami, T. G., Theilen, G. H., Dungworth, D. L., Munn, R. J., and Beall, S. G., 1967, C-type viral particles in plasma of cats with feline leukemia, *Science* **158**:1049.

Kersey, J. H., Gatti, R. A., Good, R. A., Aaronson, S. A., and Todaro, G. J., 1972, Susceptibility of cells from patients with primary immunodeficiency diseases to transformation by simian virus 40, *Proc. Natl. Acad. Sci. U.S.A.* **69**:980.

Kersey, J. H., Sabad, A., Gajl-Peczalska, K., Hallgren, H. M., Yunis, E. J., and Nesbit, M. E., 1973, Acute lymphoblastic leukemic cells with T (thymus-derived) lymphocyte markers, *Science* **182**:1355.

Klein, E., and Klein, G., 1964, Antigenic properties of lymphomas induced by the Moloney agent, *J. Natl. Cancer Inst.* **32**:547.

Kurth, R., and Bauer, H., 1973, Avian oncornavirus induced tumor antigens of embryonic and unknown origin, *Virology* **56**:496.

Kurth, R., and Bauer, H., 1975, Avian RNA tumor viruses: A model for studying tumor associated cell surface alterations, *Biochem. Biophys. Acta* **417**:1.

Laird, H. M., Jarrett, O., Crighton, G. W., and Jarrett, W. F. H., 1968, An electron microscopic study of virus particles in spontaneous leukemia in the cat, *J. Natl. Cancer Inst.* **41**:867.

Lamon, E. W., Wigzell, H., Andersson, B., and Klein, E., 1973, B lymphocytes from animals in which primary MSV tumors have regressed are active *in vitro* against target cells bearing MLV determined antigens, *Nature (London) New Biol.* **244**:209.

Lee, K. M., 1971, Comments on feline leukemia virus, *J. Am. Vet. Med. Assoc.* **158**:1037.

Livingston, D. M., and Todaro, G. J., 1973, Endogenous type C virus from a cat cell clone with properties distinct from previously described feline type C virus, *Virology* **53**:142.

Mackey, L. J., Jarrett, W. F. H., Jarrett, O., and Laird, H. M., 1972, An experimental study of virus leukemia in cats, *J. Natl. Cancer Inst.* **48**:1663.

Mackey, L., Jarrett, W., Jarrett, O., and Wilson, L., 1975*a*, B and T cells in a cat with thymic lymphosarcoma, *J. Natl. Cancer Inst.* **54**:1483.

Mackey, L., Jarrett, W., and Wilson, L., 1975*b*, A mixed-immunoglobulin rosette technique for the detection of antibody to feline oncornavirus-associated cell membrane antigen, *Cancer Res.* **35**:1064.

Mathes, L. E., Yohn, D. S., Hoover, E. A., Essex, M., Schaller, J. P., and Olsen, R. G., 1976, Feline oncornavirus associated cell membrane antigen. VI. Cytotoxic antibody in cats exposed to feline leukemia virus, *J. Natl. Cancer Inst.* **56**:1197.

McAllister, R. M., Filbert, J. E., Nicolson, M. O., Rongey, R. W., Gardner, M. B., Gilden, R. V., and Huebner, R. J., 1971, Transformation and productive infection of human osteosarcoma cells by a feline sarcoma virus, *Nature (London) New Biol.* **230**:279.

McAllister, R. M., Nicolson, M., Gardner, M. B., Rongey, R. W., Rasheed, S., Sarma, P. S., Huebner, R. J., Hatanaka, M., Oroszlan, S., Gilden, R. V., Kabigting, A., and Vernon, L., 1972, C-type virus released from cultured human rhabdomyosarcoma cells, *Nature (London) New Biol.* **235**:3.

McAllister, R. M., Nicolson, M., Gardner, M. B., Rongey, R. W., Rasheed, S., Sarma, P. S., Huebner, R. J., Hatanaka, M., Oroszlan, S., Gilden, R. V., Kabigting, A., and Vernon, L., 1973, RD-114 comparison with feline and murine type C viruses released from RD cells, *Nature (London) New Biol.* **242**:75.

McDonald, R., Wolfe, L. G., and Deinhardt, F., 1972, Feline fibrosarcoma virus quantitative focus assay, focus morphology and evidence for a "helper virus," *Int. J. Cancer* **9**:57.

McDonough, S., Larsen, S., Brodey, R. S., Stock, N. D., and Hardy, W. D., Jr., 1971, A transmissible feline fibrosarcoma of viral origin. *Cancer Res.* **31**:953.

Melnick, J. L., Altenburg, B., Arnstein, P., Mirkovic, R., and Tevethia, S., 1973, Transformation of baboon cells with feline sarcoma virus, *Intervirology* **1**:386.

Monti-Bragadin, C., and Ulrich, K., 1972, Rescue of the genome of the defective murine sarcoma virus from a non-producer hamster tumor cell lines, PM-1, with murine and feline leukemia viruses as helpers, *Int. J. Cancer* **9**:383.

Moroni, C., Robert-Guroff, M., and Martin, D., 1974, Virion and non-virion murine leukemia membrane antigens: Analysis with virus-absorbed antisera, *Intervirology* **3**:292.

Nazerian, K., 1973, Marek's disease: A neoplastic disease of chickens caused by a herpesvirus, *Adv. Cancer Res.* **17**:279.

Neiman, P. E., 1973, Measurement of RD-114 virus nucleotide sequences in feline cellular DNA, *Nature (London) New Biol.* **244**:62.

Nilsson, K., Klein, G., Henle, W., and Henle, G., 1972, The establishment of lymphoblastoid lines from adult and fetal human lymphoid tissue and its dependence on EBV, *Int. J. Cancer* **8**:443.

Noronha, F., Dougherty, E., Poco, A., Gries, C., Post, J., and Rickard, C., 1974, Cytological and serological studies of a feline endogenous C-type virus, *Arch. Gesamte Virusforsch.* **45**:735.

Notkins, A. L., Mergenhagen, S. E., and Howard, R. J., 1970, Effect of virus infection on the function of the immune system, *Annu. Rev. Microbiol.* **24:**525.

Okabe, H., Gilden, R. V., and Hatanaka, M., 1973, Extensive homology of RD 114 virus DNA with RNA of feline cell origin, *Nature (London) New Biol.* **244:**54.

Olsen, R. G., and Yohn, D. S., 1972, Demonstration of antibody in cat sera to feline oncornavirus by complement-fixation inhibition, *J. Natl. Cancer Inst.* **49:**395.

Olsen, R. G., Mathes, L. E., and Yohn, D. S., 1975, Antibody in cats to mammalian RNA-tumor virus interspecies antigens, *Cancer Res.* **35:**2580.

Olsen, R. G., Milo, G. E., Schaller, J. P., Mathes, L. E., Heding, L., and Yohn, D. S., 1976*a*, Influence of culture conditions on growth of Fl-74 cells and feline oncornavirus associated cell membrane antigen production, *In Vitro* **12:**37.

Olsen, R. G., Schaller, J. P., Hoover, E. A., and Yohn, D. S., 1976*b*, Experimental oncornavirus vaccines in the cat, in: *Comparative Leukemia Research 1975* (J. Clemmensen and D. S. Yohn, eds.), pp. 515–517, Karger, Basel.

Oshiro, L., Riggs, J., Lennette, E., and McAllister, R., 1974, Ferritin-labelled antibody study of RD-114 virus, *J. Gen. Virol.* **22:**277.

Ott, R. L., 1976, Report of the American Veterinary Medical Association Panel on Feline Leukemia, *J. Am. Vet. Med. Assoc.*, in press.

Pearson, G. R., Redmon, L. W., and Bass, L. R., 1973, Protective effect of immune sera against transplantable Moloney virus-induced sarcoma and lymphoma, *Cancer Res.* **33:**171.

Pearson, L. D., Snyder, S. P., and Aldrich, C. D., 1973, Oncogenic activity of feline fibrosarcoma virus in newborn pigs, *Am. J. Vet. Res.* **34:**405.

Penn, I., 1974, Occurrence of cancer in immune deficiencies, *Cancer* **34:**858.

Penn, I., 1975, The incidence of malignancies in transplant recipients, *Transplant. Proc.* **7:**323.

Perryman, L. E., Hoover, E. A., and Yohn, D. S., 1972, Immunological reactivity of the cat: Immunosuppression in experimental feline leukemia, *J. Natl. Cancer Inst.* **49:**1357.

Phillips, E. R., and Perdue, J. F., 1974, Ultrastructural distribution of cell surface antigens in avian tumor virus-infected chick embryo fibroblasts, *J. Cell Biol.* **61:**743.

Pope, J. H., Horne, M. K., and Scott, W., 1969, Identification of the filtrable leukocyte-transforming factor of QIMR-WIL cells as herpes-like virus, *Int. J. Cancer* **4:**255.

Prehn, R. T., 1974, Immunodulation of tumor growth, *Am. J. Pathol.* **77:**119.

Quintrell, N., Varmus, H. E., Bishop, J. M., Nicolson, M. O., and McAllister, R. M., 1974, Homologies among the nucleotide sequences of the genomes of C-type viruses, *Virology* **58:**568.

Rabin, H., Theilen, G. H., Sarma, P. S., Dungworth, D. L., Nelson-Rees, W. A., and Cooper, R. W., 1972, Tumor induction in squirrel monkeys by the ST strain of feline sarcoma virus, *J. Natl. Cancer Inst.* **49:**441.

Rickard, C. G., 1969, Feline leukemia (lymphosarcoma) Symposium 4: Discussion, *J. Small Anim. Pract.* **10:**615.

Rickard, C. G., Post, J. E., Noronha, F., and Barr, L. M., 1969, A transmissible virus-induced lymphocytic leukemia of the cat, *J. Natl. Cancer Inst.* **42:**987.

Rickard, C. G., Post, J. E., Noronha, F., and Barr, L. M., 1973, Interspecies infection by feline leukemia virus: Serial cell-free transmission in dogs of malignant lymphoma induced by feline leukemia virus, in: *Unifying Concepts of Leukemia* (R. M. Dutcher and L. Chieco-Bianchi, eds.), pp. 102–112, Karger, New York.

Riggs, J. L., McAllister, R. M., and Lennette, E. H., 1974, Immunofluorescent studies of RD-114 virus in cell culture, *J. Gen. Virol.* **25:**21.

Rogerson, P., Jarrett, W., and Mackey, L., 1975, Epidemiological studies on feline leukaemia virus infection. I. A serological survey in urban cats, *Int. J. Cancer* **15**:781.

Rohrschneider, L. R., Kurth, R., and Bauer, H., 1975, Biochemical characterization of tumor-specific cell surface antigens on avian oncornavirus transformed cells, *Virology*, in press.

Ruprecht, R. M., Goodman, N. C., and Spiegelman, S., 1973, Determination of natural host taxonomy of RNA tumor viruses by molecular hybridization: Application to RD-114, a candidate human virus, *Proc. Natl. Acad. Sci. U.S.A.* **70**:1437.

Rygaard, J., and Povlsen, C. O., 1974, The mouse mutant nude does not develop spontaneous tumors, *Acta pathol. Microbiol. Scand. Sect. B* **82**:99.

Sanford, B. H., Kohn, H. I., Daly, J. J., and Soo, S. F., 1973, Long-term spontaneous tumor incidence in neonatally thymectomized mice, *J. Immunol.* **110**:1437.

Sarma, P. S., and Log, T., 1971, Viral interference in feline leukemia-sarcoma complex, *Virology* **44**:352.

Sarma, P. S., and Log, T., 1973, Subgroup classification of feline leukemia and sarcoma viruses by viral interference and neutralization tests, *Virology* **54**:160.

Sarma, P. S., Huebner, R. J., Baskar, J. F., Vernon, L., and Gilden, R. V., 1970, Feline leukemia and sarcoma viruses: Susceptibility of human cells to infection, *Science* **168**:1098.

Sarma, P. S., Baskar, J. F., Gilden, R. V., Gardner, M. B., and Huebner, R. J., 1971a, "In vitro" isolation and characterization of the GA strain of feline sarcoma virus, *Proc. Soc. Exp. Biol. Med.* **137**:1333.

Sarma, P. S., Log, T., and Theilen, G. H., 1971b, ST feline sarcoma virus: Biological characteristics and *in vitro* propagation, *Proc. Soc. Exp. Biol. Med.* **137**:1444.

Sarma, P. S., Gilden, R. V., and Huebner, R. J., 1971c, Complement-fixation test for feline leukemia and sarcoma viruses (the cocal test), *Virology* **44**:137.

Sarma, P. S., Sharar, A. L., and McDonough, S., 1972, The SM strain of feline sarcoma virus: Biologic and antigenic characterization of virus, *Proc. Soc. Exp. Biol. Med.* **140**:1365.

Sarma, P. S., Tseng, J., Lee, Y. K., and Gilden, R. V., 1973, Virus similar to RD-114 virus in cat cells, *Nature (London) New Biol.* **244**:56.

Sarma, P. S., Sharar, A., Tseng, J., Price, P. J., and Gardner, M., 1974a, Studies on the prevalence of endogenous type C virus RD-114 in cats, *Proc. Soc. Exp. Biol. Med.* **145**:757.

Sarma, P. S., Sharar, A., Walter, V., and Gardner, M., 1974b, A survey of cats and humans for prevalence of feline leukemia-sarcoma virus neutralizing serum antibodies, *Proc. Soc. Exp. Biol. Med.* **145**:560.

Sarma, P. S., Log, T., Jain, D., Hill, P. R., and Huebner, R. J., 1975, Differential host range of viruses of feline leukemia-sarcoma complex, *Virology* **64**:438.

Schäfer, W., and Bolognesi, D. P., 1976, in: this volume, pp. 127–167.

Schäfer, W., Pister, J., Hunsmann, G., and Moennig, V., 1973, C-type viruses—evidence for the existence of different interspecies determinants, *Nature (London) New Biol.* **245**:77.

Schaller, J. P., Essex, M., Yohn, D. S., and Olsen, R. G., 1975, Feline oncornavirus-associated cell membrane antigen. V. Humoral immune response to virus and cell membrane antigens in cats injected with Gardner-Arnstein feline sarcoma virus, *J. Natl. Cancer Inst.* **55**:1373.

Schwartz, R. S., 1974, Immunosuppression and neoplasia, in: *Progress in Immunology*

II, Vol. 5 (L. Brent and J. Holborow, eds.), pp. 229–232, American Elsevier, New York.

Schneider, R., 1971, Comments on epidemiologic implications of feline leukemia virus, *J. Am. Vet. Med. Assoc.* **158**:1125.

Schneider, R., Frye, F. L., Taylor, D. O. N., and Dorn, C. R., 1967, A household cluster of feline malignant lymphoma, *Cancer Res.* **27**:1316.

Scolnick, E. M., Parks, W. P., and Livingston, D. M., 1972, Radioimmunoassay of mammalian type C viral proteins. I. Species specific reaction of murine and feline viruses, *J. Immunol.* **109**:570.

Senik, A., De Giorgi, L., Gomard, E., and Levy, J. P., 1974, Cytostasis of lymphoma cells in suspension: Probable non-thymic origin of the cytostatic lymphoid cells in mice bearing MSV-induced tumors, *Int. J. Cancer* **14**:396.

Sharma, J. M., Witter, R. L., and Purchase, H. G., 1975, Absence of age-resistance in neonatally thymectomised chickens as evidence for cell-mediated immune surveillance in Marek's disease, *Nature (London)* **253**:477.

Sherr, C. J., Lieber, M. M., Benveniste, R. E., and Todaro, G. J., 1974, Endogenous baboon type C virus (M7): Biochemical and immunological characterization, *Virology* **58**:492.

Sklar, M. D., White, B. J., and Rowe, W. P., 1974, Initiation of oncogenic transformation of mouse lymphocytes in vitro by Abelson leukemia virus, *Proc. Natl. Acad. Sci. U.S.A.* **71**:4077.

Slauson, D. O., Osburn, B. I., Shifrine, M., and Dungworth, D. L., 1975, Regression of feline sarcoma virus-induced sarcomas in dogs. 1. Morphologic investigations, *J. Natl. Cancer Inst.* **54**:361.

Snyder, S. P., 1971, Spontaneous feline fibrosarcomas: Transmissibility and ultrastructure of associated virus-like particles, *J. Natl. Cancer Inst.* **47**:1079.

Snyder, S. P., and Dungworth, D. L., 1973, Pathogenesis of feline viral fibrosarcomas: Dose and age effects, *J. Natl. Cancer Inst.* **51**:781.

Snyder, S. P., and Theilen, G. H., 1969, Transmissible feline fibrosarcoma, *Nature (London)* **221**:1074.

Snyder, S. P., Theilen, G. H., and Richards, W. P., 1970, Morphological studies on transmissible feline fibrosarcoma, *Cancer Res.* **30**:1658.

Strand, M., Wilsnack, R., and August, J. T., 1974, Structural proteins of mammalian oncogenic RNA viruses: Immunological characterization of the p15 polypeptide of Rauscher murine virus, *J. Virol.* **14**:1575.

Stutman, O., 1974, Tumor development in immunologically deficient nude mice after exposure to chemical carcinogens, in: *Proceedings of the 1st International Workshop on Nude Mice* (J. Rygaard and C. O. Povlsen, eds.), pp. 257–264, Gustav Fischer Verlag, Stuttgart.

Theilen, G. H., Kawakami, T. G., Dungworth, D. L., Switzer, J. W., Munn, R. J., and Harrold, J. B., 1968, Current status of transmissible agents in feline leukemia, *J. Am. Vet. Med. Assoc.* **153**:1864.

Theilen, G. H., Kawakami, T. G., Rush, J. D., and Munn, R. J., 1969, Replication of cat leukemia virus in cell suspension cultures, *Nature (London)* **222**:589.

Theilen, G. H., Dungworth, D. L., Kawakami, T. G., Munn, R. J., Ward, J. M., and Harrold, J. B., 1970, Experimental induction of lymphosarcoma in the cat with C-type virus, *Cancer Res.* **30**:401.

Theilen, G. H., Hall, J. G., Pendry, A., Glover, D. J., and Reeves, B. R., 1974, Tumors induced in sheep by injecting cells transformed *in vitro* with feline sarcoma virus, *Transplantation* **17**:152.

Thomas, L., 1959, Discussion, in: *Cellular and Humoral Aspects of the Hypersensitive State* (H. S. Lawrence, ed.), p. 529, Hoeber, New York.

Thompson, K. D., and Linna, T. J., 1973, Bursa-dependent and thymus-dependent "surveillance" of a virus-induced tumor in the chicken, *Nature (London) New Biol.* 245: 10–12.

Ting, C. C., Shiu, G., Rodrigues, D., and Herberman, R. B., 1974, Cell-mediated immunity to Friend virus-induced leukemia, *Cancer Res.* 34:1684.

Todaro, G. J., and Huebner, R. J., 1972, The viral oncogene hypothesis: New evidence, *Proc. Natl. Acad. Sci. U.S.A.* 69:1009.

Todaro, G. J., Tevethia, S., and Melnick, J., 1974, Isolation of an RD-114 related type-C virus from feline sarcoma virus-transformed baboon cells, *Intervirology* 1:399.

Ubertini, T., Noronha, F., Post, J. E., and Rickard, C. G., 1971, A fluorescent antibody technique for the detection of the group-specific antigen of feline leukemia virus in infected tissue-culture cells, *Virology* 44:219.

Wilson, R. E., and Penn, I., 1975, Fate of tumors transplanted with a renal allograft, *Transplant. Proc.* 7:327.

Wolfe, L. G., Smith, R. D., Hoekstra, J., Marczynska, B., Smith, R. K., McDonald, R., Northrop, R. L., and Deinhardt, F., 1972, Oncogenicity of feline fibrosarcoma viruses in marmoset monkeys: Pathologic, virologic, and immunologic findings, *J. Natl. Cancer Inst.* 49:519.

Yohn, D. S., and Olsen, R. G., 1973, Antibodies to feline oncornavirus group-specific antigens in feline sera, in: *Unifying Concepts of Leukemia* (R. M. Dutcher and L. Chieco-Bianchi, eds.), pp. 744–754, Karger, New York.

Yohn, D. S., Olsen, R. G., Schaller, J. P., Hoover, E. A., Mathes, L. E., Heding, L., and Davis, G., 1976, Experimental oncornavirus vaccines in the cat, *Cancer Res.* 36:646.

Yoshiki, T., Mellors, R. C., Hardy, W. D., Jr., and Fleissner, E., 1974, Common cell surface antigen associated with mammalian C-type RNA viruses, *J. Exp. Med.* 139:925.

Chapter 3

Intracellular and Systemic Regulation of Biologically Distinguishable Endogenous Type C RNA Viruses of Mouse Cells

Stuart A. Aaronson and John R. Stephenson

Laboratory of RNA Tumor Viruses, Viral Carcinogenesis Branch
National Cancer Institute
Bethesda, Maryland 20014

I. INTRODUCTION

The inherited basis for factors involved in leukemogenesis in mice was established many years ago with the development of inbred strains having extremely high susceptibility to the natural occurrence of leukemia (Furth *et al.*, 1933; MacDowell and Richter, 1935). The first evidence that viruses were etiologically involved in this disease was provided by Gross (1951), who demonstrated transmission of leukemia to mice by filtrates from tumors of high-leukemia-incidence strains. Subsequent studies *in vivo* have confirmed and extended these observations, documenting the intimate association of type C RNA viruses with the mouse and the etiological role of the virus in leukemia.

The question as to whether type C viruses are transmitted horizontally or vertically through infection within the reproductive tract, or genetically within the gametes themselves, has been extensively investigated in recent years. Early immunological studies demonstrated subviral expression in mouse strains which did not yield infectious virus (Huebner *et al.*, 1970). In tissue culture, evidence for the genetic transmission of the virus was provided by the discovery that mouse cells could spontaneously begin to release type C virus after growth for many generations in the absence of virus production (Aaronson *et al.*, 1969). Subsequent findings that halogenated pyrimidines could activate virus from clonal mouse cell lines of both high (Lowy *et al.*, 1971) and low (Aaronson *et al.*, 1971) leukemia incidence strains made it possible to show that endogenous type C viruses were present in an unexpressed form in every cell. The independent proof of the genetic transmission of mouse type C viral information was derived from the demonstration of nucleotide sequence homology between normal mouse-cell DNA and type C viral DNA probes prepared by reverse transcription of viral RNA (Gelb *et al.*, 1971, 1973; Chattopadhyay *et al.*, 1974). Multiple copies of virus could be detected within the high-molecular-weight cellular DNA (Gelb *et al.*, 1973). The techniques used to demonstrate genetic transmission of type C viruses in mouse cells have subsequently been useful in establishing that endogenous viruses are present in an increasing number of species. The biological functions of endogenous viruses have not, for the most part, been elucidated. The availability of inbred mouse strains with genetically defined natural incidences of disease makes the mouse a very useful experimental model with which to investigate these actions. Accumulating evidence indicates that various inbred strains possess different numbers and biological classes of endogenous viruses and regulatory factors specific to each virus. Thus it becomes feasible to investigate whether particular diseases are genetically linked to specific endogenous viruses and/or their regulatory genes. This chapter summarizes our current knowledge concerning the biological properties of endogenous mouse type C viruses and factors, both intracellular and systemic, which affect their expression.

II. EVIDENCE FOR THREE CLASSES OF BIOLOGICALLY DISTINGUISHABLE ENDOGENOUS MOUSE TYPE C VIRUSES

Studies in our laboratory, initially involving four prototype mouse strains, BALB/c, NIH Swiss, C58, and NZB, provided evidence for the existence of at least three biologically distinguishable endogenous mouse type-C viruses. These viruses can be partially discriminated on the basis of standard host range and serological tests (Table I) and by more recently developed, highly specific competition immunoassays for viral structural polypeptides (Stephenson *et al.*, 1974e; Hino *et al.*, 1976). The three viruses can also be differentiated by the manner in which the same cell regulates their expression. As shown in Table I, one class of endogenous virus preferentially replicates in NIH Swiss mouse cells and hence is termed "N-tropic." This virus can be spontaneously activated (Aaronson *et al.*, 1969) or induced by chemicals such as IdU (Lowy *et al.*, 1971; Aaronson *et al.*, 1971). Multiple loci for induction of class I virus have been demonstrated in C58 cells (Stephenson and Aaronson, 1973b), whereas only one locus for its activation exists in BALB/c cells (Stephenson and Aaronson, 1972b). Many other strains have been shown to contain one or more loci

Table 1. Properties of Endogenous Type C RNA Viruses of Normal Mouse Cells

Virus	Biological properties		Induced by[c]	
	Host range[a] (tropism)	Neutralized by normal BALB/c sera[b]	Halogenated pyrimidines	Inhibitors of protein synthesis
Class I (BALB:virus-1)	N	−	+	−
Class II (BALB:virus-2)	X	+	+	+
Class III (NIH virus)	X	+	−	−

[a]Host range is designated as NIH Swiss tropic (N) or xenotropic (X). N-tropic viruses are preferentially infectious for NIH/3T3 mouse cells, but also grow less well in BALB/3T3 mouse- or rat-derived NRK cells. X-tropic viruses are noninfectious for either mouse cell line but grow in cells of rat and human cell origin.

[b]Neutralization was performed by the focus reduction method (Aaronson and Stephenson, 1973). Briefly, around 100 focus-forming units of each type C helper virus pseudotype of KiMSV were incubated with antiserum in a volume of 0.2 ml for 30 min at 37°C. Class I viruses were assaying on NIH/3T3 cells and class II and III viruses on NRK cells. The number of KiMSV foci was scored at 7 days. At dilutions of each antiserum that inhibited the homologous reference virus by more than 95%, each test virus was either comparably inhibited (+) or inhibited by less than 10% (−).

[c]The methods used for measurement of virus activation by halogenated pyrimidines and inhibitors of protein synthesis have been described in detail previously (Aaronson and Stephenson, 1975).

for this class of endogenous virus (Rowe, 1972; Lieber et al., 1974; Stephenson et al., 1975).

A second BALB/c endogenous virus, designated "BALB:virus-2," is noninfectious for cells of most inbred strains, but replicates well in cells of several other species (Aaronson and Stephenson, 1973). BALB:virus-2 is spontaneously activated at very low frequency from BALB/c embryo cells (Aaronson and Dunn, 1974a), and its frequency of induction can be markedly increased by exposure of cells to halogenated pyrimidines (Aaronson and Stephenson, 1973; Stephenson et al., 1974b) or to inhibitors of protein synthesis (Aaronson and Dunn, 1974b) (Table I). This class of viruses can also be activated from embryo cells of many strains (Stephenson et al., 1975).

Information for a third class of endogenous virus has been shown to be present within many strains as well. In the NIH Swiss strain, for example, this virus can not be activated from embryo cells in culture by known inducers (Stephenson and Aaronson, 1972a). However, this third virus, which is also xenotropic in host range, can be isolated in vivo (Todaro et al., 1973; Stephenson et al., 1974a) or from NIH Swiss spleen cells in culture (Levy, 1973). Further, the 12,000 and 30,000 MW viral polypeptides, p12 and p30, of this virus are detectable at high levels in the absence of virus release by NIH Swiss embryo cells (Stephenson *et al.,* 1974*f*), suggesting a late block in its replication. Analysis of type C viral antigen expression by a large number of other strains indicates that information for this third virus is present in every strain so far examined (Stephenson *et al.,* 1975). Embryo cells of one strain, NZB, spontaneously generate this virus at a high level (Stephenson and Aaronson, 1974). Table II summarizes some of the inbred strains that have been studied and the endogenous viruses, whose genetic information each strain has been shown to contain.

Radioimmunological assays have provided powerful tools for distinguishing otherwise closely related type C viruses (Stephenson *et al.,* 1974*e*; Tronick *et al.,* 1974). In competition immunoassays in which antisera prepared against prototype class I, II, and III viruses are used at limiting concentration to precipitate the ^{125}I-p12 of the homologous virus, the pattern of immunological reactivity of an unknown virus makes its identification possible. As shown in Fig. 1A, a representative class I virus reacts most efficiently in the homologous BALB: virus-1 p12 assay and to a lesser extent in either BALB:virus-2 or NIH Swiss virus p12 assays. Similarly, class II (Fig. 1B) and class III (Fig. 1C) viruses in each case react most efficiently in immunoassays for their homologous viral p12. Each endogenous mouse type C virus isolate so far examined can be placed into one of the three virus classes by these immunological techniques. More recently,

Table II. Distribution of Endogenous Type C Virus Among Inbred Strains of Mice

Inbred strain	Endogenous virus class		
	I	II	III
DBA	+	+	+
CBA	+	+	+
C3H/He	+	+	+
BALB/c	+	+	+
A/He	+	+	+
C58	+	+	N.T.[a]
C57BL/6	+	+	+
C57BL/10	+	+	+
AKR	+	+	N.T.
NIH Swiss	−	−	+
SWR	−	−	+
NZB	−	−	+
NZW	+	+	N.T.

[a]Not tested.

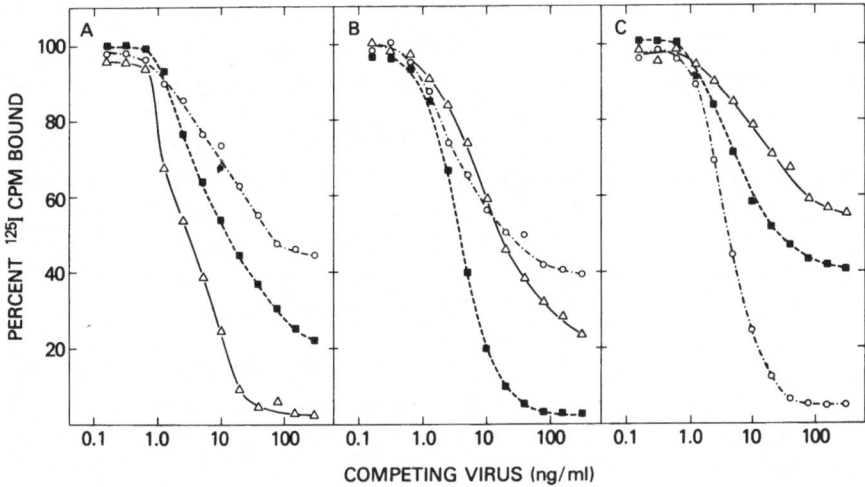

Fig. 1. Comparison of immunological reactivities of endogenous type C viruses of BALB/c and NIH Swiss mouse cells in type-specific immunoassays for the p12 virion structural polypeptide. Detergent-disrupted viruses were assayed at twofold serial dilutions by measuring their capacity to compete with ^{125}I-labeled p12 polypeptide for limiting antibody as previously described (Stephenson *et al.*, 1974*d*; Tronick *et al.*, 1974). The results are expressed as the percent of the total ^{125}I cpm in the antigen–antibody precipitate standardized to 100% in the absence of competing antigen. Reactivity was tested in the anti-AKR-MuLV:^{125}I-labeled AKR-MuLV p12 (△); anti-BALB; virus-2:^{125}I-BALB:virus-2 p12 (■); and anti-NIH Swiss virus:^{125}I-NIH Swiss virus p12 (○) type-specific competition immunoassays. Viruses tested included (A) BALB:virus-1, (B) BALB:virus-2, and (C) NIH Swiss virus.

analogous radioimmunological procedures have been developed for identification of other mouse type C viral polypeptides. These tests provide further support for the existence of three immunologically distinct classes of endogenous virus (Hino *et al.*, 1976).

III. DIFFERENTIAL ACTIVATION OF ENDOGENOUS VIRUSES

Two groups of chemicals, halogenated pyrimidines and inhibitors of protein synthesis, are highly efficient inducers of type C viruses endogenous to mouse cells (Lowy *et al.*, 1971; Aaronson *et al.*, 1971; Aaronson and Dunn, 1974*b*). Evidence that their mechanisms of action differ comes both from knowledge of their dissimilar biochemical effects and from observed differences in the virus induction response to these agents (Aaronson and Dunn, 1974*b*). This can be demonstrated by differences in the kinetics of induction of the same virus,

BALB:virus-2, from a clone of KiMSV-transformed BALB/c nonproducer cells (K-BALB) in response to iododeoxyuridine (IdU) and cycloheximide (Figs. 2 and 3). In these experiments, virus activation was measured both by the release of virus into tissue culture fluids and by the ability of activated cells to register as infectious centers on a monolayer of susceptible assay cells. Following exposure to IdU, virus release reached a peak at around 3–4 days and persisted at this level for several days (Fig. 2). The kinetics of virus induction following exposure to cycloheximide were strikingly different (Fig. 3). Virus release was maximal within the first 12 hr following drug treatment and declined rapidly thereafter. By 72 hr, virus-positive cells were no longer detectable. The fact that retreatment of the cells with cycloheximide at 72 hr caused a striking return in the level of virus activation (data not shown) indicates that differences in the actions of the two chemicals, rather than cell toxicity from drug treatment, were responsible for the much more transient virus activation observed with cyclo-heximide.

The two inducers also differ in the efficiency with which they activate different prototype endogenous viruses. To study this, mouse cell lines possessing different prototype endogenous viruese were exposed to chemicals and assayed for infectious center formation on normal rat kidney (NRK) and NIH/3T3 assay cells. Under these conditions, cells specifically activated to release xenotropic virus register as infectious centers only on NRK assay cells. In contrast, cells activated to produce class I viruses, such as BALB:virus-1 or C58-MuLV, register as virus positive on NIH/3T3 and at somewhat less efficiency on NRK. Since this latter pattern may also be observed if both mouse-tropic and xenotropic viruses are induced, virus must be propagated in each assay cell and retested for its host range and serological characteristics. Selection for growth of xenotropic virus can be enhanced further by propagation in certain lines of human cells (Stephenson et al., 1974a).

As shown in Table III, cycloheximide induced at high frequency a type C virus able to register only on NRK assay cells. The biological characteristics of this virus were found to be indistinguishable from those of BALB:virus-2. In contrast, IdU induced from the same cells viruses capable of registering on NIH/3T3 and NRK at very similar efficiencies. The serological and host range characteristics of these viruses showed them to be class I and class II viruses, respectively. While neither chemical activated detectable type C virus from NIH embryo cells (Table III), the pattern of virus induction from cells of the (NIH X BALB)F_1 hybrid generation was very similar to that observed with the inducible BALB parental strain (Table II). Cycloheximide specifically activated class II, while IdU induced both class I and II viruses.

These findings, in addition to previous studies (Aaronson and Stephenson, 1973; Aaronson and Dunn, 1974b), provide strong evidence for the differential regulation of the three endogenous virus classes. As summarized in Fig. 4, the

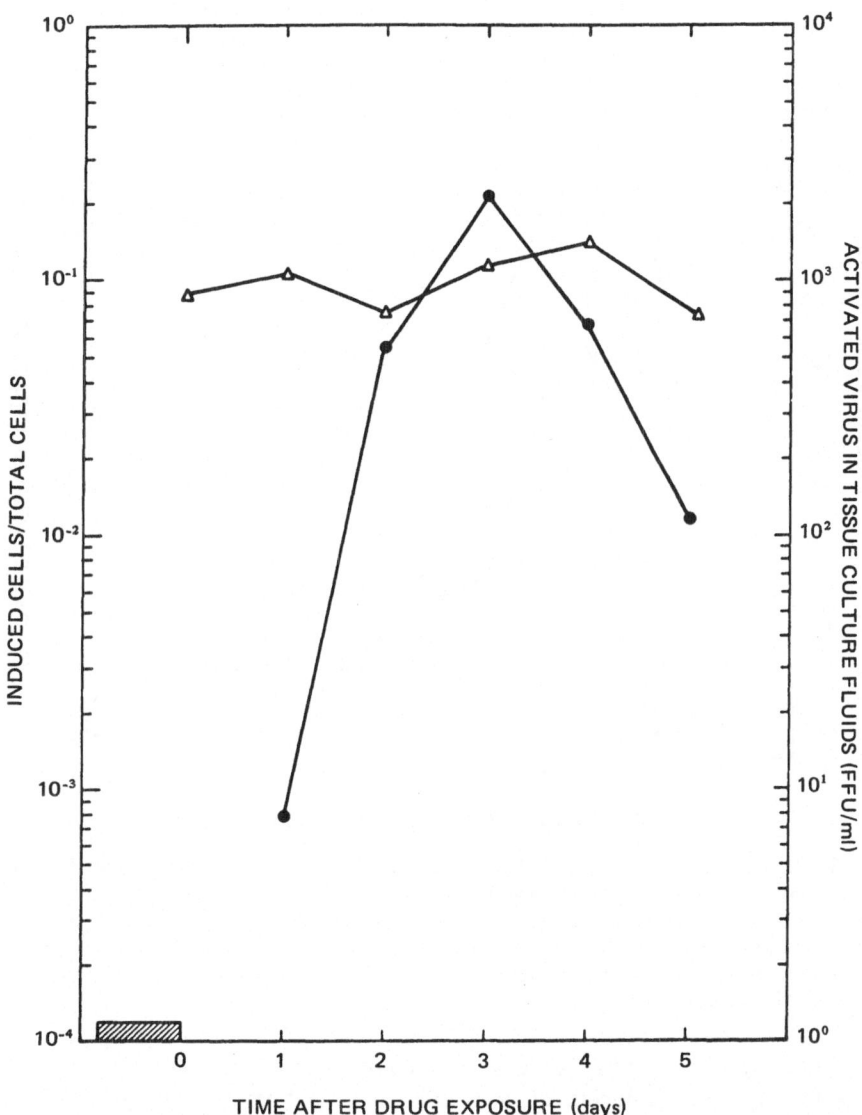

Fig. 2. Kinetics of IdU induction of K-BALB. Cultures containing 5×10^5 cells were exposed to 30 μg/ml IdU for 20 hr at 37°C and then washed twice. At subsequent 24-hr intervals, the cells were transferred for infectious center assay on NRK cells. In addition, tissue culture fluids were assayed for focus-forming virus on NRK cells. △, Induced cells/total cells; ●, activated virus/ml/10^6 cells.

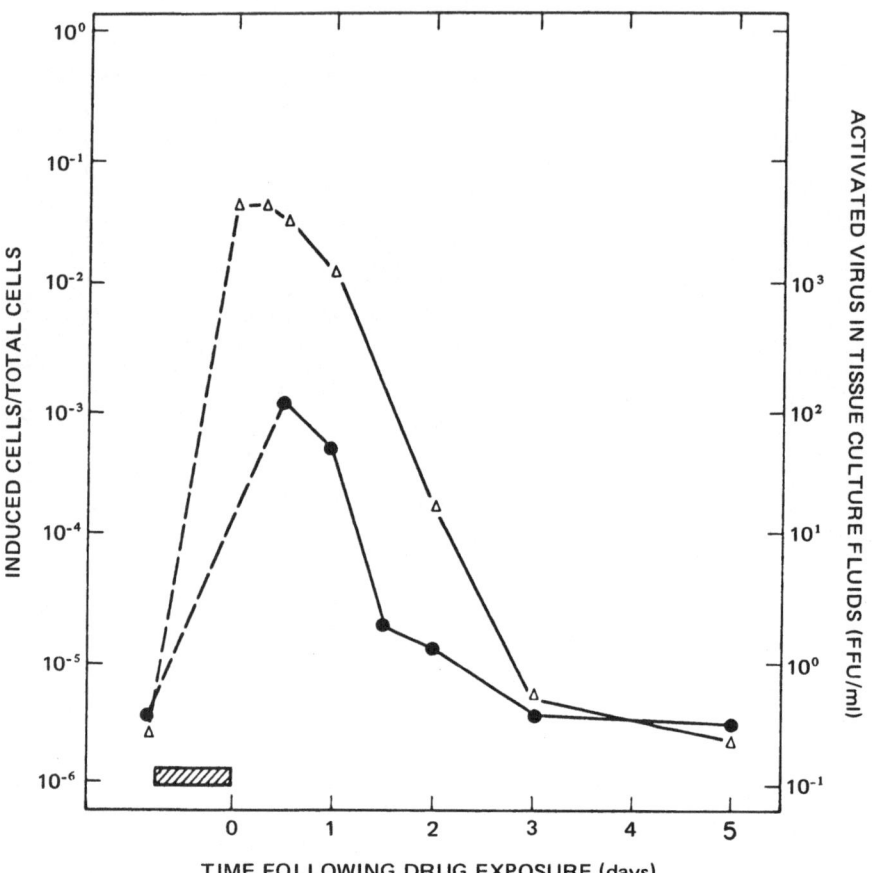

Fig. 3. Kinetics of cycloheximide induction of K-BALB. Cultures containing 5×10^5 cells were exposed to 10 μg/ml cycloheximide for 20 hr at 37°C, and then washed twice. At subsequent times, as indicated, the cells were transferred for infectious center assay on NRK cells. At 12-hr intervals for the first 48 hr, and at 24-hr intervals thereafter, tissue culture fluids were assayed for focus-forming virus on NRK cells. △, Induced cells/total cells; •, activated virus/ml/10^6 cells.

activation of class II virus is least well controlled by the cell; this virus is activated by both inducers of high efficiency, and its release can even be detected spontaneously at low frequency (Aaronson and Dunn, 1974*a*). In contrast, class I viruses, represented by C58-MuLV and BALB:virus-1, are activated at high efficiency by IdU and at much lower frequency or not at all by cycloheximide (Aaronson and Dunn, 1974*b*; Dunn *et al.*, 1975). Class III viruses of embryo cells of many strains appear to be completely resistant to induction by either class of chemicals.

IV. A GENE AFFECTING EXPRESSION OF CLASS I VIRUS

Fv-1 is a gene known to affect cell susceptibility to exogenous infection by many strains of MuLV (Odaka and Yamamoto, 1962; Axelrad, 1966; Pincus *et al.*, 1971). It appears to act at a step in virus replication beyond adsorption or penetration (Huang *et al.*, 1973; Krontiris *et al.*, 1973; Eckner, 1973). The effects of *Fv-1* on expression of class I and II viruses of BALB/c cells following IdU induction have been examined in NIH × (NIH × BALB/c)F₁ backcross embryo lines of different genotypes.

Induction of cells containing class I virus and permissive at *Fv-1* for infection by N-tropic virus results in the reproducible establishment of chronic virus production (Stephenson and Aaronson, 1972*b*; Stephenson *et al.*, 1974*b*). In contrast, persistence of this virus in *Fv-1* nonpermissive cells is much less likely. Whether this restriction pertains only to virus spread or also involves the activation process remains to be resolved. There appears to be no effect of the known alleles at *Fv-1* on the activation and persistence of class II virus. As

Table III. Induction of Different Classes of Endogenous Type C Viruses by Inhibitors of Protein Synthesis and Halogenated Pyrimidines[a]

KiMSV nonproducer clone of the following strain:	Inducer	Percent of cells registering as virus-induced on		Class of induced virus
		NRK	NIH/3T3	
BALB	Cycloheximide	5.3	<0.001	II
	IdU	3.3	2.9	I, II
NIH	Cycloheximide	<0.001	<0.001	–
	IdU	<0.001	<0.001	–
(NIH × BALB)F₁	Cycloheximide	3.1	<0.001	II
	IdU	1.8	1.7	I, II

[a]Exponentially growing cultures containing around 5×10^5 cells of each KiMSV nonproducer clone were exposed to 10 μg/ml cycloheximide or 30 μg/ml IdU for 18 hr at 37°C. The cultures were then washed twice, treated with 25 μg/ml mitomycin C for 1 hr, and transferred at tenfold cell dilutions in duplicate to petri dishes containing 10^5 NRK or NIH/3T3 cells. The latter assay cells were transferred 24 hr earlier into medium containg 2 μg/ml polybrene. Infectious centers of KiMSV-transformed cells were scored at 7–9 days as previously described (Aaronson and Dunn, 1974*a*). The percentage of virus-induced cells was calculated from the number of KiMSV infectious centers divided by the total cell number at 24 hr following transfer to an empty petri dish.

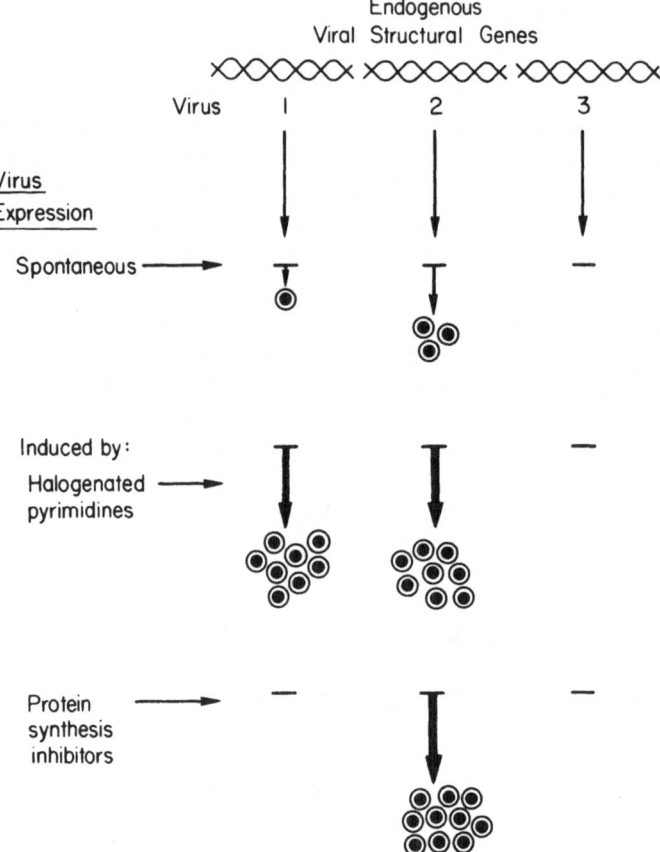

Fig. 4. Differential effects of two chemical inducers on three classes of
endogenous mouse type C viruses.

shown in Fig. 5, there were no differences in the kinetics of BALB:virus-2
activation from cells containing either $Fv-1^{nn}$ or $Fv-1^{nb}$ alleles. In neither cases
did BALB:virus-2 persist following the initial burst of chemical activation.

V. A GENE INFLUENCING THE MAGNITUDE OF RELEASE OF CLASS III
ENDOGENOUS VIRUS

Investigation of the genetic basis for the high spontaneous levels of class III
endogenous virus release by the NZB embryo cells led to findings that in crosses
with strains such as NIH Swiss, which express high levels of class III viral

antigens in the absence of detectable virus, type C virus is released at an intermediate level (Table IV). As shown in Fig. 6 in backcross and F_2 generations involving NZB and NIH Swiss strains, the pattern of virus release by cultures of individual embryos in each case is consistent with that expected for segregation of a partially dominant gene restricting spontaneous release of this virus (Stephenson and Aaronson, 1974).

VI. SUSCEPTIBILITY TO EXOGENOUS INFECTION OF MOUSE CELLS BY XENOTROPIC VIRUS

An effective restriction to virus infection can occur at the cell surface through a block to virus adsorption and/or penetration. In contrast, even dominant negative regulators such as *Fv-1,* which act intracellularly, can be overcome under certain physiological conditions (Aaronson *et al.,* 1974b). Similarly, the intrinsic mechanisms that normally restrict release of class I and II viruses be transiently overcome by treatment with chemical inducers. Findings that the murine sarcoma virus pseudotypes of xenotropic virus, which possess the xenotropic virus envelope, are absolutely restricted in their ability to induce

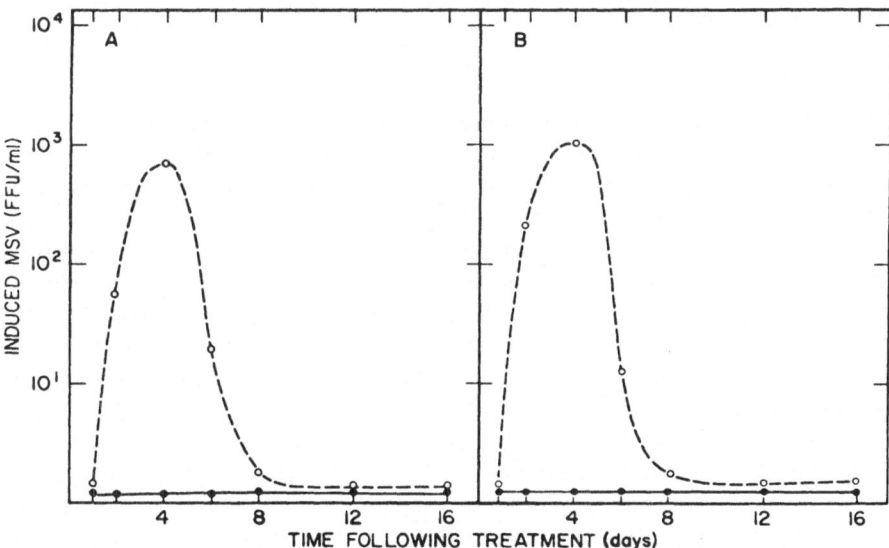

Fig. 5. Activation of KiMSV from NIH × (NIH × BALB/c)F$_1$ nonproducer clonal lines containing BALB:virus-2 alone (Stephenson *et al.,* 1974b). Cells were treated with IdU, and assayed for focus formation on NIH/3T3 (●) and NRK (○) as described in the caption of Fig. 3. The genotype at *Fv-1* was (A) *nn* and (B) *nb.*

Table IV. Neutralization of Endogenous Type C Viruses
by Sera from Different Strains of Mice

Sera from[a]	Number of sera tested	Neutralizing titer against[b]		
		BALB:virus-1	BALB:virus-2	NIH type C virus
NZB	3	<20	500–2000	1000–2000
NIH	10	<20	<20	<20
C57BL/6N	3	<20	500–2000	500–2000
C3H/HEN	3	<20	500–2000	500–2000
AKR/N	3	<20	500–2000	1000–2000
AL/N	3	<20	500–1000	500–1000
DBA/2N	3	<20	500–1000	500–1000
NZW/N	3	<20	500–1000	1000–2000
CBA/HN	3	<20	500–1000	500–1000
A/HEN	3	<20	500–1000	500–1000
C57BL/10Sn	3	<20	500–1000	500–1000
BALB/c	3	<20	500–2000	1000–2000
C58	3	<20	1000–2000	500–2000

[a]Sera were from mice at 2–3 months of age.
[b]Neutralization tests were performed as described in footnote b of Table I. Results are presented as the reciprocal of the highest serum dilution giving 67% or greater reduction in the number of MSV foci when tested against approximately 100 FFU of the appropriate MuLV pseudotype of KiMSV.

focus formation in cells of most inbred mouse strains (Aaronson and Stephenson, 1973) strongly suggested that restriction to xenotropic virus infection might occur at an early step involving virus absorption/penetration or integration within the cell genome.

Recently, in tests of many strains, including wild mice of various sources, embryo cells from wild mice provided by Dr. J. Parker (Microbiological Associates, Bethesda, Md.) have been found to be susceptible to focus formation by MSV pseudotypes of xenotropic virus. Further, embryo cells derived from genetic crosses between mouse strains such as NIH Swiss or BALB/c and the wild mouse are similarly susceptible. These results suggest that the wild mouse possesses a dominant gene conferring susceptibility at an early step in xenotropic virus infection. To further test this hypothesis, the pattern of segregation of virus susceptibility to xenotropic virus infection must be examined in backcross and F_2 generations. The preliminary evidence, however, would argue that a major factor responsible for the "xenotropic" host range of class II and III endogenous viruses and a very important factor in controlling the expression of these viruses may be the lack of accessible surface receptors for xenotropic virus infection in cells of most inbred mouse strains.

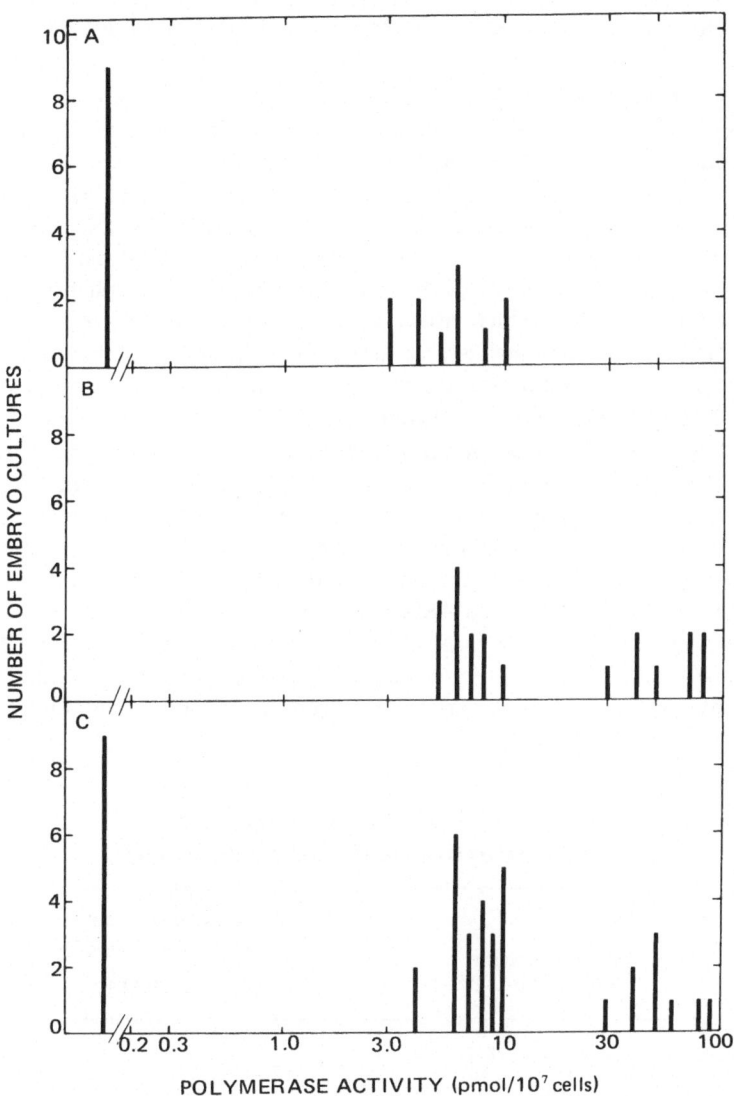

Fig. 6. Spontaneous virus release by cell lines derived from individual embryos of genetic crosses between NIH and NZB mice. Culture fluids from exponentially growing cultures were concentrated one-thousandfold and assayed for poly(rA)·oligo(dT) synthesis by methods described previously (Stephenson and Aaronson, 1972b). Results are expressed as the number of embryo lines of each genotype with the indicated levels of reverse transcriptase activity (pmol [³H]TMP incorporated per 10⁷ cells).

VII. HIGH-TITERED NEUTRALIZING ACTIVITY DIRECTED AGAINST XENOTROPIC VIRUS IN NORMAL MOUSE SERA

It has been reported that mouse sera contain antibodies that precipitate AKR MuLV (Ihle *et al.,* 1973). Further, antibody–viral antigen complexes can be detected in the kidneys of some mouse strains (Oldstone *et al.,* 1972). These findings suggest that the mouse possesses natural immunity to its endogenous type C RNA viruses. Sera of many but not all mouse strains also possess very high-titered neutralizing activity specifically directed against both classes of xenotropic endogenous virus (Table IV) (Aaronson and Stephenson, 1974). Findings that the cell in which virus is grown does not markedly alter its pattern of reactivity and that normal sera of several other species including goat, rabbit, and human show no inhibitory activity against mouse xenotropic virus confirm further the highly virus-specific nature of the inhibitor activity (data not shown). In an attempt to correlate serum immunoprecipitating and neutralizing activities, the abilities of mouse serum fractions containing IgG and IgM to neutralize xeno-tropic virus and to precipitate AKR MuLV were tested. Lee *et al.* (1974) reported that the serum fraction containing IgM possessed xenotropic virus-neutralizing activity while both mouse IgM and IgG fractions were able to precipitate radioactively labeled AKR MuLV.

More recent studies performed in collaboration with Dr. Michael Potter, NCI, have indicated that antisera prepared against purified IgM synthesized by mouse myeloma cells do not remove the serum inhibitory activity under condi-

Table V. Properties of Natural Virus Inhibitory Activity in Normal Mouse Serum[a]

Neutralizing activity removed by	Serum obtained from	
	NZB	BALB/c
Dialysis	−	−
RNAse	−	−
DNAse	−	−
Pronase	+	+

[a]Neutralization was performed by the focus-reduction techniques described in footnote *b* of Table I. Sera were exposed to RNAse (100 μg/ml), DNAse (50 μg/ml), or pronase (50 μg/ml) for 30 min at 37°C. The pronase-treated serum was extracted twice with phenol and the phenol removed by Sephadex G-50 chromatography. Results are expressed as (+), greater than 90% removal of neutralizing activity and (−), less than 10% removal of neutralizing activity.

tions where more than 95% of labeled marker mouse IgM was precipitated from the same serum. These results led to an attempt to further characterize the serum inhibitor. As shown in Table V, the inhibitor is nondialyzable, is not removed by RNAse or DNAse treatment, but is destroyed by pronase, indicating that it is a protein. Further, the inhibitor elutes in the void of Sephadex G-200 under nondenaturing conditions and migrates in the same region as radioactively labeled marker mouse IgM on DEAE-cellulose. Whether the inhibitor represents a class of antibodies distinct from IgG and IgM, an IgM not precipitable under the conditions utilized, or a completely different molecule is not yet known. In any case, it provides a striking example of a systemic mechanism for inhibition of the expression of an endogenous virus. Further understanding of its action may lead to methods for specific inhibition of other type C viruses as well.

VIII. ACTIVATION OF TYPE C VIRUSES FROM LYMPHOID CELLS FOLLOWING ANTIGENIC STIMULATION

Previous studies have shown that immune stimulation as in the graft-versus-host reaction and mixed lymphocyte cultures can lead to release of either mouse cell-tropic (Hirsch et al., 1972) or xenotropic virus (Sherr et al., 1974). Thus, it was reasoned that appropriate antigenic stimuli of a more defined nature might elicit type C virus from lymphoid cells. To examine this question, spleen cells from BALB/c mice were placed in tissue culture and exposed to a wide variety of lymphocyte mitogens. Treated spleen cells were then cocultivated with assay cells permissive for mouse cell-tropic and xenotropic viruses, respectively.

As shown in Table VI, exposure to one mitogen, lipopolysaccharide (LPS), was associated with a specific and very marked stimulation of xenotropic virus production (Greenberger et al., 1975a). Immunological analysis of this virus indicates that it is indistinguishable from BALB:virus-2. A number of other mitogens, including concanavalin A and phytohemagglutinin, that are at least as active in causing blastogenesis are much less effective or completely inactive as virus inducers (Greenberger et al., 1975a). Similar observations using biochemical methods of virus detection have recently been reported by Moroni et al. (1975).

Unlike BALB/c spleen cells, BALB/c embryo fibroblasts are not inducible by LPS. These findings suggest that the differentiated state of the cell may also play an important role in endogenous virus regulation. The mechanisms involved in virus activation by LPS remain to be elucidated. Nonetheless, the fact that an agent as ubiquitous as this bacterial component can activate type C virus indicates that exposure to chemical agents that are a natural part of the environment may drastically alter the level of endogenous viral expression.

Table VI. Influence of *in Vitro* Immunological Activation
on Recovery of Type C Virus from BALB/c Spleen Cells

Treatment	Animal No.	Rescue of KiMSV ($\log_{10}$ FFU/ml) following cocultivation with[a]		Blastogenesis[b] (cpm incorporated) [³H]-thymidine × 10³
		K-NRK	K-NIH	
Control	1	<0.0	<0.0	3.4
	2	0.3	<0.0	0.9
	3	<0.0	<0.0	1.4
Lipopolysaccharide	1	2.4	<0.0	14.0
	2	2.8	<0.0	17.0
	3	2.3	<0.0	8.1

[a]Spleen cell cultures were prepared from individual 2-month-old BALB/c mice. Response to specific mitogens was determined by treatment of 3.0×10^7 nucleated spleen cells with lipopolysaccharide (50 μg/ml). After 2 days incubation, each of the above treated and untreated control cultures was washed in medium and assayed for virus release by measuring rescue of focus-forming virus from K-NIH and K-NRK as described previously (Greenberger *et al.*, 1975a).

[b]Spleen cell blastogenesis after 2 days *in vitro* exposure to mitogens was measured as previously described (Greenberger *et al.*, 1975a). Results are expressed as cpm [³H]thymidine incorporated per 10^6 spleen cells and represent mean values from two separate determinations.

IX. BIOLOGICAL FUNCTIONS OF ENDOGENOUS TYPE C VIRUSES

The above studies summarize some of the current investigations in this laboratory concerning endogenous mouse type C viruses, their differential cellular regulation, and the influence of systemic factors on their expression. A major biological question regarding these viruses concerns their actions in the host. In this regard, it is now firmly established that at least one endogenous virus is oncogenic. C58-MuLV, induced in tissue culture from virus-negative cells, causes lymphatic leukemia in NIH Swiss mice, a strain characterized by a very low incidence of naturally occurring leukemia (Stephenson *et al.*, 1974c). Thus there can be little question that the class I endogenous virus of C58 mouse cells is etiologically linked to the development of leukemia in that strain. There is also evidence that inoculation of the class I virus of BALB/c cells causes hematological abnormalities in susceptible mice (Greenberger *et al.*, 1975b). Further, in more recent studies, measurement of endogenous virus expression in genetic crosses involving the high leukemia incidence AKR strain has shown a positive correlation between the magnitude of class I virus release in the young animal and the subsequent development of leukemia (Lilly *et al.*, 1975).

The pathogenicity of class II and III endogenous viruses has been more difficult to study because these viruses lack infectivity for inbred mouse strains. Here, a genetic approach should aid in developing an understanding of their actions. *In vivo* characterization of genetic crosses between appropriate strains may make it possible to correlate the occurrence of particular disease with the presence of specific xenotropic endogenous viruses and/or regulatory genes influencing their expression.

Current evidence indicates that endogenous type C viruses have existed in many species over a long period of evolution (Benveniste and Todaro, 1974). Therefore, some selective advantage for their presence would be expected. For example, if increased expression of type C virus antigens occurred as a result of malignant transformation, immune surveillance mechanisms might be more likely to eliminate the altered cells. In fact, in the mouse, replication of type C virus in tumor cells has been shown to enhance the probability of tumor rejection (Stephenson and Aaronson, 1972c; Greenberger and Aaronson, 1973). Roles for endogenous viruses in processes including cellular differentiation and information transfer are also possible (Huebner *et al.*, 1970). In the process of studies aimed at investigating the biological functions of endogenous viruses, it is hoped that systematic study of the mechanisms by which the host affects their expression may aid in understanding the molecular processes involved in gene regulation.

X. REFERENCES

Aaronson, S. A., 1971, Chemical activation of focus-forming virus from nonproducer cells transformed by murine sarcoma virus, *Proc. Natl. Acad. Sci. U.S.A.* **68**:3069.

Aaronson, S. A., and Dunn, C. Y., 1974a, Endogenous C-type viruses of BALB/c cells: Frequencies of spontaneous and chemical induction, *J. Virol.* **13**:181.

Aaronson, S. A., and Dunn, C. Y., 1974b, High frequency C-type virus induction by inhibitors of protein synthesis, *Science* **183**:422.

Aaronson, S. A., and Stephenson, J. R., 1973, Independent segregation of loci for activation of biologically distinguishable RNA C-type viruses in mouse cells, *Proc. Natl. Acad. Sci. U.S.A.* **70**:2055.

Aaronson, S. A., and Stephenson, J. R., 1974, Widespread natural occurrence of high-titered neutralizing antibodies to a specific class of endogenous mouse C-type virus. *Proc. Natl. Acad. Sci. U.S.A.* **71**:1957.

Aaronson, S. A., and Stephenson, J. R., 1975, Differential cellular regulation of three distinct classes of type-C RNA viruses endogenous to mouse cells, *Cold Spring Harbor Symp. Quant. Biol.* **39**:1129.

Aaronson, S. A., and Weaver, C. A., 1971, Characterization of murine sarcoma virus (Kirsten) transformation of mouse and human cells, *J. Gen. Virol.* **13**:245.

Aaronson, S. A., Hartley, J. W., and Todaro, G. J., 1969, Mouse leukemia virus: "Spontaneous" release by mouse embryo cells after long-term *in vitro* cultivation, *Proc. Natl. Acad. Sci. U.S.A.* **64**:87.

Aaronson, S. A., Todaro, G. J., and Scolnick, E. M., 1971, Induction of C-type viruses from clonal lines of virus-free BALB/3T3 cells, *Science* **174**:157.

Aaronson, S. A., Anderson, G. R., Dunn, C. Y., and Robbins, K. C., 1974*a*, Cycloheximide induction of type-C RNA virus: Increased expression of virus-specific RNA, *Proc. Natl. Acad. Sci. U.S.A.* **71**:3941.

Aaronson, S. A., Stephenson, J. R., and Greenberger, J. S., 1974*b*, Cellular replication and persistence of inducible RNA type C viruses, *J. Virol.* **13**:1404.

Axelrad, A., 1966, Genetic control of susceptibility to Friend leukemia virus in mice: Studies with the spleen focus assay method, *Natl. Cancer Inst. Monogr.* **22**:619.

Benveniste, R. E., and Todaro, G. J., 1974, Evolution of C-type viral genes: Inheritance of exogenously acquired viral genes, *Nature (London)* **252**:456.

Benveniste, R. E., Lieber, M. M., and Todaro, G. J., 1974, A distinct class of inducible murine type-C virus that replicates in the rabbit SIRC cell line, *Proc. Natl. Acad. Sci. U.S.A.* **71**:602.

Chattopadhyay, S. K., Lowy, D. R., Teich, N. M., Levine, A. S., and Rowe, W. P., 1974, Evidence that the AKR murine-leukemia-virus genome is complete in DNA of the high-virus AKR mouse and incomplete in the DNA of the "virus-negative" NIH mouse, *Proc. Natl. Acad. Sci. U.S.A.* **71**:167.

Dunn, C. Y., Aaronson, S. A., and Stephenson, J. R., 1975, Interactions of chemical inducers and steroid enhancers of endogenous mouse type C RNA viruses, *Virology* **66**:579.

Eckner, R. J., 1973, Helper-dependent properties of Friend spleen focus-forming virus: Effect of the *Fv-1* gene on the late steps of virus synthesis, *J. Virol.* **12**:523.

Furth, J., Seibold, H. R., and Rathbone, R. R., 1933, Experimental studies on lymphomatosis of mice, *Am. J. Cancer* **19**:521.

Gelb, L. D., Aaronson, S. A., and Martin, M. A., 1971, Heterogeneity of murine leukemia virus *in vitro* DNA; detection of viral DNA in mammalian cells, *Science* **172**:1354.

Gelb, L. D., Milstien, J. B., Martin, M. A., and Aaronson, S. A., 1973, Characterization of murine leukemia virus-specific DNA present in normal mouse cells, *Nature (London) New Biol.* **244**:76.

Greenberger, J. S., and Aaronson, S. A., 1973, *In vivo* inoculation of RNA C-type viruses inducing regression of experimental solid tumors, *J. Natl. Cancer Inst.* **51**:1935.

Greenberger, J. S., Phillips, S. M., Stephenson, J. R., and Aaronson, S. A., 1975*a*, Induction of mouse type-C RNA virus by lipopolysaccharides and concanavalin A, *J. Immunol.* **115**:317.

Greenberger, J. S., Stephenson, J. R., Moloney, W. C., and Aaronson, S. A., 1975*b*, Different hematoligic diseases induced by type-C viruses chemically activated from embryo cells of different mouse strains, *Cancer Res.* **35**:245.

Gross, L., 1951, Pathogenic properties, and "vertical" transmission of the mouse leukemia agent, *Proc. Soc. Exp. Biol. Med.* **78**:342.

Hino, S., Stephenson, J. R., and Aaronson, S. A., 1976, Radioimmunoassays for the 70,000-molecular-weight glycoproteins of endogenous mouse type-C viruses: Viral antigen expression in normal mouse tissues, *J. Virol.* **18**:933.

Hirsch, M. S., Phillips, S. M., Solnick, C., Black, P. H., Schwartz, R. S., and Carpenter, C. B., 1972, Activation of leukemia viruses by graft-versus-host and mixed lymphocyte reactions *in vitro*, *Proc. Natl. Acad. Sci. U.S.A.* **69**:1069.

Huang, A. S., Besmer, P., Chu, L., and Baltimore, D., 1973, Growth of pseudotypes of vesicular stomatitis virus with N-tropic murine leukemia virus coats in cells resistant to N-tropic viruses, *J. Virol.* **12**:659.

Huebner, R. J., Kelloff, G. J., Sarma, P. S., Lane, W. T., and Turner, H. C., 1970, Group-specific antigen expression during embryogenesis of the genome of the C-type

RNA tumor virus: Implications for ontogenesis and oncogenesis, *Proc. Natl. Acad. Sci. U.S.A.* **67**:366.

Ihle, J. N., Yurconic, M., Jr., and Hanna, M. G., Jr., 1973, Autogenous immunity to endogenous RNA tumor virus: Radioimmune precipitation assay of mouse serum antibody levels, *J. Exp. Med.* **138**:194.

Ihle, J. N., Hanna, M. G., Jr., Roberson, L. E., and Kenney, F. T., 1974, Autogenous immunity to endogenous RNA tumor virus: Identification of antibody reactive to select viral antigens, *J. Exp. Med.* **139**:1568.

Klement, V., Nicolson, M. O., and Huebner, R. J., 1971, Rescue of the genome of focus-forming virus from rat nonproductive lines by 5'-bromodeoxyuridine, *Nature (London) New Biol.* **234**:12.

Krontiris, T., Soeiro, R., and Fields, B. N., 1973, Host range restriction of Friend leukemia virus. Role of the viral outer coat, *Proc. Natl. Acad. Sci. U.S.A.* **70**:2549.

Lee, J. C., Hanna, M. G., Jr., Ihle, J. N., and Aaronson, S. A., 1974, Autogenous immunity to endogenous RNA tumor virus: Differential reactivities of immunoglobulins M and G to virus envelope antigens, *J. Virol.* **14**:773.

Lieber, M. M., Sherr, C. J., and Todaro, G. J., 1974, S-tropic murine type-C viruses: Frequency of isolation from continuous cell lines, leukemia virus preparations and normal spleens, *Int. J. Cancer* **13**:587.

Lilly, F., Duran-Reynals, M. L., and Rowe, W. P., 1975, Correlation of early leukemia virus titer and H-2 type with spontaneous leukemia of the BALB/c x AKR cross: A genetic analysis, *J. Exp. Med.* **141**:882.

Levy, J. A., 1973, Xenotropic viruses: Murine leukemia viruses associated with NIH Swiss, NZB, and other mouse strains, *Science* **182**:1151.

Levy, J. A., and Pincus, T., 1970, Demonstration of biological activity of a murine leukemia virus of New Zealand Black mice, *Science* **170**:326.

Lowy, D. R., Rowe, W. P., Teich, N., and Hartley, J. W., 1971, Murine leukemia virus: High-frequency activation *in vitro* by 5-iododeoxyuridine and 5-bromodeoxyuridine, *Science* **174**:155.

MacDowell, E. C., and Richter, M. N., 1935, Mouse leukemia, IX. The role of heredity in spontaneous cases, *Arch. Pathol.* **20**:709.

Meier, H., Taylor, B. A., Cherry, M., and Huebner, R. J., 1973, Host-gene control of type-C RNA tumor virus expression and tumorigenesis in inbred mice, *Proc. Natl. Acad. Sci. U.S.A.* **70**:1450.

Mellors, R. C., Aoki, T., and Huebner, R. J., 1969. Further implication of murine leukemia-like virus in the disorders of NZB mice, *J. Exp. Med.* **129**:1045.

Moroni, C., Schumann, G., Robert-Guroff, M., Suter, E. R., and Martin, D., 1975, Induction of endogenous murine C-type virus in spleen cell cultures treated with mitogens and 5-bromo-2'-deoxyuridine, *Proc. Natl. Acad. Sci. U.S.A.* **72**:535.

Odaka, T., and Yamamoto, T., 1962, Inheritance of susceptibility to Friend mouse leukemia virus, *Jpn. J. Exp. Med.* **32**:405.

Oldstone, M. B., Aoki, T., and Dixon, F. J., 1972, The antibody response of mice to murine leukemia virus in spontaneous infection: Absence of classical immunological tolerance, *Proc. Natl. Acad. Sci. U.S.A.* **69**:134.

Pincus, T., Rowe, W. P., and Lilly, F., 1971, A major genetic locus affecting resistance to infection with murine leukemia viruses. II. Apparent identity to a major locus described for resistance to Friend murine leukemia virus, *J. Exp. Med.* **133**:1234.

Rowe, W. P., 1972, Studies of genetic transmission of murine leukemia virus by AKR mice. I. Crosses with $Fv-1^n$ strains of mice, *J. Exp. Med.* **136**:1272.

Rowe, W. P., Hartley, J. W., and Bremner, T., 1972, Genetic mapping of a murine leukemia virus-inducing locus of AKR mice, *Science* **178**:860.

Sherr, C. J., Lieber, M. M., and Todaro, G. J., 1974, Mixed splenocyte cultures and graft-versus-host reactions selectively induce an "S-tropic" murine type C virus, *Cell* 1:55.

Strand, M., and August, J. T., 1973, Structural proteins of oncogenic ribonucleic acid viruses: Interspec II, a new interspecies antigen, *J. Biol. Chem.* 248:5627.

Stephenson, J. R., and Aaronson, S. A., 1972*a*, Genetic factors influencing C-type RNA virus induction, *J. Exp. Med.* 136:175.

Stephenson, J. R., and Aaronson, S. A., 1972*b*, A genetic locus for inducibility of C-type virus in BALB/c cells: The effect of a nonlinked regulatory gene on detection of virus after chemical activation, *Proc. Natl. Acad. Sci. U.S.A.* 69:2798.

Stephenson, J. R., and Aaronson, S. A., 1972*c*, Antigenic properties of murine sarcoma virus-transformed BALB/3T3 nonproducer cells, *J. Exp. Med.* 135:503.

Stephenson, J. R., and Aaronson, S. A., 1973*a*, Expression of endogenous RNA C-type virus group specific antigens in mammalian cells, *J. Virol.* 12:564.

Stephenson, J. R., and Aaronson, S. A., 1973*b*, Segregation of genetic loci for virus inducibility in high and low leukemia incidence strains of mice, *Science* 180:865.

Stephenson, J. R., and Aaronson, S. A., 1974, Demonstration of a genetic factor influencing spontaneous release of a xenotropic virus of mouse cells, *Proc. Natl. Acad. Sci. U.S.A.* 71:4925.

Stephenson, J. R., Aaronson, S. A., Arnstein, P., Huebner, R. J., and Tronick, S. R., 1974*a*, Demonstration of two immunologically distinct xenotropic RNA type-C viruses of mouse cells, *Virology* 61:244.

Stephenson, J. R., Crow, J. D., and Aaronson, S. A., 1974*b*, Differential activation of biologically distinguishable endogenous mouse type-C RNA viruses: Interaction with host cell regulatory factors, *Virology* 61:411.

Stephenson, J. R., Greenberger, J. S., and Aaronson, S. A., 1974*c*, Oncogenicity of an endogenous C-type virus chemically activated from mouse cells in culture, *J. Virol.* 13:237.

Stephenson, J. R., Tronick, S. R., and Aaronson, S. A., 1974*d*, Isolation from BALB/c mouse cells of a structural polypeptide of a third endogenous type-C virus, *Cell* 3:347.

Stephenson, J. R., Tronick, S. R., and Aaronson, S. A., 1974*e*, Analysis of type specific antigenic determinants of two structural polypeptides of mouse RNA C-type viruses, *Virology* 58:1.

Stephenson, J. R., Tronick, S. R., Reynolds, R. K., and Aaronson, S. A., 1974*f*, Isolation and characterization of C-type viral gene products of virus negative mouse cells, *J. Exp. Med.* 139:427.

Stephenson, J. R., Reynolds, R. K., Tronick, S. R., and Aaronson, S. A., 1975, Distribution of three classes of endogenous type-C RNA viruses among inbred strains of mice, *Virology* 67:404.

Taylor, B. A., Meier, H., and Myers, D. D., 1971, Host-gene control of C-type RNA tumor virus: Inheritance of the group specific antigen of murine leukemia virus, *Proc. Natl. Acad. Sci. U.S.A.* 68:3190.

Todaro, G. J., Arnstein, P., Parks, W. P., Lennette, E. H., and Huebner, R. J., 1973, A type-C virus in human rhabdomyosarcoma cells after inoculation into NIH Swiss mice treated with antithymocyte serum, *Proc. Natl. Acad. Sci. U.S.A.* 70:859.

Tronick, S. R., Stephenson, J. R., and Aaronson, S. A., 1974, Comparative immunologic studies of primate RNA C-type viruses: Radioimmunoassay for a low molecular weight polypeptide of woolly monkey leukemia virus, *Virology* 57:347.

Chapter 4

Mammalian C-Type Oncornaviruses: Relationships between Viral Structural and Cell-Surface Antigens and Their Possible Significance in Immunological Defense Mechanisms

Werner Schäfer

Max-Planck-Institut für Virusforschung
Tübingen, Germany

and

Dani P. Bolognesi

Duke University Medical Center
Department of Surgery
Durham, North Carolina 27710

I. INTRODUCTION *

Over the past several years, there has been a coordinated effort between our research groups and those of P. Fischinger (Bethesda, Md.), F. de Noronha (Ithaca, N.Y.), and J. Ihle and M. Hanna, Jr. (Frederick Cancer Research Center) to study the various properties of mammalian C-type viruses. Our main intentions were: (1) To clarify the morphology of the virion; (2) to isolate its

---

*Abbreviations: FeLV, feline leukemia virus (Rickard); FLV, Friend MuLV; GALV, gibbon ape lymphoma virus; GLV, Gross MuLV; gp45, gp 71, FLV, glycoproteins; HA, hemagglutination; IEM, immunoelectron microscopy; MuLV, murine leukemia virus; MuX, murine xenotropic C virus; PAS, periodic acid-Schiff reagents; p10–p31, FLV proteins (number indicates molecular weight $\times$ 10^3); p.i., post infection; RIA, radioimmunoassay; RLV, Rauscher MuLV; SDS PAGE, sodium dodecylsulfate–polyacrylamide gel electrophoresis; SSV-SSAV, simian sarcoma–simian sarcoma associated virus; UA, uranyl acetate staining.

constituent proteins and glycoproteins; and (3) to characterize the structural components in biochemical, biological, and seroimmunological terms. In most of these studies, Friend leukemia virus (FLV) was employed as a model for murine viruses and the Rickard leukemia virus (FeLV) for feline agents. For both systems, suspension cultures were developed (Schäfer and Seifert, 1968; Seifert et al., 1975; Rickard et al., 1969) which produce the large quantities of virus necessary for this work. Other mammalian C-type viruses were also included in some of the studies dealing with viral structure and their serological relationship to the murine and feline viruses.

In this chapter, emphasis will be placed on the immunological aspects of the major viral structural components. Our emphasis on this topic stems from recent studies where the major viral glycoprotein and its antiserum were successfully employed in the immunoprophylaxis and immunotherapy of virus infection and leukemia.

II. MORPHOLOGY OF MAMMALIAN C-TYPE VIRUSES

Visualization of the morphology of mammalian C-type viruses by electron microscopy has been generally impaired because of their labile structure. Standard virus purification procedures, particularly centrifugation in density gradients, which do not overtly affect various measurable properties of these agents, noticeably alter key morphological aspects of the virus structure. Foremost among these is the loss of knoblike components on the virus surface (Nermut et al., 1972; Witter et al., 1973a). There are various electron microscopic preparation procedures employed to study the fine structure of C-type viruses, but negative staining with phosphotungstic acid (PTA) is not recommended because it introduces artifacts in the inner structure of the virus particle. In order to minimize these problems, we have utilized relatively gentle procedures to concentrate and purify the virus. When material from FLV and FeLV suspension cultures was used we obtained pure preparations of intact virus as illustrated in Fig. 1. Instead of PTA, virus was negatively stained with uranyl acetate (Nermut et al., 1972). A more detailed visualization of the virus surface morphology was achieved by freeze-drying and shadowing (Nermut et al., 1972; see below). The surface architecture of the virus core could also be seen in this manner, although intact cores were difficult to isolate. The best core preparations were derived after treating the virus with cold ether (Lange et al., 1973; see below).

On the basis of these studies, various substructures of the virus could be identified. The surface of the particle consists of a lipid bilayer derived from the host cell from which project the loosely attached surface knobs and within which lies the virus core. The outer shell of the core is composed of hexagonally

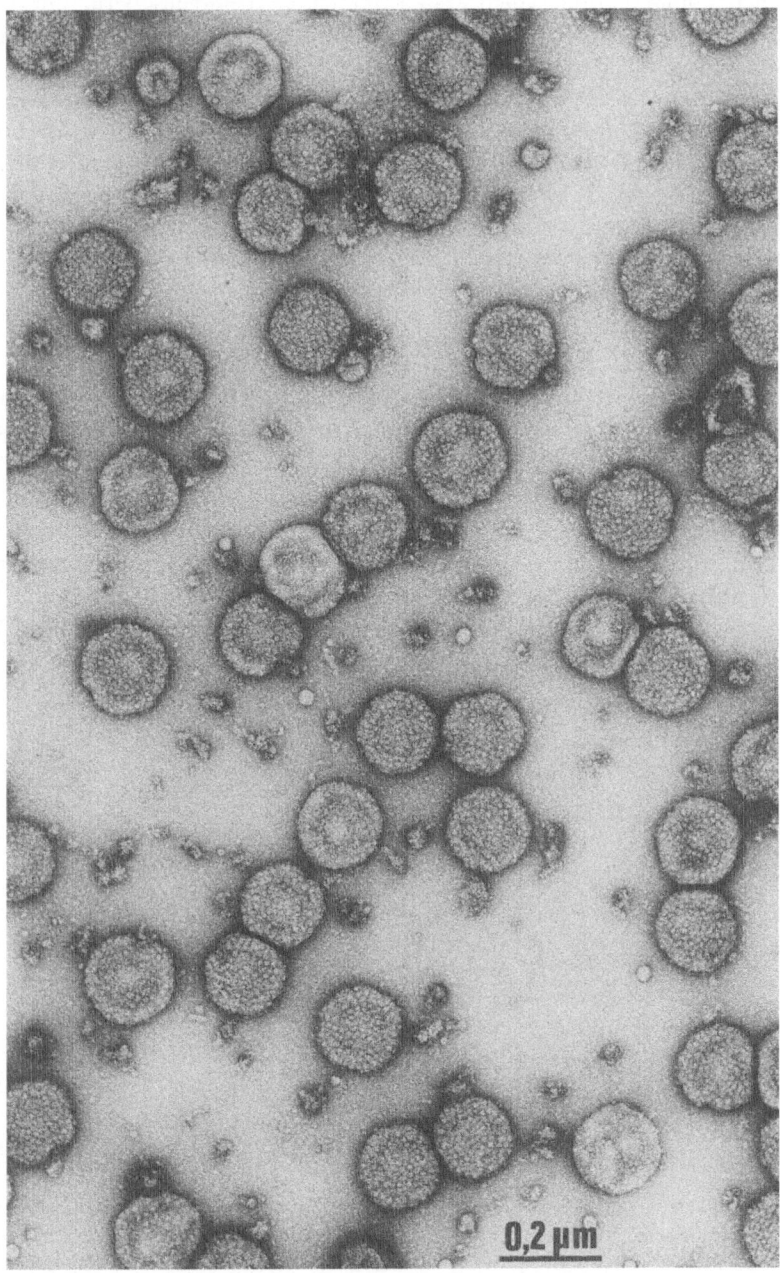

Fig. 1. Purified FLV stained with uranyl acetate.

arranged subunits within which lies an internal electron-dense structure (nucleoid), consisting of a filamental strand in the form of a spiral. Electron micrographs of the actual structures are shown in Fig. 2.

Electron microscopic studies with other mammalian C-type viruses demonstrated a strong morphological similarity to FLV (see Figs. 3 and 4 for porcine and bovine viruses) (Schäfer et al., 1975a). One distinguishing feature of these agents is the ease by which the knobs become dissociated from the viral envelope. The strongest association between a virus particle and the surface projections which we have noted thus far occurs with the porcine C-type virus (Moennig et al., 1974a).

III. ISOLATION AND PHYSICOCHEMICAL CHARACTERIZATION OF STRUCTURAL POLYPEPTIDES OF MURINE AND FELINE VIRUSES

Analysis of the Friend virus proteins and glycoproteins by SDS PAGE is illustrated in Fig. 5. Five major components designated on the basis of their chemical properties and molecular weight (p, protein; gp, glycoprotein; number is molecular weight $\times$ 10^{-3}) are indicated as p10, p12, p15, p31, and gp71 (Green et al., 1973; Moennig et al., 1973, 1974b; August et al., 1974; Schäfer et

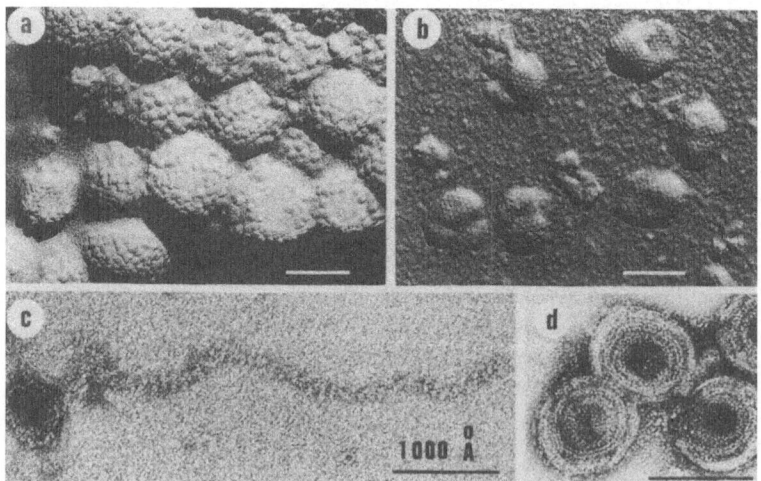

Fig. 2. Electron micrographs of FLV. (a) Knobs on the viral surface (freeze-drying plus shadowing). (b) Isolated cores flattened during preparation (freeze-drying plus shadowing). (c) Virus core releasing internal filament (uranyl acetate). (d) Internal filament in situ in the virion (uranyl acetate, longer treatment).

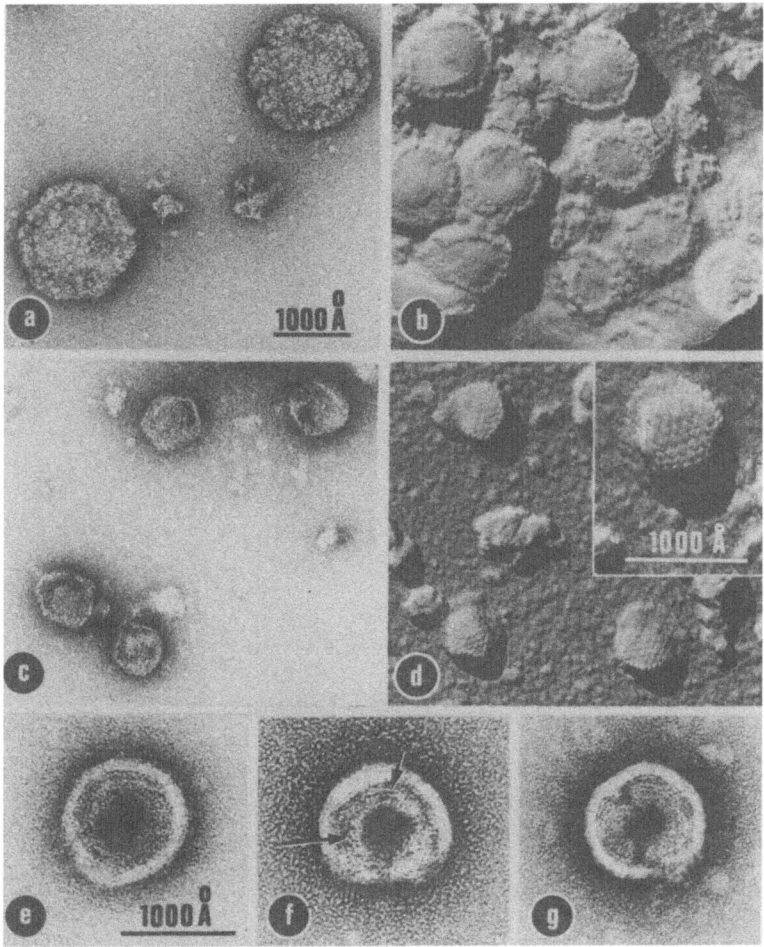

Fig. 3. C-type particle from pig. (a) Virions with knobs on surface (uranyl acetate). (b) Virions with knobs on surface (freeze-drying, shadowing). (c) Isolated cores (uranyl acetate). (d) Isolated cores (freeze-drying, shadowing). (e,f,g) Internal filament *in situ* (uranyl acetate).

al., 1969, 1975*b*). To distinguish the p15 described here from a p15 molecule described by other authors, it will be designated as p15(E) because of its location on the virus envelope (see below). The molecular weight of the protein components was determined by gel filtration in guanidine hydrochloride (GuHCl) (Fig. 6), whereas that of the major glycoprotein (gp71) was obtained from its mobility in SDS PAGE (Moennig *et al.*, 1974*b*). In addition a minor

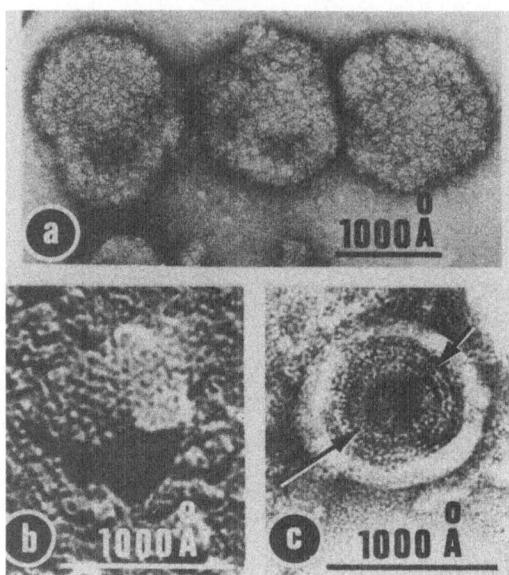

Fig. 4. Bovine C-type particles (Courtesy of Drs. Über-schär and Frank). (a) Virions with knobs on surface (uranyl acetate). (b) Isolated core (freeze-drying, shadowing). (c) Internal filament *in situ* (uranyl acetate).

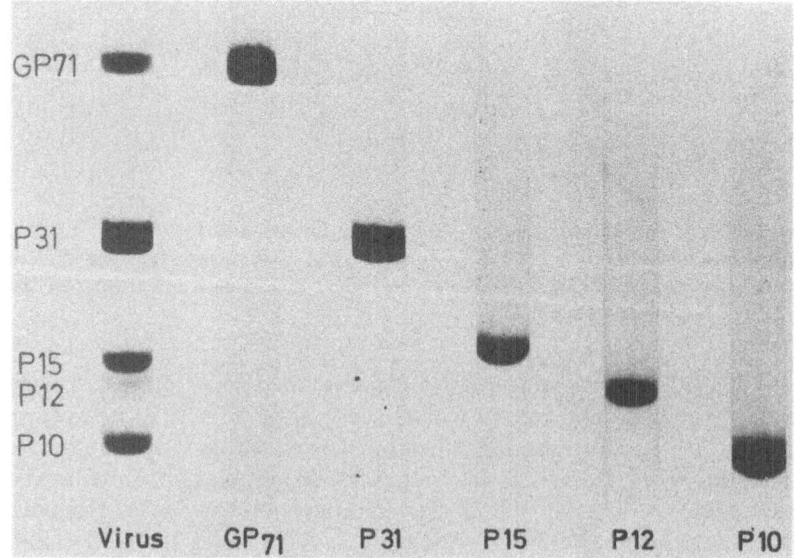

Fig. 5. SDS PAGE of whole FLV and its isolated major polypeptides.

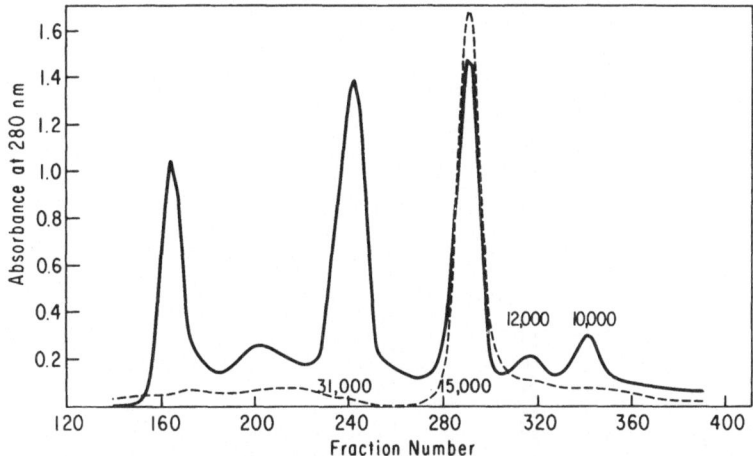

Fig. 6. Gel filtration of FLV polypeptides in GuHCl. Dotted line indicates position of purified p15(E).

glycoprotein (gp45) was revealed by analysis of [³H]glucosamine and [¹⁴C]amino acid labeled virus in SDS PAGE (Fig. 7) and a polypeptide distinguishable from p15 and p15(E) was found in the 15,000-molecular-weight peak from GuHCl which remains to be characterized (Fig. 8). Finally, studies by Moennig and Schäfer (unpublished) uncovered yet another component from Tween-ether degraded FLV which migrated more rapidly than p10 (Fig. 7 and 9). This component (designated p<10) possesses some but not all of the antigenic activity in common with p31 and seems to represent a breakdown product of it, possibly resulting from proteolytic digestion. A similar phenomenon could also account for the cross-reactivity between p10 and p12 reported by Parks et al. (1974, 1975), which has not as yet been observed by other workers.

Those components which are present in larger quantities, namely p10, p12, p15(E), p31, and gp71 of FLV, were isolated and investigated in more detail (Green et al., 1973; Moennig et al., 1974b; Schäfer et al., 1975b). Gel filtration in GuHCl combined with ion exchange chromatography was employed to isolate p10, p12, p15(E), and p31. The p31 molecule was also obtained from RLV and FLV by nondenaturing procedures (Schäfer et al., 1969) and compared to the renatured product from GuHCl. Nondenaturing procedures were used for gp71 isolation, including osmotic shock to release the antigen, followed by affinity chromatography on Con A Sepharose, and gel filtration (Moennig et al., 1974b). The purified component consisted of a single molecule on the basis of various physicochemical analyses. Recently we have been able to show that renaturation of gp71 from GuHCl also yields a serologically active molecule which behaves similarly to the nondenatured molecule in radioimmunoassay analysis (Bolognesi et al., unpublished).

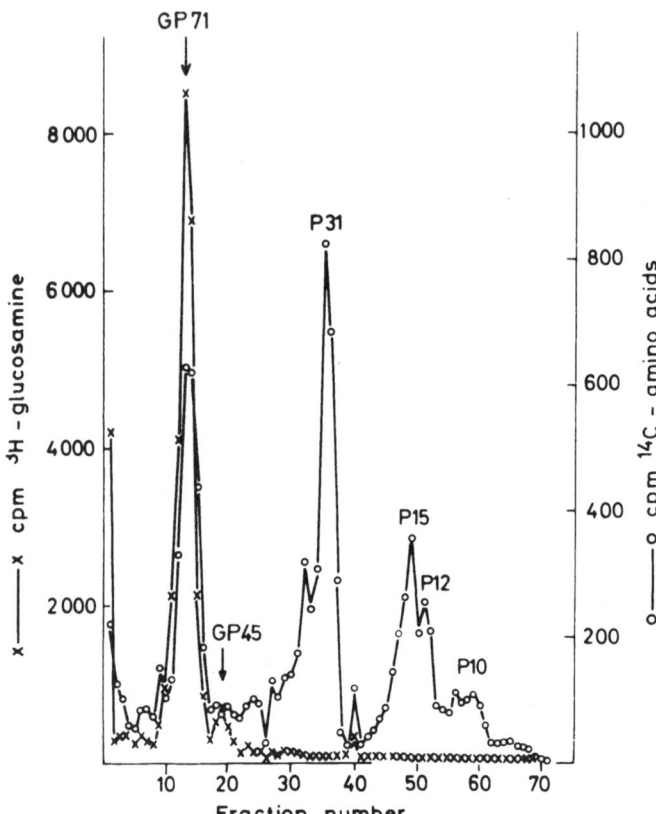

Fig. 7. SDS PAGE of FLV labeled with [³H]glucosamine and
[¹⁴C]amino acids.

Some of the biochemical characteristics of individual virus components have
also been determined. As indicated in Table I, p10 is a strongly basic
protein which is closely associated with the virus RNA. The p12 component
reveals unique staining properties with Coomassie blue (red instead of blue) and
was found to be associated with small quantities of carbohydrate. Whether it
represents an additional glycoprotein remains to be determined. The p15(E)
component shows a strong tendency to aggregate in dilute salt solutions. Recent
work indicates that it possesses a hydrophobic tail (presumably the part of the
molecule embedded in the viral membrane) which forms micelles with the
detergent sodium deoxycholate (DOC) (R. Webster, personal communication).
In fact, 0.1–0.4% DOC is required to keep this component in solution, and
fortunately the presence of the detergent does not affect its serological properties. Recent studies with anti-p15(E) serum strongly suggest that a component

isolated earlier which aggregated strongly in detergent-free solutions, forming ringlike structures [designated component X (Schäfer *et al.*, 1972*b*)] may, in fact, represent p15(E). The major viral structural component, p31, which comprises about 50% of the virus protein, is weakly basic. Detailed analyses of its chemical properties have been carried out by Gilden and co-workers (Oroszlan *et al.*, 1974) and will not be discussed here. The principal viral glycoprotein, gp71, consists of about 20% by weight of carbohydrate, most of which is glucosamine (unpublished). The *N*-terminal amino acid of FLV gp71 is phenylalanine (unpublished). Recent studies to determine the role of carbohydrate in various properties of gp71 indicated that by treatment with protease-free glycosidase enzymes it was possible to remove over 60% of the carbohydrate (Bolognesi *et al.*, 1975*a*). This produced a molecule which migrated 10% more rapidly in SDS PAGE than native gp71. The serological or biological properties with the exception of HA of the molecule (see below) were not detectably affected by the removal of the carbohydrate (Bolognesi *et al.*, 1975*a*; unpublished), suggesting a minor role for the sugars, perhaps merely to protect the protein moiety from protease digestion.

In our studies, FeLV revealed structural components similar to those of FLV (Green *et al.*, 1973; Schäfer *et al.*, 1971*a*). However, some relative differ-

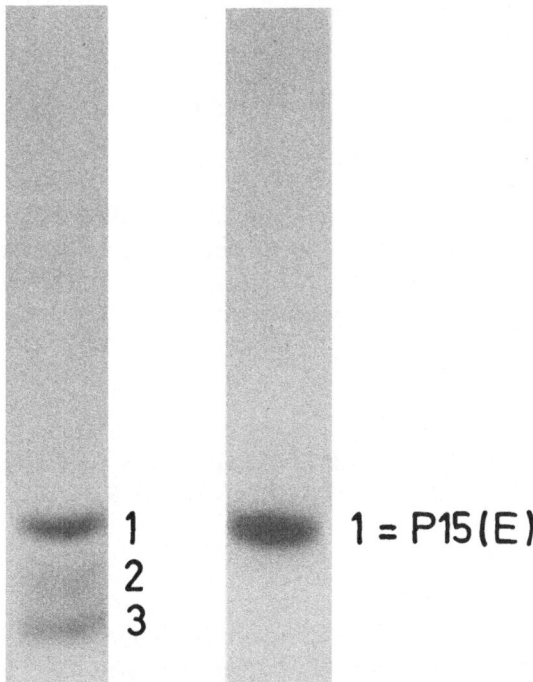

Fig. 8. SDS PAGE of FLV p15 fraction from GuHCl. In addition to p15(E), two further proteins are recognizable.

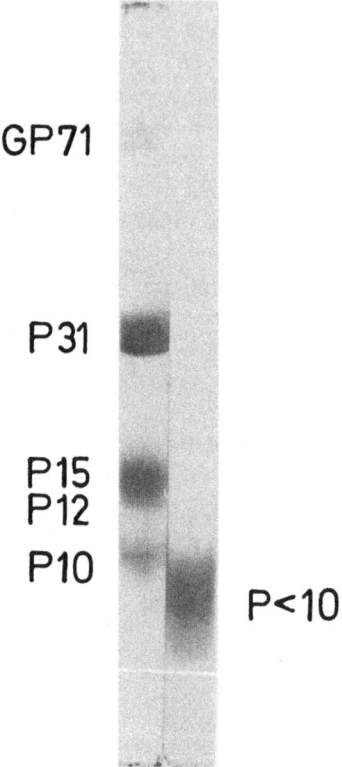

GP71

P31

P15
P12

P10

P<10

Fig. 9. SDS PAGE of whole FLV and
isolated p<10.

ences in migration properties of its components in SDS PAGE, notably p12, were observed. Initially p10 and p30 of FeLV were isolated in nondenatured form (Schäfer *et al.*, 1971*a*), but subsequently by the GuHCl method (Green *et al.*, 1973). The p12 and p15 components were obtained exclusively by the latter procedure (Green *et al.*, 1973).

IV. ANTIGENIC AND OTHER BIOLOGICAL PROPERTIES OF THE STRUCTURAL POLYPETIDES

A. FLV

The availability of the major FLV structural components in larger quantities and in purified form made it possible to prepare potent, highly specific antisera in rabbits and goats. With these and other sera prepared against disrupted virus particles, the antigenic properties of the individual molecules were examined in detail by *immunodiffusion* (Green *et al.,* 1973; Hunsmann *et al.,* 1974; Schäfer and de Noronha, 1971; Schäfer and Seifert, 1968; Schäfer *et al.,* 1970, 1971*b,* 1972*a,b,* 1973*a,b,* 1975*b*) and the findings are summarized in Fig. 10 and Table I. Various serological specificities were found which are defined as follows: (1) *type*-specific determinants are those found only in a single virus serotype; (2) *group*-specific are those determinants shared by various serotypes within a single species; and (3) *interspecies* determinants are those which are shared among viruses originating from different species (e.g., murine, feline, simian).

In our immunodiffusion tests, the lower molecular weight polypeptides displayed unique serological properties: (1) *p12* revealed only type determinants (Fig. 10b); (2) *p10* reacted group specifically (Fig. 10a); and (3) *p15(E)* was represented exclusively by interspecies determinants (shared with FeLV p15) (Fig. 10c,h), which operationally behave as group-specific in the murine system. Tronick *et al.* (1973) found minor group-specific determinants in RLV p12 using a radioimmunoassay (RIA) technique. Strand *et al.* (1974) described a p15 molecule from RLV which possessed mainly type-specific determinants and is

Table I. Properties of Friend Virus Proteins

Proteins	Chemical properties	Hemag-glutination activity	Interfering activity	Neutralizing antibody (absorption /induction)	Antigenicity		
					Type	Group (species)	Interspecies
p10	Strongly basic protein	−	−	−	−	+	−
p12	Acidic protein	−	−	−	+	−[a]	−
p15(E)	Hydro-phobic protein	−	−	− (+)[b]	−	−	+
p31	Basic protein	−	−	−	−[c]	+	+ (a+b)
gp71	Glyco-protein	+	+	+	+	+	+

[a]Minor group reactivity found with RLV-p12 by Tronick *et al.* (1973).
[b]Antiserum inactivates in C'-dependent reactions MuX and FeLV.
[c]Minor type reactivity found with RLV-p31 by Strand and August (1975).

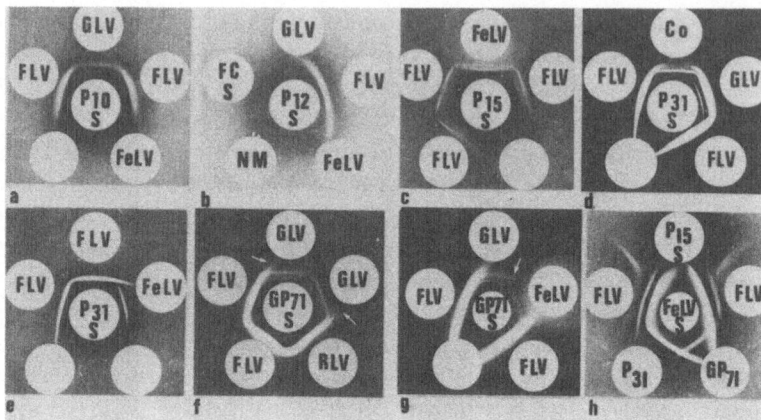

Fig. 10. Ouchterlony tests with antisera against isolated FLV polypeptides. Abbreviations: S, respective antiserum; FCS, fetal calf serum; NM, normal mouse cell extract; Co, cores isolated from FLV. For further abbreviations, see abbreviations footnote to the Introduction. (a) p10 serum showing group reactivity. (b) p12 serum showing type reactivity. (c) p15(E) serum showing interspecies reactivity with FeLV (full identity). (d) p31 serum showing group reactivity. (e) p31 serum showing interspecies reactivity with FeLV. (f) gp71 serum showing group (line with GLV) and type [spurs with FLV-RLV (arrows)] reactivities. (g) gp71 serum showing type (FLV spur against GLV), group [separate line (arrow) with GLV], and interspecies (line with FeLV) reactivities. (h) Demonstration of three interspecies components in FLV by FeLV antiserum and their identification by isolated FLV polypeptides and component specific antiserum [p15-S = p15(E) serum], respectively.

thought to represent the Friend-Moloney-Rauscher (FMR) antigen. Other studies suggest that the FMR antigen is localized in the interior of the particle somewhere between the viral envelope and the nucleoid (Friedman *et al.,* 1974). The properties of the FMR component fit best with those of the molecule we have designated as FLV p12 (Schwarz *et al.,* 1976). Regarding p15(E), the extent of interspecies specificity of the molecule is not yet established. Thus far, cross-reactivities in complement fixation (CF) have been found with feline (FeLV), rat (RaLV), hamster (HaLV), and to a minor degree with simian (SSV-SSAV) C-type viruses.

The major structural protein, *p31,* possesses multiple serological determinants including mainly group, some interspecies (Fig. 10d,e,h), and, according to Strand and August (1974), a minor type-specific determinant. More detailed serological investigation by immunodiffusion (Schäfer *et al.,* 1973*b*) demonstrated that the interspecies region of p31 consists of at least two subdeterminants (a and b) where (a) is found in p31 of classical feline viruses and those of small rodents, but not in the respective p31 molecules of endogenous cat (RD-114), woolly monkey (SSV-SSAV), gibbon ape (GaLV), or pig viruses. In contrast, subdeterminant (b) was detectable in all mammalian C-type viruses studied but does not extend to the avian C-type agents. Similar analyses of p31 by RIA confirmed the immunodiffusion analyses and revealed yet a further subdeterminant which is present in most mammalian C-type viruses but was not found in endogenous cat and baboon viruses (Sherr *et al.*, 1975; Strand and August, 1975).

The *gp71* glycoprotein of FLV also possesses multiple antigenic determinants. In contrast to p31, the primary determinant is type specific, and lesser amounts of group and interspecies reactivity are present (Fig. 10f,g,h). Similar results were reported for the RLV glycoproteins, gp69/71 (Strand and August, 1974). The interspecies cross-reactivity pattern of FLV gp71 is similar to that of subdeterminant (a) of p31 when analyzed by complement fixation (Hunsmann *et al.*, 1974). With more sensitive competition RIA minor relationships were also established with pig virus, SSV-SSAV, and GALV but not with endogenous cat or baboon viruses (unpublished). It is of interest that interspecies serological determinants similar to those of p31(a) and gp71 are found in the reverse transcriptases of the respective viruses (Scolnick *et al.*, 1972). The restricted distribution of certain interspecies antigenic determinants to C-type viruses of small rodents and classical feline viruses suggests that these are probably characteristic of the rodent agents and appear in the classical feline viruses as a result of horizontal transmission. Since subdeterminant (b) (Schäfer *et al.*, 1973b, 1975a) of p31 is present in many, if not all, mammalian C-type viruses, it would appear to represent the most conserved sequence in terms of the evolution of these agents. These conclusions are supported by hybridization analyses carried out by Benveniste and Todaro (personal communication).

Because the murine agents employed are not cloned viruses, one could imagine that the group reactivity of gp71 could be due to the presence of other agents in the FLV stock. Two observations, however, which argue against this are that (1) the p12 molecule in FLV reacts exclusively in a type-specific fashion (Fig. 10b) (Green *et al.*, 1973) and (2) no xenotropic murine virus could be isolated from the culture used for production of FLV (Fischinger *et al.*, 1976). Furthermore, recent studies with gp71 molecules of other viruses showed that even among the murine agents, in particular between endogenous viruses and FMR agents, there were differences in the murine-specific as well as interspecies determinants of gp71 (Ihle *et al.*, 1976c). The significance of these findings is under investigation.

Antibodies which are capable of *neutralizing* virus infectivity are clearly of interest for many reasons. Of the various virus structural components, only gp71 is able to elicit classical neutralizing antibodies (Hunsmann *et al.*, 1974; Schäfer *et al.*, 1975a), that is, antibodies which are able to neutralize virus in the absence of complement (C'). Heat-inactivated anti-gp71 serum was able to neutralize homologous MuLV serotypes (FLV, RLV) with a high titer, and, in addition, neutralized the heterologous Gross leukemia virus (GLV) serotype, although to a somewhat lower titer. Thus type- as well as group-specific determinants on gp71 are reactive in virus neutralization in a C′-independent reaction.

On the other hand, if C′ is present an inactivating effect of the anti-gp71 serum on C-type viruses of other mammalian species, such as FeLV and possibly SSV-SSAV, is also observed (Fischinger et al., 1976). Surprisingly, a similar C′-dependent inactivation was also observed if anti-p15(E) serum was reacted with an endogenous murine xenotropic virus (MuX) or with FeLV, but not with FLV or GLV (Fischinger et al., 1976). With both sera, the C′-dependent inactivation could be specifically inhibited by absorption with the respective purified viral component, indicating that the targets for neutralization are indeed determinants on gp71 and p15(E). One could postulate that this type of serum reactivity is initiated by C′-dependent lysis of the virus (virolysis) or a similar effect on the target cell. If the C′-dependent reaction is indeed virolysis, it is reasonable to assume that portions of p15(E) and the interspecies determinant of gp71 are situated on the viral envelope and accessible to antibody (see below).

It is of interest that the anti-p15(E) serum inactivates FeLV and MuX, but not the ecotropic murine viruses (e.g., FLV, GLV), which share p15(E) antigenic determinants with FeLV and MuX. Our interpretation of this phenomenon is that the effect depends on the accessibility of p15(E) to the antibody. It is possible that in MuX and FeLV the p15(E) is not masked by other viral envelope components (e.g., gp71), as might be the case with FLV and GLV (see below and Fig. 15).

An additional property associated with gp71 which may be of biological significance is its capacity to *hemagglutinate* red blood cells (Table I). Initially these activities could be detected using the virus particles. Treatment with neuraminidase or a combination of neuraminidase and phospholipase C, however, was required to obtain the hemagglutination reaction (HA) (Schäfer and Szántó, 1969). Subsequently, Schäfer et al. (1972b) and Witter et al. (1973a,b) were able to show that the hemagglutinating principle was associated with a viral component migrating like gp71 on SDS PAGE which displayed type, group, and interspecies reactivity. If gp71 was released from the virion, the HA activity was lost, but could be restored to the liberated molecules after treatment with group-specific anti-MuLV serum (indirect HA) (Witter et al., 1973b; Moennig et al., 1973). When treated in this manner, highly purified FLV gp71 likewise revealed high HA activity. These results suggested that monovalent nonhemagglutinating units were rendered multivalent by cross-linking antibody molecules and were thereby capable of HA activity. A similar phenomenon was observed with an adenovirus substructure (Rosen, 1960).

As with other C-type viruses, an *interference* phenomenon is observed with MuLV (Sarma et al., 1967). However, in contrast to avian viruses, different serotypes of MuLV, such as FLV and GLV, compose a single interference group.

Examination of the isolated FLV structural components for interference capacity indicated that only gp71 was reactive (Hunsmann *et al.*, 1974; Schäfer *et al.*, 1975*a*) (Table I). As little as 10 ng of the purified glycoprotein was sufficient to produce a 50% interference of 100 FLV-PFU (by XC test) on 10^6 target cells. As expected, infection by FLV and GLV were affected in a similar manner by FLV gp71.

B. FeLV

The proteins isolated from FeLV have not been studied as extensively as those of FLV, and its major glycoprotein has yet to be isolated in amounts sufficient for a thorough characterization. A general similarity was observed between the corresponding murine and feline components. Within the feline system, p10 could be shown to possess group-specific reactivity. However, this was demonstrable only if FeLV p10 was isolated following Tween-ether degradation (Schäfer and de Noronha, 1971; Schäfer *et al.*, 1971*a*) but not after GuCHl treatment (Green *et al.*, 1973). The reactivity of FeLV p12 was not investigated in detail. For FeLV p15, it could be shown that this polypeptide represents the interspecies counterpart of FLV p15(E) (Schäfer *et al.*, 1975*b*). As was the case for FLV p31, FeLV p30 reveals type, group, and interspecies reactivity. However, in this case the interspecies antigen(s) would appear to comprise a larger portion of the serological determinants of the molecule. Moreover, the type specificity, detectable in MuLV p31 only by RIA, could be demonstrated in FeLV p30 by immunodiffusion and this also appears to be more prominent (Green *et al.*, 1973).

From the results described in this section, it can be seen that most reactivities which are of special interest with regard to viral biological functions are associated with gp71 (see also Table I) and possibly the other viral envelope constituents [p15(E) and gp45]. In order to better understand the function of the various virion components in virus–host interactions, especially the immunological phenomena, their arrangement in the virion is discussed in more detail in the next section.

V. LOCALIZATION OF THE VIRION PROTEINS AND GLYCOPROTEINS IN THE PARTICLE STRUCTURE

Some indications of the organization of the various components in the virion could be obtained from the immunobiological behavior of the intact particles. Additional information has been obtained by selectively removing distinct viral surface structures or by isolating the virus core and the ribonucleoprotein complex. Finally, immunoelectron microscopy (IEM) of virus-producing cells with component-specific antisera has provided further insights.

With regard to *gp71*, all activities associated with the molecule could also be demonstrated using intact virus, indicating that this component resides on the surface of the particle (Witter *et al.,* 1973*a*; Schäfer *et al.,* 1975*a*; Hunsmann *et al.,* 1974). This view was substantiated when removal of the surface knobs by treating them with bromelain (Figs. 11 and 12) resulted in loss of HA activity

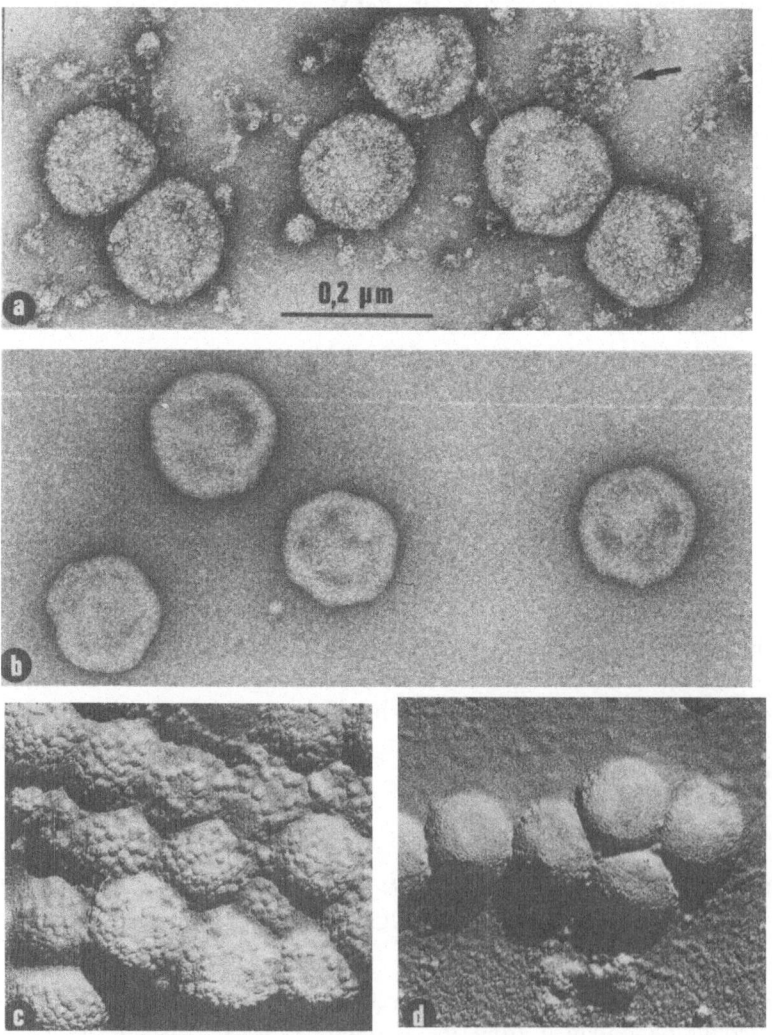

Fig. 11. Effect of bromelain treatment on FLV demonstrated by electron microscopy. (a,c) Before treatment. (b,d) After treatment. (a,b) Uranyl acetate. (c,d) Freeze-drying, shadowing.

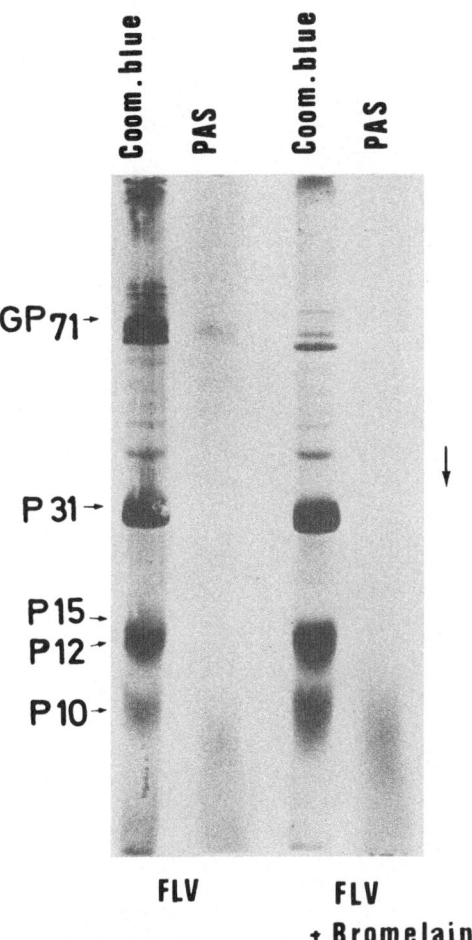

Fig. 12. SDS PAGE of untreated and bromelain-treated FLV. By bromelain treatment, only PAS-stainable, carbohydrate-containing gp71 was removed.

and the capacity to absorb neutralizing antibody. In addition, virus infectivity was lost, indicating that gp71 plays an important role in initiating the infectious process, probably in the attachment of the virus to the host cell. Furthermore, isolated viral cores were found to be free of gp71 following analysis of SDS PAGE (Fig. 13) (Lange *et al.*, 1973). On the basis of these findings, it was concluded that gp71 is situated in the knobs on the virus particle surface and such a superficial arrangement could, in fact, be demonstrated by IEM using anti-gp71 serum (see below, Fig. 18) (Schwarz *et al.*, 1976).

Analysis of the isolated cores in SDS PAGE likewise indicated that *p15(E)* is lacking or present in only very minor amounts (Fig. 13) (Bolognesi *et al.*, 1973;

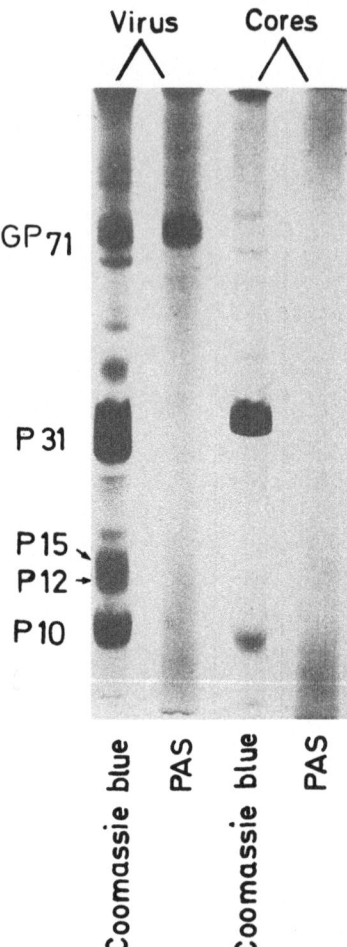

Fig. 13. SDS PAGE of FLV cores isolated after
treating the virus with cold ether.

Lange *et al.*, 1973). Recent evidence indicates that the p15 species in the core is real but represents a different component from p15(E). The p15(E) is most likely situated in the viral envelope. Its tendency to aggregate in aqueous solutions, but not in the presence of detergent, is reminiscent of typical membrane proteins which possess hydrophobic regions. Furthermore, antiserum prepared against it precipitates density-gradient-purified virions (Ihle *et al.*, 1975). In IEM, however, it was accessible to specific antibody in some (Ihle *et al.*, 1976*f*) but not all virus strains studied (see below) (Schwarz *et al.*, 1976). Accessibility to antibody in certain viruses could also be demonstrated with the C′-dependent neutralizing capacity of anti-p15(E) serum, as mentioned previously. These results can best be explained if one assumes that p15(E) is a constituent of the viral envelope with part of the polypeptide embedded in the outer virus membrane and the remainder exposed on the exterior of the virus. However, in some C-type viruses it may be masked by the presence of the glycoprotein knobs. Just how densely the knobs are packed on the surface of freshly produced intact FLV is illustrated in Fig. 14. Removal of these knobs during virus purification or by spontaneous release from certain viruses (e.g., MuX, FeLV) may result in the observed reactivity with p15(E) antibody. It is tempting to suggest that p15(E) represents the molecule which anchors gp71 to the virus surface, analogous to the spike glycoprotein (gp35) of avian oncornaviruses (Bolognesi *et al.*, 1972).

The *p12* polypeptide is probably situated at or near the viral surface, although it is clearly not exposed on the virus exterior (Bolognesi *et al.*, 1973; Friedman *et al.*, 1974; Hunsmann *et al.*, 1976). Like p15(E), no significant amounts of p12 were detectable by SDS PAGE in isolated cores (see Fig. 13) (Bolognesi *et al.*, 1973; Lange *et al.*, 1973). Intact viruses do not react with anti-p12 serum either in neutralization, in absorption of antibody, or in IEM (Fig. 19) (Green *et al.*, 1973; Hunsmann *et al.*, 1976; Schwarz *et al.*, 1976).

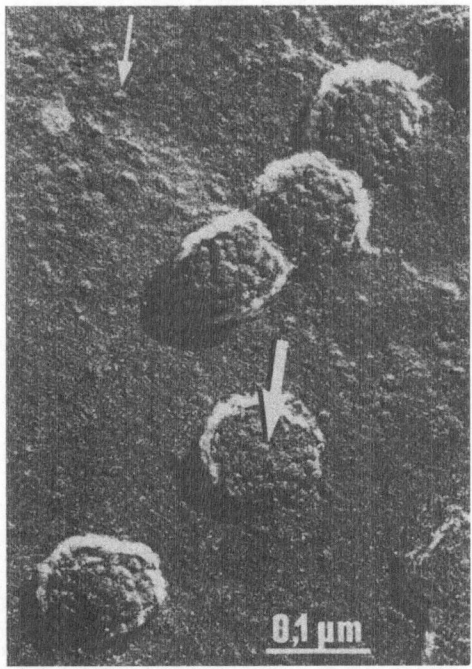

Fig. 14. Electron micrograph of a replica of the surface of a FLV-producing cell. Note densely packed knobs on budding particles. Similar structures visible also on nonbudding areas (small arrow).

However, degraded virus was found to bind p12-specific antibodies intensively (Hunsmann *et al.,* 1976).

Investigation of isolated cores (Fig. 13) leaves little doubt that *p31* and *p10* are its major constituents (Bolognesi *et al.,* 1973; Lange *et al.,* 1973). The p10 component is the most basic protein of the virus and apparently forms the internal filament togeιner with the viral RNA and reverse transcriptase (Bolognesi *et al.,* 1973; Lange *et al.,* 1973; Schäfer *et al.,* 1975a). Although some p31 was found to be associated with the isolated high density nucleoid structure (Bolognesi *et al.,* 1973; Schäfer *et al.,* 1975a), most of it apparently resides in the core shell which is represented by hexagonally arranged subunits. As was expected, neither anti-p10 nor anti-p31 sera neutralized the virus or reacted with the viral surface in IEM (Schwarz *et al.,* 1976). The detailed characteristics of the 15,000-dalton polypeptide present in low amounts in the virus core (Bolognesi *et al.,* 1973) remains to be determined. Our concept of the organization of the virus in terms of its constituent parts is illustrated in the model presented in Fig. 15.

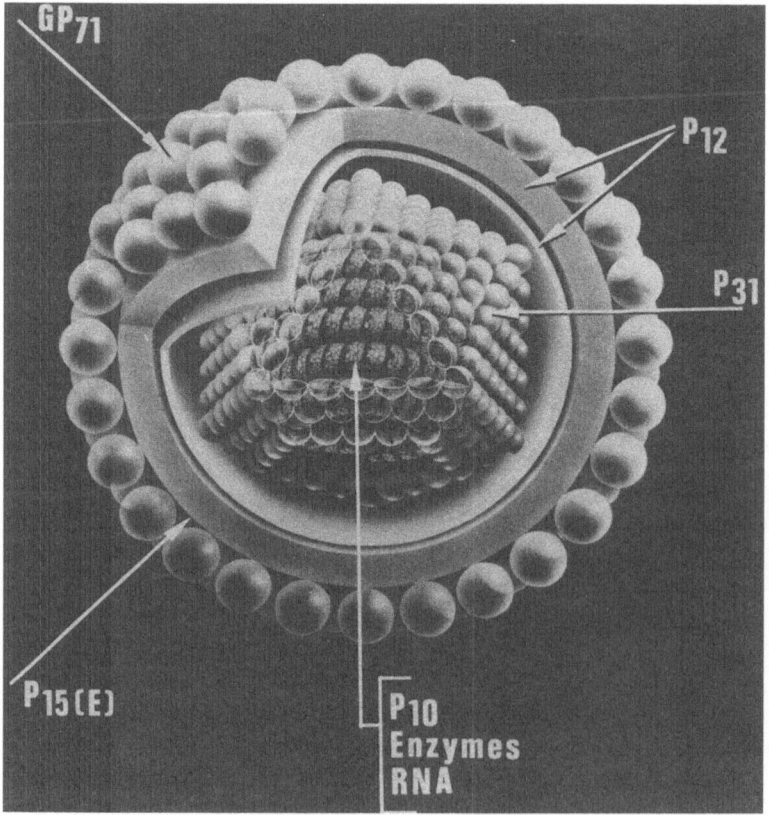

Fig. 15. Model of MuLV Friend.

VI. VIRAL STRUCTURAL ANTIGENS ON THE CELL SURFACE

In order to evaluate which of the viral structural antigens are accessible to antibody on the cell surface and could be used as targets for immunological attacks on virus producing and/or transformed cells, cytotoxic and IEM studies with component-specific antisera were performed.

From the work described above regarding the virus particle structure, gp71 was considered as the most likely candidate for a cell-surface target. Initial studies by Grant et al. (1974) indicated that, in addition to gp71, p31, and p10, antigens were detectable on the surface of virus-producing cells. The presence of a p31 antigen on the cell surface was also reported by other authors (Yoshiki et al., 1974). However, the significance of p31 antigen on the cell surface is not entirely clear. It could be shown by Grant et al. (1974) that after addition of isolated p31 to normal cells this material can become attached and act as a cytotoxic target. In this regard, it was suggested that the viral internal proteins (p31 and p10) on the cell surface probably represent material from disrupted virus and/or cells which is passively adsorbed. Interestingly, recent studies showed that these components could indeed be found in soluble form in supernatants from virus-releasing cell cultures (Bolognesi et al., 1975b), while Del Villano et al. (1975) have found that soluble virus-like antigens can occur naturally in vivo as well.

More comprehensive analyses of expression of C-type virus antigens on the cell surface, with both cytotoxic and IEM analyses, were carried out by Hunsmann et al. (1976) and Schwarz et al. (1976). These authors employed component-specific antisera which were carefully absorbed with normal antigens to investigate normal cells from STU mice, STU cells infected with FLV and GLV, murine sarcoma virus–transformed nonproducer cells (K-BALB, MS85, and HT-1), FeLV-producing cells, and monkey cells producing SSV-SSAV and GAL virus. Antisera to FLV p10, p15, and p30 were tested on all these cells and found to react only with a single murine cell line (Eveline) which produces large amounts of FLV. Another cell producing the same virus, but in lower amounts, was not reactive.

In contrast, gp71 antigen was found on all FLV- and GLV-producing mouse cells, as well as on FeLV-producing cat cells (Figs. 16, 17, and 18). Although the titer of the FLV-gp71 serum for cat cells was relatively low and its activity demonstrable only by cytotoxicity, the result was highly reproducible. However, normal STU cells, as well as the non-virus-producing MSV-transformed cells and cells infected with simian viruses, did not yield a clear positive reaction with anti-gp71 serum. The electron microscopic studies (Fig. 18) indicated that gp71 antigen is distributed on infected murine cells in a fashion similar to the glycoprotein antigen of avian C-type viruses (Gelderblom et al., 1972), namely, on the surface of budding and released virus particles, as well as on nonbudding areas of the cell membrane. No difference in the distribution in type- and

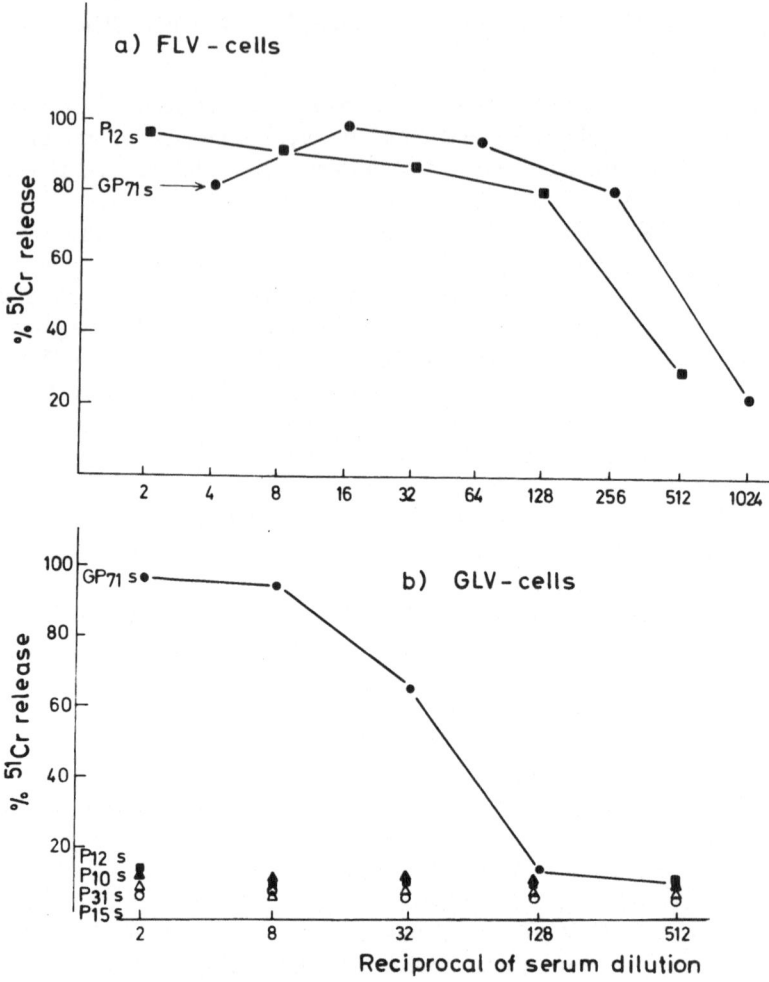

Fig. 16. ^{51}Cr-release tests with FLV- (a) and GLV- (b) producing murine cells using FLV-p12 and FLV-gp71 antisera. p12 serum lyses only FLV cells. gp71 serum lyses GLV cells as well.

group-specific determinants was observed. From these results, it was concluded that type, as well as group and interspecies, determinants of gp71 are expressed in reactive form on the surface of virus-producing cells. The interspecies reactivity of anti-gp71 serum with feline-virus-producing cells and lack of activity with simian virus-producing cells are consistent with the gp71 antigenic pattern observed in other serological tests (see above).

A further integral constituent on the surface of certain murine virus producing cells is the *p12* antigen. As in other serological assays with this component, it displayed a high degree of type specificity in cytotoxic and IEM analyses (Figs. 16 and 19). Furthermore, it was found exclusively on nonbudding areas of the cell membrane (Fig. 19a). The lack of reactivity of budding or mature virus with anti-p12 serum contrasts with its expression on other areas of the cell membrane and suggests that, as in the case of p15(E), p12 may be masked by the virus glycoprotein knobs. Alternatively, after inclusion in the particle, it may be localized beneath the virus envelope. Why the p15(E) was not detectable on

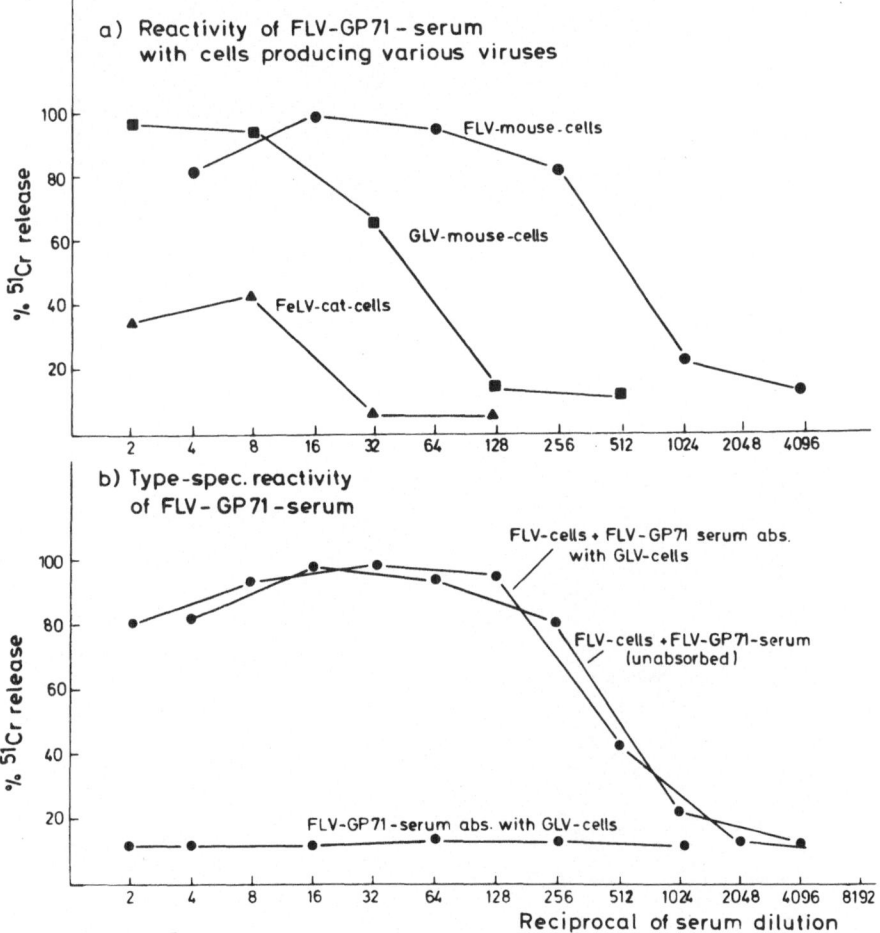

Fig. 17. (a) ⁵¹Cr-release tests with FLV-, GLV-, and FeLV- (cat cells) producing cells. FLV-gp71 serum lyses all three cell types. (b) ⁵¹Cr-release tests with FLV- and GLV-producing cells using gp71 serum before and after absorption with GLV cells. Evidence for presence of *type*-specific cytotoxic antibody.

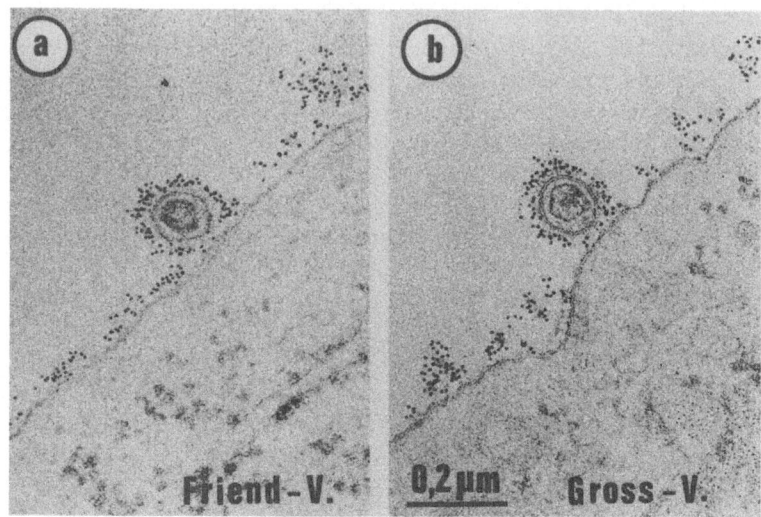

Fig. 18. IEM with FLV- (a) and GLV- (b) producing STU mouse cells using
FLV-gp71 serum.

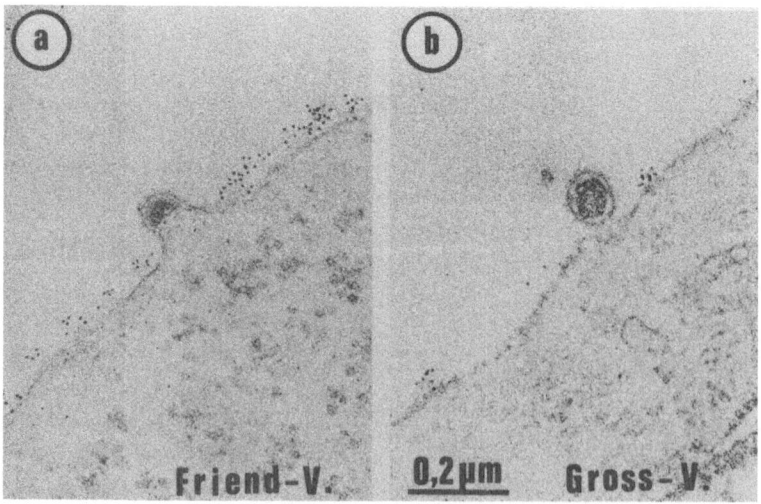

Fig. 19. IEM with FLV- (a) and GLV- (b) producing STU mouse cells using
FLV-p12 serum.

the cell surface by these assays is not clear. The possibility exists that, in contrast to p12 and gp71, this component is restricted to the budding areas and, as suggested previously, is prevented in the systems studied from reacting with the antisera because of the presence of the viral glycoprotein knobs.

In earlier studies by other investigators, a series of cell-surface and soluble antigens associated with murine leukemias have been described (for review, see Bauer, 1974). It was possible that at least some of these are related to the structural antigens of the virus. The well-studied *viral envelope antigens* share many properties in common with gp71. Like the latter, such antigens possess type- and group-specific reactivities and are found on the viral and cellular membranes or as soluble antigens in mouse plasma. The occurrence of such soluble antigens may be considered analogous to the *in vitro* release of gp71 from the virus or the infected cell (Bolognesi *et al.*, 1975*b*).

A further well-studied antigen which may be related to gp71 is the G_{IX} *differentiation marker*. In the mouse, this is associated with naturally occurring Gross virus and is detectable as a surface antigen on virus-producing cells as well as on non-virus-producing thymocytes of certain mouse strains. Soluble G_{IX} was also found in the mouse plasma. Experimental evidence for an antigenic relationship between G_{IX} and gp71 was obtained by Obata *et al.* (1975), Tung *et al.* (1975), and Del Villano *et al.* (1975). That gp71 can be expressed similarly to G_{IX} on normal murine cells was shown by Grant *et al.* (1974). Normal C57BL/6 mouse cells could be shown to express gp71 in the absence of detectable p31 antigen either on the cell surface or within the cell (Grant *et al.*, 1974). These studies and those of other authors (Bilello *et al.*, 1974) led to the concept of noncoordinate expression of the murine viral antigens similar to the expression of chicken factor (chf) in avian cells (Hanafusa *et al.*, 1973). Recently, chf has been shown to be represented, at least in part, by the major glycoprotein, gp85, of avian C-type viruses (Halpern *et al.*, 1975).

Other leukemia cell-surface antigens include the *FMR antigen* and its analogue, the Gross cell-surface antigen (GCSA). These are highly specific for the respective virus group and are not observed in the absence of virus production. As mentioned above, Friedman *et al.* (1974) recently provided evidence that the FMR antigen corresponds to a type-specific viral structural antigen which is located between the surface and the nucleoid of the virion. This conclusion was reached, since degraded but not intact virus was able to absorb antibody directed against it. Immunoelectron microscopy studies by Aoki *et al.* (1972) detected the FMR antigen on nonbudding areas of the cell membrane but not on budding virions. All of these properties are shared by p12 of FLV as has been described above. Additionally, F. Lilly (personal communication) recently found that this viral component absorbs an appreciable portion of the cytotoxic activity from a standard anti-FMR serum. Therefore, at least part of the FMR antigenic reactivity is represented by FLV-p12. The remainder might be associated with the type-specific p15 described by Strand *et al.* (1974), unless these are in fact one and the same molecule.

These observations indicate that at least some of the well-studied cell-surface antigens are represented by viral structural components. Others, such as the tumor-specific cell-surface antigens (TSSA), which have also been detected on non-virus-producing cells such as K-BALB and MS85 (Aoki *et al.*, 1973), have no apparent relationship to any of the structural antigens examined thus far since no activity was obtained with any of the component-specific antisera on these cells. In the avian system, TSSA has been identified as a nonstructural but possible virus-coded glycoprotein (Bauer, 1974).

VII. AUTOGENOUS IMMUNITY IN MICE TO VIRAL STRUCTURAL ANTIGENS

For a long time it was thought that mice were immunologically tolerant to C-type viral structural antigens, based primarily on studies with p31. As a result of the pioneer work of Hanna, Ihle, and co-workers (for review, see Ihle *et al.*, 1975*b*), an autogenous immunity in inbred mouse strains to several surface components of endogenous viruses has been demonstrated. Normal mouse sera were capable of precipitating radioactively labeled AKR virus in the presence of antibody against mouse serum globulins. Analysis of the immune complexes obtained revealed three prominent virus components migrating similarly to gp71, gp45, and p15(E), respectively. Using the viral components and/or the mono-specific antisera described above, two of these could indeed be shown to represent gp71 and p15(E) (Ihle *et al.*, 1975*a*, 1976). Separate analyses indicated that with many inbred mouse strains (Ihle *et al.*, 1976*e*) an inverse relationship exists between the gp71 and p15(E) antibody titers and the incidence of leukemia in the mouse. However, strains like NIH, where endogenous virus is not expressed, were antibody negative as well as leukemia negative. From such results, it would appear that a genetically controlled immune surveillance system against the virus is operative, which may be influential also in regulating leukemia development. The experiments described in the sections which follow are an attempt to artificially enhance the host immune surveillance by both vaccination with purified antigens as well as treatment with their respective antibody.

VIII. IMMUNOGENIC POTENCY OF ISOLATED VIRAL PROTEINS AND GLYCOPROTEINS

On the basis of the studies presented, those antigens expressed on the virus surface as well as on the surface of the cell were considered the most promising candidates for immunization trials. Nevertheless, all of the structural viral antigens were included in our studies. STU mice were vaccinated with 110–120 μg of each of the major structural components in the presence of Freund's incomplete adjuvant. One week after the booster, mice were challenged by intraperitoneal (i.p.) injection with a high dose (10^5 mouse ID_{50}) of spleen-derived cell-free FLV or RLV. Four weeks after infection, some of the mice were sacrificed, the spleens taken, and their weights registered. Virus content in some of the spleens were determined by the XC test.

Photographs of the spleens from such experiments are presented in Figs. 20 and 21 and indicate that vaccination with gp71 was the most effective in this regard (Hunsmann *et al.,* 1975; Schäfer *et al.,* 1976). The spleens of the gp71-immunized mice were nearly normal in size and contained either none or relatively low amounts of infectious virus. Preliminary studies showed that some effect was also observed with p15(E) immunization (Fig. 21), the significance of

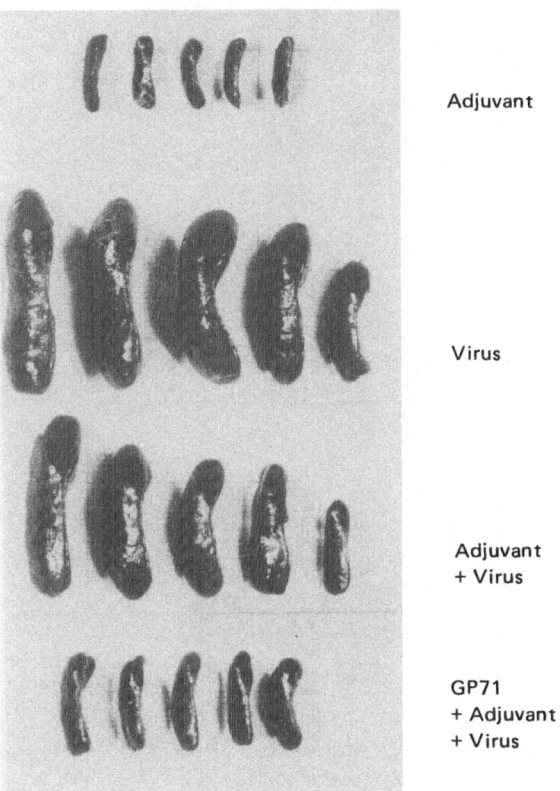

Adjuvant

Virus

Adjuvant
+ Virus

GP71
+ Adjuvant
+ Virus

Fig. 20. Immunization of mice with FLV gp71. Spleens 4 weeks after challenge with FLV.

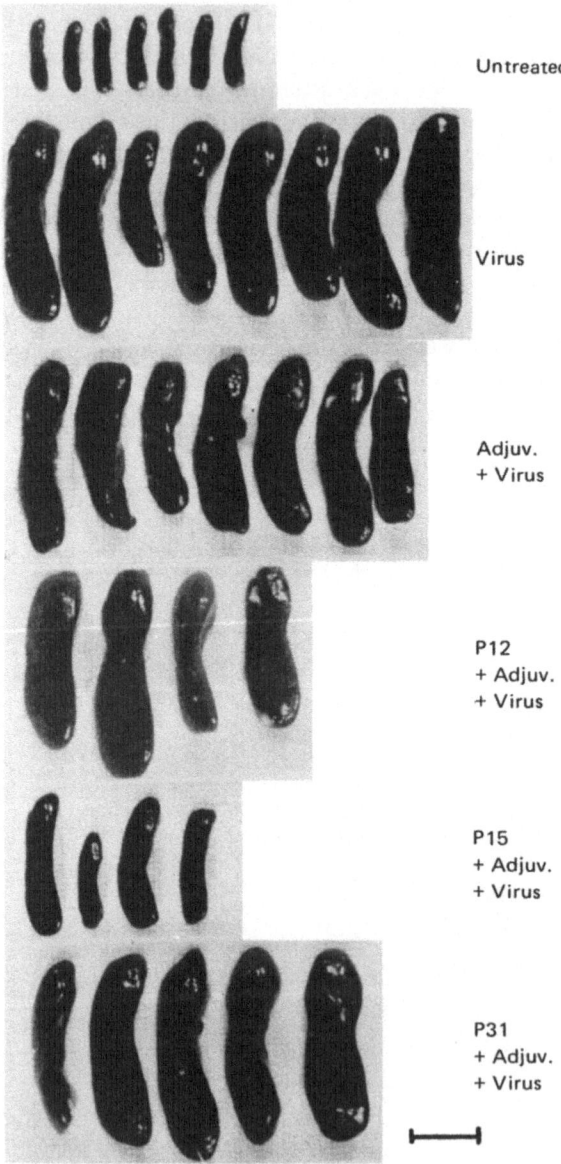

Fig. 21. Immunization of mice with vaccines prepared with FLV proteins other than gp71.

which is being investigated. In contrast, no demonstrable protection was obtained with p12-immunization, possibly because this component is inaccessible in the virus particle. As expected, immunization with the internal p31 and p10 (not shown) antigens likewise had no effect. These studies show that at least two of the structural components on the virion surface which were found to elicit autogenous immunity in mice (Ihle *et al.*, 1976e), namely, gp71 and p15(E), might be used to artifically stimulate the immune response of the host against C-type virus infection and subsequent leukemia development. Interestingly, no immunity to gp71 was observed if Freund's adjuvant was replaced with aluminum hydroxide, indicating an important role for the adjuvant in this process.

Whereas the exact mechanism of gp71-induced immunity to C-type virus leukemias remains to be defined, extensive studies have been carried out in collaboration with Ihle and co-workers (Frederick, Md.) to determine the immune response of the mouse to the purified gp71 antigen (Ihle *et al.*, 1976a,b). BALB/c and C57BL/6 mice were injected with 20–30 μg of FLV-gp71 by the subcutaneous (S.C.) (with Freund's complete adjuvant) and/or intravenous (i.v.) routes (without adjuvant). Both strains developed humoral antibodies as well as cellular immunity, but the mode of immunization influenced the outcome considerably. Best results were obtained with the s.c. route followed by an i.v. booster.

The humoral antibodies were detected by RIA, as well as by a C'-dependent microcytotoxicity assay. In BALB/c mice, this immune response was *type-specific*. In C57BL/6 mice, vaccination with gp 71 stimulated the immune response which is directed against its endogenous virus. Thus a secondary consequence of immunization with FLV-gp71 was the enhancement of antibodies directed against a Gross-type gp71, in addition to antibodies specific for FMR gp71 determinants. Competition assays were performed to demonstrate that *two classes* of antibodies existed, each of which was type-specific for the respective gp71.

Differences in the two strains were also observed in the cellular immune response. In BALB/c mice, cytotoxic lymphocytes and lymphocytes which could be stimulated to undergo blastogenesis with gp71 were found. The cytotoxic lymphocytes exhibited group specificity in that they lysed both FMR- and Gross-virus-infected target cells. In contrast, C57BL/6 mice did not exhibit cytotoxic lymphocytes, although gp71-specific blastogenesis was demonstrated. Whether or not the activation of the endogenous virus antigen expression or parameters such as the H-2 haplotype (Zinkernagel and Doherty, 1975) are responsible for this effect is unknown. However, the humoral immune response, as well as the blastogenic activity, were considerably stronger in C57BL/6 than in BALB/c mice.

In addition to the gp71-type-specific antibodies, a broad reacting antibody activity was detected in the immunized C56BL/6 mice by radioimmunoprecipitation assays against intact viruses. Preliminary studies indicate that such anti-bodies are directed against p15(E) of the endogenous Gross-type virus of C57BL/6 mice. Similar antibodies also exist in natural sera of older mice (see above), and because of their broad reactivities these antibodies may be impor-tant for recognition of heterologous viruses.

These results show that various factors are important for successful immuni-zation of mice with gp71 including the antigenic dose, its method of immuniza-tion (i.e., route and use of adjuvant), as well as the particular mouse strain used. The studies in C57BL/6 mice, for example, where immunization with gp71 activates the expression of an endogenous virus function, indicate that care should be taken before a general application of this procedure is considered. This notion is underscored by recent findings indicating that immunization of AKR mice with FLV-gp71 results in enhancement of leukemia and earlier death of the animals (Ihle et al., 1976b).

IX. SEROIMMUNOTHERAPY OF C-TYPE VIRUS INFECTIONS

It might well be that the dangers posed by active immunization with gp71 do not apply in the treatment of infected animals with specific antisera to this component. Furthermore, serum therapy would be more likely to warrant consideration for eventual application in treatment of human leukemic diseases.

The following schedule was employed in the studies to be described (Huns-mann et al., 1975; Schäfer et al., 1976): Twelve-week-old STU mice were infected i.p. with about 10^5 mouse ID_{50} doses of FLV or RLV. Intraperitoneal injection of the goat anti-gp71 serum or the respective IgG was begun between 6 and 7 days after virus inoculation. The serum treatment was continued for 7–14 days and as much as 2.8–4.0 ml was inoculated per mouse. Some of the mice were sacrificed 4 weeks after infection and their spleens weighed, while others were maintained for several months with their blood smears examined at various times after treatment. Thus far, antisera to FLV-gp71 and FLV-p12 were employed, and similar studies with anti-p15(E) serum are in progress.

No therapeutic effect was observed using anti-p12 serum in this protocol. However, goat anti-gp71 serum was clearly effective against FLV and RLV infections (Figs. 22 and 23). Extracts from three of the spleens of mice infected with RLV revealed no infectious virus (two mice) or barely detectable amounts (one mouse). That this protection was mediated by antibody and not by other components in the goat serum could be shown in experiments in which elec-trophoretically homogeneous IgG from the anti-gp71 serum was similarly ad-ministered to the mice. In these studies the animals were observed for much longer periods. In one test, eight of ten mice treated with anti-gp71 IgG have continued to survive for over 5 months while all ten untreated control mice and

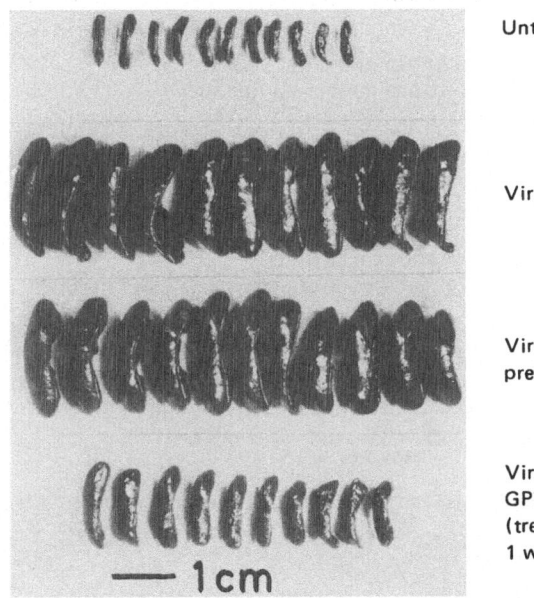

Untreated mice

Virus

Virus +
preimmune-serum

Virus +
GP71 antiserum
(treatment start.
1 week post inf.)

Fig. 22. Serum therapy of FLV infection of mice with FLV-gp71 goat serum.
Spleens 4 weeks after infection.

all mice (ten) treated with corresponding amounts of normal goat IgG died 2–2½ months after virus infection (Fig. 24). In a second experiment where larger amounts of IgG were employed, all seven mice treated with anti-gp71 IgG survived (now 4 months p.i.). A closer examination of all surviving mice showed that most of them had a nearly normal blood picture and no detectable virus in the serum. Subsequent studies have shown that for long-term survival, IgG rather

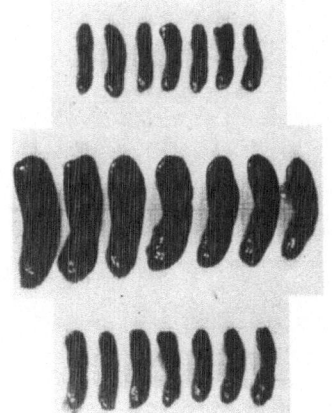

Untreated mice

Virus + normal serum

Virus + GP71 antiserum
(treatment started 6 days
p.i. with RLV)

Fig. 23. As Fig. 22, but RLV infection.

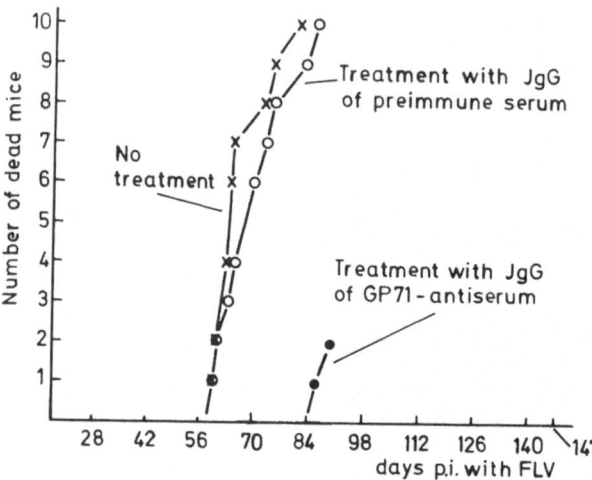

Fig. 24. Serum therapy of FLV infection of mice with IgG from FLV-gp71 goat serum. Survival of treated mice (from day 6–20 p.i. 7 × 0.4 ml i.p.).

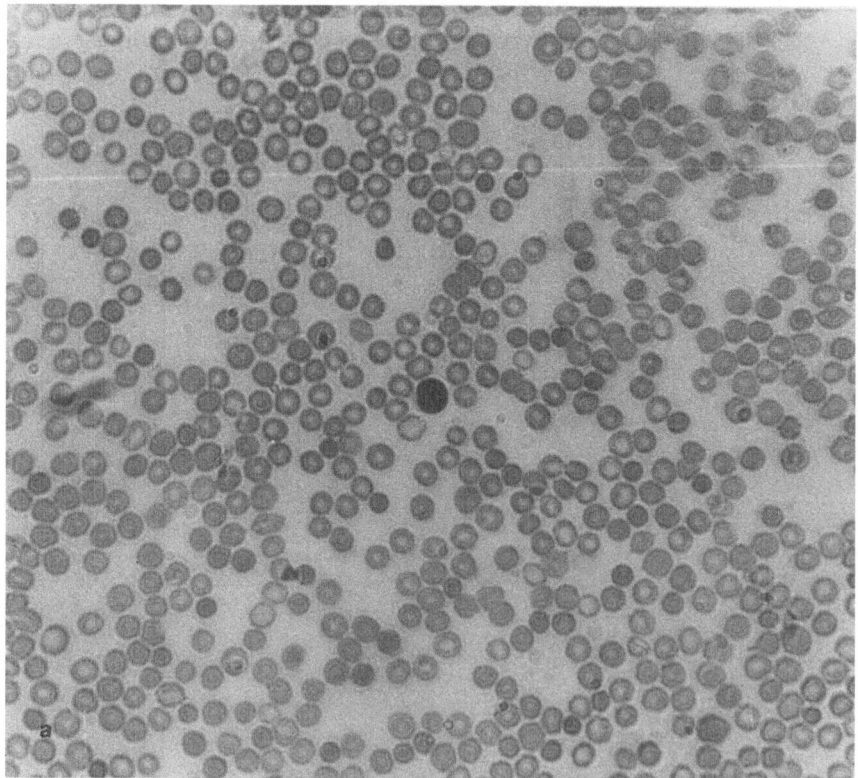

Fig. 25. Blood films of anti-FeLV (a) and normal control serum (b) treated FLV-infected mice. Start of treatment 4 days p.i.; blood films 4 weeks p.i.

than whole serum must be administered. Furthermore, an important consequence of the serotherapy protocol employed is the development of a host-immune response against the infecting virus which itself may be responsible for the long-term protection achieved.

The serotherapeutic regimen described above would be especially useful if it could be applied to virus-induced leukemias of other animal species. For anti-FLV gp71 serum, such a prospect was promising since this antiserum is effective in C'-dependent virus inactivation and cytotoxicity via its interspecies determinant, in addition to its other antigenic sites (see above). In order to explore this possibility a preliminary experiment with FeLV-infected kittens was initiated in collaboration with F. de Noronha, Cornell University (in preparation). The data thus far available (Schäfer *et al.*, 1976) show that two of four 6-month-old kittens which were infected with FeLV and 6 days later treated with anti-gp71 serum (6ml/kitten) for a period of 11 days were free of infectious virus. In

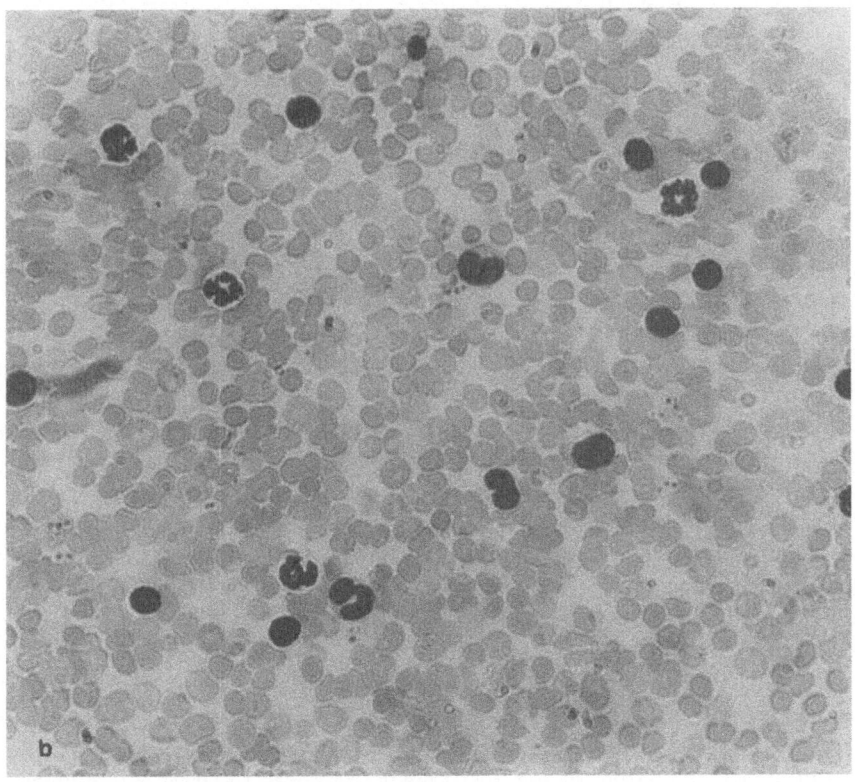

Fig. 25(b).

contrast, all six control kittens treated with normal serum contained large amounts of virus in their buffy coat cells. In a reciprocal experiment, mice infected with murine FLV were treated with a potent antiserum to FeLV prepared in goats. This serum cross-reacts prominently in immunodiffusion tests with the interspecies determinants of MuLV p15, p30, and gp71 (Fig. 10h). As judged from the reduction in spleen size in comparison to controls (not shown), some therapeutic effect was achieved. The same conclusion can be drawn from the examination of blood smears (Fig. 25), where a nearly normal distribution was seen at 4 weeks post infection in contrast to controls. Thus *interspecies* reactivity seems to be functional also for immunotherapy.

To our knowledge, these results represent the first clear evidence that virus-induced leukemias can be influenced therapeutically by antibody against a purified viral structural component. Clearly the mechanism of this immunity is of major interest. The effect could be either on the virus, the target cells, or, more likely, both. If the activity is directed solely against the virus, its value would be primarily for leukemias resulting from horizontal transmission of virus, such as feline leukemia. If either active or passive immunization is effective on target cells, it might be applicable to endogenous leukemias such as those in AKR mice. Studies are in progress to resolve these questions.

X. CONCLUDING REMARKS

With the isolation of the major viral polypeptides from a model murine C-type virus and the preparation of the corresponding component-specific antisera, powerful experimental tools have been obtained which permit a more thorough study of the immunological consequences of virus infection, and an immunoprophylactic and therapeutic approach to virus-induced diseases.

However, these questions cannot be approached unambiguously without consideration of the presence of endogenous virus activity. Studies by Lerner and colleagues (Lerner *et al.*, 1976) indicate that viral gene expression, particularly in the form of gp71-like molecules occurs in certain tissues of the mouse even during normal embryo development. It is of obvious importance to determine the function of these glycoproteins not only because they might play important roles in differentiation, but because their presence might lead to other pathogenic phenomena in the host. In particular, "autoimmune diseases" (Mellors *et al.*, 1971) appear to be caused by immune complexes with the virus antigens which can be easily shed by the particle or the infected cell (Bolognesi *et al.*, 1975b). Moreover, the presence of such components in large quantities may influence the nature of the host immune response to virus or immunizing antigens.

The work of Ihle, Hanna, and co-workers (Ihle *et al.*, 1976*e*) has shown that autogenous immunity to certain viral antigens, one of which is the Gross-type gp71, could be detected in sera from normal inbred mice. This concept was further supported by a recent finding showing that the precipitation of purified Gross-type gp71 occurs by various normal mouse sera or their immunoglobulins (Ihle *et al.*, 1976*c*). How such antibodies can exist in free form in the presence of large amounts of similar glycoprotein antigens is a challenging and provocative question. However, it is becoming apparent that most free natural mouse antibodies possess a very narrow specificity and perhaps recognize only subdeterminants of these glycoproteins which are highly type specific.

The ability to successfully vaccinate STU mice with purified FLV gp71 against FLV- and RLV-induced leukemia reinforces the notion that the mouse can respond in some fashion to at least a portion of the viral glycoprotein. Our studies indicate that this response is largely *type-specific* for FLV gp71 and therefore similar to the reactivity of natural immune sera, which is type specific for endogenous virus glycoproteins. The artificially induced immune response is apparently directed not only against the virus but also against infected leukemic cells as suggested by the presence of cytotoxic antibodies and lymphocytes in BALB/c mice. The absence of prominent neutralizing antibodies for FLV or RLV also imply that other activities are involved in the protection observed following gp71 immunization. However, it was noted that similar immunization in other mouse strains, notably C57BL/6 and AKR, led to an enhanced expression of antigen of the endogenous virus and possibly the virus itself and a separate immune response against it. These observations preclude a general application of active immunization with gp71 and restrict it to those mouse strains where endogenous agents are not expressed or easily induced.

Our studies indicated that it was also possible to treat FLV- or RLV-infected STU mice with anti-gp71 serum prepared in goats or rabbits as a preventive measure against leukemia. Because this serum has broad reactivity, it can be applied to homologous as well as certain heterologous virus-induced leukemias. Furthermore, this treatment may be more applicable to mouse strains where immune stimulation of endogenous virus as a result of active immunization is detrimental to the host. Interestingly, none of the treated STU mice have thus far exhibited *pathological* immune complex disease symptoms which might have been expected if large amounts of endogenous cross-reacting gp71 molecules were present. It is evident that more mouse strains, as well as other species, need to be examined to determine the generality of the endogenous expression of gp71-like molecules.

On the basis of our preliminary studies with active immunization with gp71 or serum treatment with gp71 antiserum, several aspects require further investigation in order to determine the limits of applicability of these regimens for immunoprophylaxis and therapy of C-type virus-induced diseases. For active immunization, it is important to determine (1) the mechanism of the protection observed, as well as the primary target against which it is directed (i.e., virus, cell, or both); (2) the mechanism of endogenous virus activation in some mouse strains occurring as a result of immune stimulation with gp71; and (3) applicability of other viral antigens, particularly p15(E), to which the mouse responds with group-specific reactivity. With regard to serum treatment, the following questions require clarification: (1) What is the mechanism which leads to successful immunotherapy with anti-gp71 serum? (2) Is it possible to develop a protocol which can suppress and eradicate more advanced stages of leukemia?

As suggested by our studies, immunogens obtained from a C-type virus of one species can be used for prophylactic and possibly therapeutic regimens in another species. It is therefore important to know to what extent mammalian C-type viruses are related by such antigens. Our approach to this question is to define these relationships on a more solid basis and to search for the least common denominator, i.e., the interspecies region of gp71 which is shared among the viruses of various species. If linear protein or glycopeptide sequences can be found which constitute specific interspecies determinants as suggested by recent studies with p30 (Oroszlan *et al.,* 1975), their isolation in immunologically active form might provide safer and more powerful reagents than those prepared against the entire gp71 molecule. In this regard, the p15(E) component may, in fact, represent an antigen of this type, and its role in immunity is therefore under investigation.

The immunotherapeutic regimens applied to animal leukemias carry important implications for similar studies with leukemias in man. It should be noted in this regard that we have dealt exclusively with highly purified components which are free of genetic material. Furthermore, since single antigens are used, it permits one to study unambiguously the beneficial as well as the detrimental effects (e.g., activation of endogenous virus, blocking antibody) of the immunization. Similar application to humans can occur only when leukemia-specific antigens can be identified, and isolated, and powerful antisera are prepared against them. Our recent findings, in collaboration with T. Mohanakumar and R. Metzgar, indicate that some serological cross-reactivity exists between mammalian C-type virus antigens and surface antigens of human leukemia cells (Metzgar *et al.,* 1976*a,b*) which may provide a vehicle to this end.

ACKNOWLEDGMENTS

We are grateful to our co-workers who have participated in these studies over the years and to the technical and clerical staffs of our respective laboratories who have contributed much to our efforts. The electron micrographs were provided by Drs. H. Frank and H. Schwarz.

XI. REFERENCES

Aoki, T., Herberman, R. B., Johnson, P. A., Liu, M., and Sturm, M. M., 1972, Wild-type Gross leukemia virus: Classification of soluble antigens (GSA), *J. Virol.* **10**:1208–1219.

Aoki, T., Stephenson, J. R., and Aaronson, S. A., 1973, Demonstration of a cell-surface antigen associated with murine sarcoma virus by immunoelectron microscopy, *Proc. Natl. Acad. Sci. U.S.A.* **70**:742–746.

August, J. T., Bolognesi, D. P., Fleissner, E., Gilden, R., and Nowinski, R. C., 1974, A proposed nomenclature for the virion proteins of oncogenic RNA viruses, *Virology* **60**:595–601.

Bauer, H., 1974, Virion and tumor cell antigens of C-type RNA tumor viruses, in: *Advances in Cancer Research,* Vol. 20, p. 275, Academic Press, New York.

Bilello, J. A., Strand, M., and August, J. T., 1974, Murine sarcoma virus gene expression: Transformants which express viral envelope glycoprotein in the absence of the major internal protein and infectious particles. *Proc. Natl. Acad. Sci. U.S.A.* **71**:3234–3238.

Bolognesi, D. P., Bauer, H., Gelderblom, H., and Hüper, G., 1972, Polypeptides of avian RNA tumor viruses. IV. Components of the viral envelope, *Virology* **47**:551–556.

Bolognesi, D. P., Luftig, R., and Shaper, J. H., 1973, Localization of RNA tumor virus polypeptides. I. Isolation of further virus substructures, *Virology* **56**:549–564.

Bolognesi, D. P., Collins, J. J., Leis, J. P., Moennig, V., Schäfer, W., and Atkinson, P. H., 1975a, Role of carbohydrate in determining the immunochemical properties of the major glycoprotein of Friend leukemia virus, *J. Virol.* **16**:1453–1463.

Bolognesi, D. P., Langlois, A. J., and Schäfer, W., 1975b, Polypeptides of mammalian oncornaviruses. IV. Structural components of murine leukemia virus released as soluble antigens in cell culture, *Virology* **68**:550–555.

Del Villano, B. C., Nave, B., Croker, B. P., Lerner, R. A., and Dixon, F. J., 1975, The oncornavirus glycoprotein gp69/71: A constituent of the surface of normal and malignant thymocytes, *J. Exp. Med.* **141**:172–187.

Fischinger, P. J., Schäfer, W., and Bolognesi, D. P., 1976, Neutralization of homologous and heterologous oncornaviruses by antisera against the p15(E) and gp71 polypeptides of Friend murine Leukemia virus, *Virology* **71**:169–184.

Friedman, M., Lilly, F., and Nathenson, S. G., 1974, Cell surface antigen induced by Friend murine leukemia virus is also in the virion, *J. Virol.* **14**:1126–1131.

Gelderblom, H., Bauer, H., and Graf, T., 1972, Cell-surface antigens induced by avian RNA tumor viruses: Detection by immunoferritin technique, *Virology* **47**:416–425.

Grant, J. P., Bigner, D. D., Fischinger, P. J., and Bolognesi, D. P., 1974, Expression of murine leukemia virus structural antigens on the surface of chemically induced murine sarcomas, *Proc. Natl. Acad. Sci. U.S.A.* **71**:5037–5041.

Green, R. W., Bolognesi, D. P., Schäfer, W., Pister, L., Hunsmann, G., and de Noronha, F., 1973, Polypeptides of mammalian oncornaviruses. I. Isolation and serological analysis of polypeptides from murine and feline C-type viruses, *Virology* **56**:565–579.

Halpern, M. S., Bolognesi, D. P., Friis, R. R., and Mason, W. S., 1975, Expression of the major viral glycoprotein of avian tumor virus in cells of chf(+) chicken embryos, *J. Virol.* **15**:1131–1140.

Hanafusa, H., Aoki, T., Kawai, S., Miyamoto, T., and Wilsnack, R. E., 1973, Presence of antigen common to avian tumor viral envelope antigen in normal chick embryo cells, *Virology* **56**:22–32.

Hunsmann, G., Moennig, V., Pister, L., Seifert, E., and Schäfer, W., 1974, Properties of mouse leukemia viruses. VIII. The major viral glycoprotein of Friend leukemia virus: Seroimmunological, interfering and hemagglutinating capacities, *Virology* **62**:307–318.

Hunsmann, G., Moennig, V., and Schäfer, W., 1975, Properties of mouse leukemia viruses. IX. Active and passive immunization of mice against Friend leukemia with isolated viral gp71 glycoprotein and its corresponding antiserum, *Virology* **66**:327–329.

Hunsmann, G., Claviez, M., Moennig, V., Schwarz, H., and Schäfer, W., 1976, Properties of mouse leukemia viruses. X. Occurrence of viral structural antigens on the cell surface as revealed by a cytotoxicity test, *Virology* **69**:157–168.

Ihle, J. N., Hanna, M. G., Jr., Schäfer, W., Hunsmann, G., Bolognesi, D. P., and Huper G., 1975, Polypeptides of mammalian oncornaviruses. III. Localization of p15 and reactivity with natural antibody, *Virology* **63**:60–67.

Ihle, J. N., Lee, J. C., Hanna, M. G., Jr., Collins, J. J., Bolognesi, D. P., Fischinger, P. J., Moennig, V., and Schäfer, W., 1976a, Characterization of the immune response to the major glycoprotein (gp71) of Friend leukemia virus. I. Response in BALB/c mice, *Virology*, in press.

Ihle, J. N., Collins, J. J., Lee, J. C., Fischinger, P. J., Pazmino, N., Moennig, V., Schäfer, W., Hanna, M. G., Jr., and Bolognesi, D. P., 1976b, Characterization of the immune response to the major glycoprotein (gp71) of Friend leukemia virus. III. Influence on endogenous MuLV-mediated pathogenesis, *Virology*, in press.

Ihle, J. N., Denny, T. P., and Bolognesi, D. P., 1976c, Purification and serological characterization of the major envelope glycoprotein from AKR murine leukemia virus and its reactivity with autogenous immune sera from mice, *J. Virol.* **17**:727–736.

Ihle, J. N., Lee, J. C., Hanna, M. G., Jr., Collins, J. J., Bolognesi, D. P., Fischinger, P. J., Pazmino, N., Moennig, V., and Schäfer, W., 1976d, Characterization of the immune response to the major glycoprotein (gp71) of Friend leukemia virus. II. Response in C57BL/6 mice, *Virology*, in press.

Ihle, J. N., Lee, J. C., and Hanna, M. G., Jr., 1976e, Characterization of natural antibodies in mice to endogenous leukemia virus, in: *The Biology of Radiation Carcinogenesis* (J. M. Yuhan, R. W. Tennant, and J. D. Regan, eds.), pp. 261–273, Raven Press, New York.

Ihle, J. N., Lee, J. C., Longstreth, J., and Hanna, M. G., Jr., 1976f, Characterization of virion and cell surface reactivities of natural immune sera to murine leukemia viruses, in: *Tumor Viruses and Immunity* (R. Crowell, H. Friedman, and J. E. Prier, eds.), pp. 197–214, University Park Press, Baltimore.

Lange, J., Frank, H., Hunsmann, G., Moennig, V., Wollmann, R., and Schäfer, W., 1973, Properties of mouse leukemia viruses. VI. The core of Friend virus; isolation and constituents, *Virology* **53**:457–462.

Lerner, R. A., Wilson, C. B., Del Villano, B. C., McConahey, P. J., and Dixon, F. J., 1976, Endogenous oncornaviral gene expression in adult and fetal mice: Quantitative, histologic, and physiologic studies of the major viral glycoprotein, gp70, *J. Exp. Med.* **143**:155–166.

Mellors, R. C., Shirai, T., Aoki, T., Huebner, R. J., and Krawczynski, K., 1971, Wild-type Gross leukemia virus and the pathogenesis of the glomerulonephritis of New Zealand mice, *J. Exp. Med.* **133**:113–132.

Metzgar, R. S., Mohanakumar, T., and Bolognesi, D. P., 1976a, Relationships between membrane antigens of human leukemia cells and oncogenic RNA virus structural components, *J. Exp. Med.* **143**:47–63.

Metzgar, R. S., Mohanakumar, T., and Bolognesi, D. P., 1976b, Antigenic relationships between murine, feline and primate RNA tumor viruses and membrane antigens of human leukemic cells, in: *Comparative Leukemia Research,* pp. 549–554, Karger, Basel, in press.

Moennig, V., Hunsmann, G., and Schäfer, W., 1973, Partielle Reinigung und biologischserologische Charakterisierung kohlenhydrathaltiger Komponenten aus Präparaten von Friend-Leukämie-Virus, *Z. Naturforsch* **28c**:785–788.

Moennig, V., Frank, H., Hunsmann, G., Ohms, P., Schwarz, H., Schäfer, W., and Strand-ström, H., 1974a, C-type particles produced by a permanent cell line from a leukemic pig. II. Physical, chemical and serological characterization of the particles, *Virology* 57:179–188.

Moennig, V., Frank, H., Hunsmann, G., Schneider, I., and Schäfer, W., 1974b, Properties of mouse leukemia viruses. VII. The major viral glycoprotein of Friend leukemia virus, Isolation and physicochemical properties, *Virology* 61:100–111.

Nermut, M. V., Frank, H., and Schäfer, W., 1972, Properties of mouse leukemia viruses. III. Electron microscopic appearance as revealed after conventional preparation techniques as well as freeze-drying and freeze-etching, *Virology* 49:345–358.

Obata, Y., Ikeda, H., Stockert, E., and Boyse, E. A., 1975, Relation of G_{1X} antigen of thymocytes to envelope glycoprotein of murine leukemia virus, *J. Exp. Med.* 141: 188–197.

Oroszlan, S., Gilden, R. V., and Sallay, S., 1975, Immunochemistry of a synthetic undeca-peptide of mammalian type C virus major internal protein, in: *First Chemical Congress of the North American Continent, Mexico City, Mexico,* in press.

Oroszlan, S., Summers, M. R., Foreman, C., and Gilden, R. V., 1974, Murine type-C virus group-specific antigens: Interstrain immunochemical, biophysical, and amino acid se-quence differences, *J. Virol.* 14:1559–1574.

Parks, W. C., Scolnick, E. M., Noon, M. C., and Watson, C. J., 1974, Immunological cross-reactions between two low-molecular-weight polypeptides from a murine type-C virus, *J. Virol.* 14:430–433.

Parks, W. C., Noon, M. C., Gilden, R., and Scolnick, E. M., 1975, Serological studies with low-molecular-weight polypeptides from the Moloney strain of murine leukemia virus, *J. Virol.* 15:1385–1395.

Rickard, C. G., Post, J. E., de Noronha, F., and Barr, L. M., 1969, A transmissible virus-induced lymphocytic leukemia of the cat, *J. Natl. Cancer Inst.* 42:987–1014.

Rosen, L., 1960. A hemagglutination-inhibition technique for typing adenoviruses, *Am. J. Hyg.* 70:120–128.

Sarma, P. S., Cheong, M. P., Hartley, J. W., and Huebner, R. J., 1967, A viral interference test for mouse leukemia viruses, *Virology* 33:180–184.

Schäfer, W., and de Noronha, F., 1971, A test system for identification of the antigen shared by leukemia viruses of the cat and other mammalian species. *J. Am. Vet. Med. Assoc.* 158:1092–1098.

Schäfer, W., and Seifert, E., 1968, Production of a potent complement-fixing murine leukemia virus-antiserum from the rabbit and its reactions with various types of tissue culture cells, *Virology* 35:323–328.

Schäfer, W., and Szántó, J., 1969, Studies on mouse leukemia viruses. II. Nachweis eines virusspezifischen Hamagglutinins, *Z. Naturforsch.* 24b:1324–1331.

Schäfer, W., Anderer, F. A., Bauer, H., and Pister, L., 1969, Studies on mouse leukemia viruses. I. Isolation and characterization of a group-specific antigen, *Virology* 38: 387–394.

Schäfer, W., Lange, J., Pister, L., Seifert, E., de Noronha, F., and Schmidt, F. W., 1970, Vergleichende serologische Untersuchungen über Leukämieviren: Eine Komplement-bindungsreaktion zum Nachweis der bei Leukämieviren verschiedener Säuger vorkom-menden gemeinsamen antigenen Komponente, *Z. Naturforsch.* 25b:1029–1036.

Schäfer, W., Lange, J., Bolognesi, D. P., de Noronha, F., Post, J. E., and Rickard, C. G., 1971a, Isolation and characterization of two group-specific antigens from feline leuke-mia virus, *Virology* 44:73–82.

Schäfer, W., de Noronha, F., Lange, J., and Bolognesi, D. P., 1971b, Comparative studies on group-specific antigens of RNA-leukemia viruses, in: *The Biology of Oncogenic Viruses* (Proc. 2nd Le Petit Colloquium, Paris, 1970), pp. 116–123, North-Holland, Amsterdam.

Schäfer, W., Fischinger, P. J., Lange, J., and Pister, L., 1972a, Properties of mouse leukemia viruses. I. Characterization of various antisera and serological identification of viral components, *Virology* 47:197–209.

Schäfer, W., Lange, J., Fischinger, P. J., Frank, H., Bolognesi, D. P., and Pister, L., 1972b, Properties of mouse leukemia viruses. II. Isolation of viral components, *Virology* 47:210–228.

Schäfer, W., Hunsmann, G., Moennig, V., Wollmann, R., Pister, L., Deinhardt, F., and Hoekstra, J., 1973a, Nachweis verschiedener antigener Determinanten vom interspecies Typ in RNS-Tumorviren (C-Typ) der Säuger: Vergleichende serologische Untersuchung von Viren mehrerer Tierarten und von einem als Menschenvirus deklarierten Isolat, *Z. Naturforsch.* 28c:214–222.

Schäfer, W., Pister, L., Hunsmann, G., and Moennig, V., 1973b, Comparative serological studies on type C viruses of various mammals, *Nature (London) New Biol.* 245:75–77.

Schäfer, W., Demsey, A., Frank, H., Hunsmann, G., Lange, J., Moennig, V., Pister, L., Bolognesi, D. P., Green, R. W., Luftig, R. B., Shaper, J., and Hüper, G., 1975a, Morphological, chemical and antigenic organization of mammalian C-type viruses, in: *Comparative Leukemia Research 1973* (Y. Ito and R. M. Dutcher, eds.), pp. 497–515, Karger, Basel.

Schäfer, W., Hunsmann, G., Moennig, V., de Noronha, F., Bolognesi, D. P., Green, R. W., and Hüper, G., 1975b, Polypeptides of mammalian oncornaviruses. II. Characterization of a murine leukemia virus polypeptide (p15) bearing interspecies reactivity, *Virology* 63:48–59.

Schäfer, W., Claviez, M., Frank, H., Hunsmann, G., Moennig, V., Schwarz, H., Thiel, H. J., Bolognesi, D. P., Green, R. W., Langlois, A. J., Fischinger, P. J., and de Noronha, F., 1976, Mammalian C-type oncornaviruses. Relationships between structural virus and cell surface antigens and their possible significance in immunological defense mechanisms, in: *Comparative Leukemia Research 1976* (J. Clemmensen, ed.), pp. 88–96, Karger, Basel.

Schwarz, H., Hunsmann, G., Moennig, V., and Schäfer, W., 1976, Properties of mouse leukemia viruses. XI. Immunoelectron microscopic studies on viral structural antigens on the cell surface, *Virology* 69:169–178.

Scolnick, E. M., Parks, W. P., Todaro, G. J., and Aaronson, S. A., 1972, Immunological characterization of primate C-type virus reverse transcriptases, *Nature (London) New Biol.* 235:35–40.

Seifert, E., Claviez, M., Frank, H., Hunsmann, G., Schwarz, H., and Schäfer, W., 1975, Properties of mouse leukemia viruses. XII. Produktion grösserer Mengen von Friend-Virus durch eine permanente Zell-Suspensions-Kultur (Eveline-Suspensions-Zellen), *Z. Naturforsch.* 30c:698–700.

Sherr, C. J., Fedele, L. A., Benveniste, R. E., and Todaro, G. J., 1975, Interspecies antigenic determinants of the reverse transcriptases and p30 proteins of mammalian type C viruses, *J. Virol.* 15:1440–1448.

Strand, M., and August, J. T., 1974, Structural proteins of mammalian oncogenic RNA viruses: Multiple antigenic determinants of the major internal protein and envelope glycoprotein, *J. Virol.* 13:171–180.

Strand, M., and August, J. T., 1975, Structural proteins of mammalian RNA tumor viruses: Relatedness of the interspecies antigenic determinants of the major internal protein, *J. Virol.* 15:1332–1341.

Strand, M., Wilsnack, R., and August, J. T., 1974, Structural proteins of mammalian oncogenic RNA viruses: Immunological characterization of the p15 polypeptide of Rauscher murine virus, *J. Virol.* **14**:1575–1583.

Tronick, S. R., Stephenson, J. R., and Aaronson, S. A., 1973, Immunological characterization of a low molecular weight polypeptide of murine leukemia virus, *Virology* **54**:199–206.

Tung, J.-S., Vitetta, E., Fleissner, E., and Boyse, E. A., 1975, Biochemical evidence linking the $G_1 x$ thymocyte surface antigen to the gp69/71 envelope glycoprotein of murine leukemia virus, *J. Exp. Med.* **141**:198–205.

Witter, R., Frank, H., Moennig, V., Hunsmann, G., Lange, J., and Schäfer, W., 1973*a*, Properties of mouse leukemia viruses. IV. Hemagglutination assay and characterization of hemagglutinating surface components, *Virology* **54**:330–345.

Witter, R., Hunsmann, G., Lange, J., and Schäfer, W., 1973*b*, Properties of mouse leukemia viruses. V. Hemagglutination-inhibition and indirect hemagglutination tests, *Virology* **54**:346–358.

Yoshiki, T., Mellors, R. C., Hardy, Jr., W. D., and Fleissner, E., 1974, Common cell surface antigen associated with mammalian C-type RNA viruses, *J. Exp. Med.* **139**:925–942.

Zinkernagel, R. M., and Doherty, P. C., 1975, H-2 compatibility requirement for T-cell-mediated lysis of target cells infected with lymphocytic choriomeningitis virus. Different cytotoxic T-cell specificities are associated with structures coded for in H-2K or H-2D, *J. Exp. Med.* **141**:427–436.

Chapter 5

Natural Immunity to Endogenous Oncornaviruses in Mice

James N. Ihle and M. G. Hanna, Jr.

Basic Research Program
NCI Frederick Cancer Research Center
Frederick, Maryland 21701

I. INTRODUCTION

Murine C-type viruses have been etiologically linked to spontaneous leuke-mias in mice (Gross, 1951). These viruses are endogenous in mice and are vertically transmitted (Huebner and Todaro, 1969; Rowe *et al.*, 1971; Aaronson *et al.*, 1971). A number of biologically distinguishable C-type viruses occur naturally in various strains of mice. Ecotropic viruses, which include the AKR or Gross-type viruses, are capable of replicating in mouse cells. These viruses have been further differentiated by their preference for replication in various mouse cells into N- or B-tropic viruses (Pincus *et al.*, 1971), although by hybridization experiments the N and B viruses are closely related (Callahan *et al.*, 1974). Xenotropic viruses are characterized by their ability to replicate in cells of other species (Levy, 1973). Two groups of xenotropic viruses have been identified by serological techniques (Stephenson *et al.*, 1974) and by hybridization experi-ments (Callahan *et al.*, 1975). The xenotropic viruses are only partially related to the ecotropic viruses, as determined by hybridization (Callahan *et al.*, 1974), and to date have not been implicated in any spontaneous neoplasia of mice.

The expression of endogenous leukemia viruses can be detected in most strains of mice. In high leukemic strains, such as AKR, virus expression and infectious virus can be detected throughout life, and increase with age (Rowe and Pincus, 1972). Genetic crosses of AKR mice with low lymphoma strains have demonstrated a correlation between virus expression and the incidence of spontaneous leukemias (Meier *et al.*, 1973; Lilly *et al.*, 1975). Strains such as

BALB/c have low or nondetectable levels of virus expression early in life, and have moderate levels of lymphoma late in life. The level of virus expression in this strain increases with age until, at the age of 18–24 months, 60% of the animals are virus positive (Peters *et al.*, 1972). Some strains of mice, such as the NIH/Swiss, SWR/J, and 129, show levels of incomplete virus expression, but have never yielded infectious ecotropic virus.

A number of genetic loci have been identified which influence virus expression. The *Fv-1* locus, defined initially by Lilly and Pincus (1973), has been extensively examined and appears to influence the ability of N- or B-tropic endogenous viruses to infect and replicate. The *Fv-1* gene product can be identified in cellular extracts (Tennant, 1974) but has not been completely characterized. Rowe (1972) has worked extensively on the genetics of virus expression in AKR mice and has defined two loci, *Akv-1* and *Akv-2*. *Akv-1* has been mapped on chromosome 7, and in recent experiments has been shown to be the genetic locus of at least a portion of the viral genome (Chattopadhyay *et al.*, 1975). *Akv-2* is felt to be a second identical locus of the viral genome, although this has not been substantiated.

It had initially been suggested that mice are immunologically tolerant to the endogenous C-type viruses because of the widespread occurrence of these viruses and their spontaneous expression, particularly in fetal tissues (Old *et al.*, 1968; Huebner *et al.*, 1971). However, other investigators postulated that there was a lack of immunological tolerance because of the chronic deposition of immune complexes in kidneys of mice from NZB (Mellors *et al.*, 1971), AKR (Oldstone *et al.*, 1972), RFM (Hanna *et al.*, 1973; Clapp and Yuhas, 1973), and B6C3F$_1$ strains of mice (Ihle *et al.*, 1973; Batzing *et al.*, 1974). Two of these studies also noted an inverse correlation of immune complex nephritis and lymphoid neoplasia (Hanna *et al.*, 1973; Clapp and Yuhas, 1973), suggesting that an immune response to endogenous leukemia viruses may be involved in the regulation of spontaneous leukemias and radiation-induced leukemias. Reactivity of antibodies with specificity for the virion reverse transcriptase has also been suggested from studies of kidney eluates of AKR mice (Hollis *et al.*, 1974). Similarly, the detection of widespread neutralizing activity in sera from normal mice has been correlated with a specific immune response (Aaronson and Stephenson, 1974), although recent evidence suggests that this neutralization is not due to a classical immunoglobulin (Levy *et al.*, 1975). Other recent results have suggested that natural cell-mediated immunity to antigens associated with endogenous murine leukemia viruses may exist (Hirsch *et al.*, 1975).

During the past 3 years, our laboratory has concentrated on the analysis of the natural humoral immune response to endogenous C-type virus in mice. This report is an overall synopsis of our results and interpretations regarding the functional role of autogenous immunity to endogenous MuLV AKR and the possible correlation of this host response to virus-mediated pathogenesis.

II. WIDESPREAD OCCURRENCE OF NATURAL ANTIBODIES TO MuLV

The existence of antibodies in mice, specific for endogenous leukemia viruses, was first clearly demonstrated with a sensitive and quantitative radio-immune precipitation assay (Ihle *et al.*, 1973). The techniques were comparable to those initially used to detect antibodies against polio virus (Gerloff *et al.*, 1962), except for the use of [³H] leucine-labeled C-type viruses. The assay and a discussion of the factors which influence it have been published (Ihle *et al.*, 1973). The most important consideration, however, is the purity and integrity of the radioactively labeled virus. In general, banded and/or rebanded viruses purified after *in vivo* labeling have been used. Attempts to use viruses iodinated *in vitro* have generally been unsuccessful due to the degradation of the virus. Virus preparations which have been frozen-thawed more than once have not been used.

The specificity of the assay has also been examined (Ihle *et al.*, 1973) and is further demonstrated by the results shown in Fig. 1. For these experiments, a

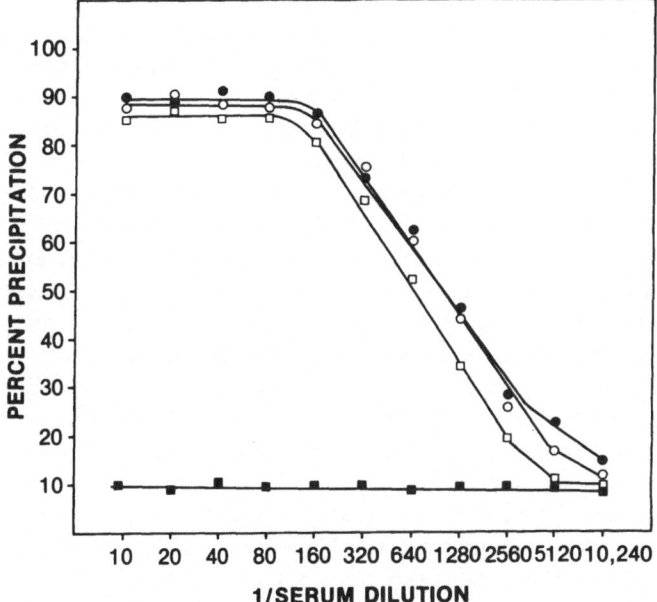

Fig. 1. Radioimmune precipitation assays of B6C3F₁ sera. Sera from 1.5-year B6C3F₁ were titered against labeled AKR MuLV. •, Normal sera; ■, sera absorbed with AKR MuLV; ○, sera absorbed with mammary tumor virus; ◻, immunoglobulins prepared from these sera. Normal rabbit and hamster sera were titered as control sera and yield curves comparable to ■.

pool of serum derived from B6C3F$_1$ [(C57BL/6 × C3H/Anf)F$_1$] mice and a [^{3}H] leucine-labeled virus, purified from a clone of AKR mouse embryo fibroblasts which spontaneously activated virus replication, was used. The titer of this serum, which is defined as the reciprocal of the serum dilution giving 50% precipitation of the labeled virus, is approximately 1280. In contrast, sera from other species, including normal rabbit and hamster sera, fail to precipitate any virus. Total immunoglobulins prepared by 50% ammonium sulfate precipitation retain all the activity of the serum. The specificity for C-type viruses is indicated by the ability to absorb all the precipitating activity with AKR C-type viruses but not with purified mouse mammary tumor virus. Consequently, these techniques provide a quantitative and sensitive assay for the presence of antibodies specific for C-type viruses.

Using this assay, Ihle *et al.* (1973) and Nowinski and Kaehler (1974) examined a variety of strains of mice for antibodies specific for the AKR virus. Typical results are shown in Table I. When titers are examined for strain and age, considerable variation is seen in a number of parameters of the response. Optimal titers for a particular strain are usually observed by approximately 1 year of age. Several strains, such as AKR, NIH/Swiss, and SWR/J, have very low titers or no titers against this virus throughout life. In contrast, strains such as STU and an F$_1$ hybrid, B6C3F$_1$, have high titers. A number of strains, such as C57BL/6 and C3H/Anf, have intermediate titers.

Many factors contribute to the differences in the titers among strains. Since the radioimmune precipitation assay measures free antibodies, the titers may be a function of the level of virus burden. In particular, previous studies have shown the existence of antibodies specific for C-type virus in kidneys of AKR mice (Batzing *et al.*, 1974), demonstrating that, even in strains having continuously high levels of virus expression, no immunological tolerance exists. Therefore, the failure to detect titrable antibodies in this strain is probably a consequence of persistant viremia. This is compatible with the observation that, in general, leukemic animals have low or nondetectable levels of free antibody. Strains such as NIH/Swiss, SWR/J, and 129 also have either extremely low titers or no demonstrable antibodies. In contrast to the AKR strain, these mice lack an endogenous, ecotropic virus, which accounts for the lack of immune stimulation and thus antibody. This is substantiated by the observation that immunization of these mice with formalinized MuLV vaccines induces a strong humoral immune response. These data also suggest that expression of the ecotropic endogenous virus is required for an immune response, as discussed in greater detail below.

The variations that occur among those strains which have demonstrable antibody levels may be linked to the relative levels of endogenous virus expression or may be caused by other factors, such as a genetically defined immune response to viral antigens. To establish the basis of these variations, spleens from

Table I. Strain and Age Distribution of Natural Antibodies to Endogenous Ecotropic Leukemia Virus

Strain	Radioimmune precipitation titers						Tumor-bearing animals
Months of age:	0–3	3–6	6–9	9–12	12–18	18–24	
(C57BL/6 × C3H/An)F$_1$	0–640[a]	640–1280	640–1280	640–1280	1280–5120	1280	
STU	–	640–1280	–	5120–10240			0
AKR/J	0–40	0–40	0–40	0–40	–	–	
RF	0–80	0–320	80–320	80–320	–	–	
BALB/c	0–160	0–160	160–640	160–640			
C57BL/6	0–160	160–640	320–1280	320–1280	–	–	
C3H/An	0–160	0–160	160–640	160–640	–	–	
129	–	0–80	–	0–80		–	
SWR/J	–	0–80	–	0–80			
NIH	–	0–80	–	0–80	–		
(BALB/c × DBA/2)F$_1$	0–320	–	320–640	320–640	320–640	320–640	0

[a]Titers were determined by radioimmune precipitation assay with [³H]leucine-labeled AKR virus from individual serum samples and pooled sera.

individual mice of known antibody titers were examined for the level of virion p30 by competition radioimmunoassays. These experiments have demonstrated that different strains of mice may have very comparable spleen levels of p30, but have significant differences in titers of antiviral antibodies. However, among the strains examined, mice that developed an autogenous immune response have generally higher levels of p30 than mice that do not have antibodies. Therefore, there appears to be a relationship between the amount of virus expression, as detected by competition radioimmune precipitation assays for p30, and the induction of an immunological response. However, little correlation is apparent between this expression and the ultimate antiviral titer in these strains.

The possibility that genetic factors control the immune response of mice to virion proteins has been suggested by Lilly (1966, 1972), Lilly and Pincus (1973), and Lilly et al. (1975). This work has defined a genetic locus, *Rgv-1*, which influences susceptibility to Gross virus infection and which has been mapped in the H-2 region. *Rgv-1* may be identical or related to the *Ir-1* gene function controlling the immune response to various antigens. The characteristics of the *Rgv-1* locus are compatible with an immune function; its influence is most striking at intermediate levels of virus expression and can only be demonstrated *in vivo*. This is in contrast to the *Fv-1* function and *Akv-1* and *Akv-2*. Experiments are currently in progress to further examine this possibility. These data should be significant in terms of defining the *Rgv-1* function and examining the influence of an immune response to regulate leukemia-virus-induced pathogenesis.

The age-dependent differences in antibody titer have several significant characteristics and implications. In general, antibody titers in all strains are initially low after birth, and these antibodies are maternally derived (Ihle et al., 1973; Nowinski and Kaehler, 1974). These antibodies are observed only in neonates from virus-positive, antibody-positive females, and their presence is highly dependent on the age of the mother. The influence of maternal antibody on virus expression in several strains is currently being examined. After the neonatal period, the development of antibody appears to be related to the expression of the endogenous virus. This is emphasized in Fig. 2, which shows the results of experiments in which individual animals were examined, according to age, for the presence of antiviral antibodies. The most striking observation is the age and rate differences among strains at which the mice develop an immune response to the virus. Strains such as C57BL/6 and BALB/c are generally negative until late in life. In contrast, the F_1 hybrid, B6C3F$_1$, and C3H/Anf develop antibody titers early in life. These observations as noted above are consistent with the observation that an antibody response occurs as a consequence of virus expression, although more extensive examination is needed to definitively relate the initiation of antibody production to the expression of virus. These data also suggest that the immune response can be used as a very

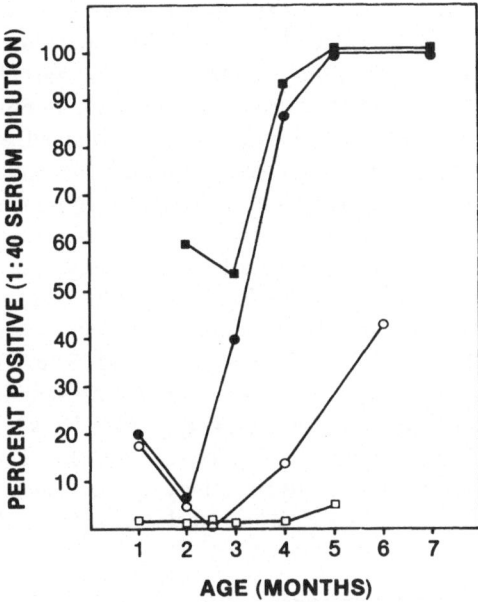

Fig. 2. Age dependence of antibody appearance.
Sera were obtained from male mice of various
strains at the indicated ages and were reacted with
labeled AKR MuLV at a dilution of 1:40. Sera
were considered positive if greater than 15% of the
labeled virus was precipitated. The strains examined included C3H/Anf (■), B6C3F$_1$ (●), C57BL/6
(○), and BALB/c (□).

sensitive measure of *virus expression* independent of more time-consuming
assays which measure infectious virus.

III. CHARACTERIZATION OF THE IMMUNE RESPONSE

The efficiency of an immune response might be dependent on a number of
factors other than quantitative differences. Therefore, it becomes imperative to
characterize the immune response with respect to the specific viral antigens
involved, as well as the immunoglobulin specificity of these reactions. The
techniques used have been described in detail (Ihle *et al.*, 1974). Briefly,
[^{3}H] leucine-labeled virions are disrupted with detergent and high salt, diluted to
reduce salt and detergent concentrations, and reacted with the test sera. Immune
complexes are precipitated with an antiglobulin, washed, disrupted with a buffer

containing sodium dodecyl sulfate (SDS), and analyzed by polyacrylamide gel electrophoresis. Detailed adherence to the published procedure is required, since considerable aggregation of virion protein can occur, particularly at elevated temperatures, which gives rise to spurious results. Also, unless viruses are grown in cells of the species from which the serum is obtained, similar artifactual results can be observed. The latter results presumably reflect a nonspecific heterophile immune-type reaction to normal cellular components on the virion acquired during budding from the cell.

The results of the immune precipitation assay using normal B6C3F$_1$ serum from 1-year-old animals are shown in Fig. 3. With this sera, gel profiles having radioactive peaks at positions corresponding to molecular weights of 68,000, 43,000, and 15,000 have been consistently observed. The 68,000 and 43,000 molecular weight components can be labeled with glucosamine and correspond to the virion glycoproteins, gp71 and gp43 (Ihle *et al.*, 1974). The specificity of these reactions has been examined in a variety of ways (Ihle *et al.*, 1974). Figure 4 further confirms the results of this specificity by showing competition experiments using monospecific antisera. When labeled virions are disrupted, reacted

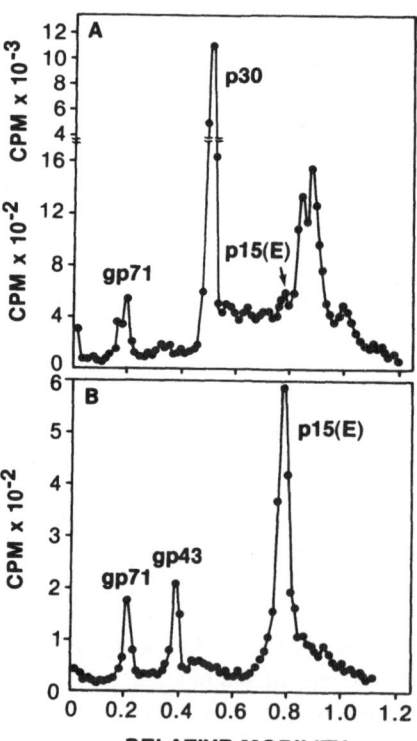

Fig. 3. Immune precipitation of disrupted labeled AKR MuLV. Sera from 1.5-year B6C3F$_1$ mice were reacted at a 1:20 dilution with 2 × 10^5 cpm of disrupted labeled AKR MuLV in 0.2 ml. The immune complexes were precipitated with an antiglobulin serum and the precipitates were electrophoresed on SDS polyacrylamide gels (B). In A, the profile obtained with the disrupted virus is shown for comparison.

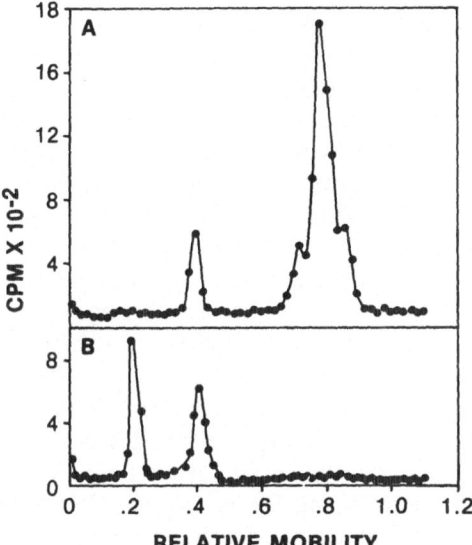

Fig. 4. Immune precipitation competitions with labeled AKR MuLV. Sera from B6C3F₁ mice were reacted with labeled AKR MuLV as in Fig. 3, except that a 1:50 dilution of antisera to Friend MuLV gp71 (A) or p15(E) (B) was reacted with the disrupted virus 1 hr at 37°C prior to the addition of the normal mouse sera.

with monospecific rabbit antiserum to gp71, and then reacted with B6C3F₁ serum followed by rabbit anti-mouse γ-globulin serum, the resulting immune precipitates contain only p15(E) and gp43. Similarly, competition with a monospecific rabbit antiserum to p15(E) specifically blocks precipitation of the 15,000 molecular weight component. These results demonstrate that the 68,000 molecular weight component is gp71 and that the 15,000 molecular weight component is p15(E). Furthermore, the results suggest that each virion component is precipitated as a distinct antigen, not as a complex.

The existence of gp43 has been somewhat ambiguous. Polyacrylamide gel profiles of disrupted virions generally lack a gp43 component. Consequently, the appearance of a gp43 in immune precipitates may have been considered to be a breakdown of gp71. The above competition experiments, however, are not consistent with this hypothesis and the lack of competition for precipitation of gp43 by antisera to gp71 suggests that this is a serologically *unique* virion glycoprotein. The basis of the inability to observe gp43 on SDS polyacrylamide gels appears to be due to aggregation. In particular, profiles obtained with disrupted [³H]glucosamine-labeled virus characteristically have a major peak at

68,000 molecular weight, a peak migrating with the dye, and considerable radioactivity which does not enter the gel. The radioactivity migrating with the dye can be removed by acetone precipitation of the virus prior to electrophoresis and presumably represents a glycolipid fraction. Similar profiles have also been observed after treating the virus with other disrupting agents such as urea or guanidine hydrochloride. Curiously, however, immune precipitation with B6C3F$_1$ serum has consistently given profiles with little radioactivity at the top of the gel and a peak at 43,000 molecular weight. It is therefore felt that gp43, although a unique glycoprotein, normally exists as an aggregate and, consequently, does not migrate into the gel. This aggregate may correspond to a glycoprotein fraction with a molecular weight of 100,000 as detected by gel filtration in guanidine hydrochloride (Nowinski et al., 1972).

The p15(E) component observed in immune precipitates with normal mouse sera has been shown by the previously mentioned data, as well as by additional experiments (Ihle et al., 1975b), to correspond to the p15(E) protein purified by Schäfer et al. (1975) from Friend leukemia virus. This polypeptide has been demonstrated to be a virion envelope component common to a number of mammalian C-type viruses. Serological analysis has revealed a high degree of cross-reactivity of this component among these viruses. Strand et al. (1974) have also described the purification of a p15 virion component from Rauscher virus. A number of important characteristics indicate that this protein is unique from p15(E). The Rauscher p15 is an internal virion component, although it may be expressed on the cell surface of infected cells. This antigen also appears to be type specific and probably is the FMR type-specific antigen previously described by cytotoxicity assays (Strand et al., 1974). The difference in these antigens is further suggested by the studies of Ikeda et al. (1975) which have shown the coexistence of p15 and p15(E) in a number of viruses and have emphasized the commonality of the p15(E) component.

The specific immune response to the viral glycoprotein is of particular importance. Structurally, this component is the major virion envelope component detected by lactoperoxidase iodination of intact virions (Witte et al., 1973). It is also expressed as a cell-surface component of infected and/or transformed cells (discussed below). Consistent with these observations, heterologous antisera to this component have been shown to have high neutralizing activities against the virus (Steeves et al., 1974) and are cytotoxic to cells replicating the virus (Grant et al., 1974). These observations provide a spectrum of biological activities associated with an immune response to this component, but as noted later, are not always manifested in autogenous immune sera.

Although the preceding techniques provide a method to measure immunological reactions to the virus and provide an indirect way of determining the specificity of the immune response, it is obviously desirable to confirm these reactions by radioimmune precipitation assays of purified proteins. Attempts to titer natural sera against purified, iodinated p15(E) from Friend leukemia virus have been made; however, no significant precipitation has been obtained thus far. Failure in this attempt could be due to destruction of the confirmational properties of the protein required for immunoprecipitation by natural sera by purification of the antigen by repeated chromatography in guanidine hydrochloride. Furthermore, this component tends to aggregate; thus the immune precipitation assays are run in deoxycholate, which could similarly interfere with recognition.

The reaction of autogenous immune sera with purified gp71 from Rauscher and AKR virus is shown in Fig. 5. Sera from $B6C3F_1$ mice have a high titer against the AKR MuLV gp71 and a low titer against Rauscher MuLV gp71. Comparable results have also been obtained with autogenous immune sera from other strains of mice (Ihle *et al.*, 1976*b*). The type specificity of these autogenous immune sera for the AKR MuLV gp71 suggests that the virus inducing

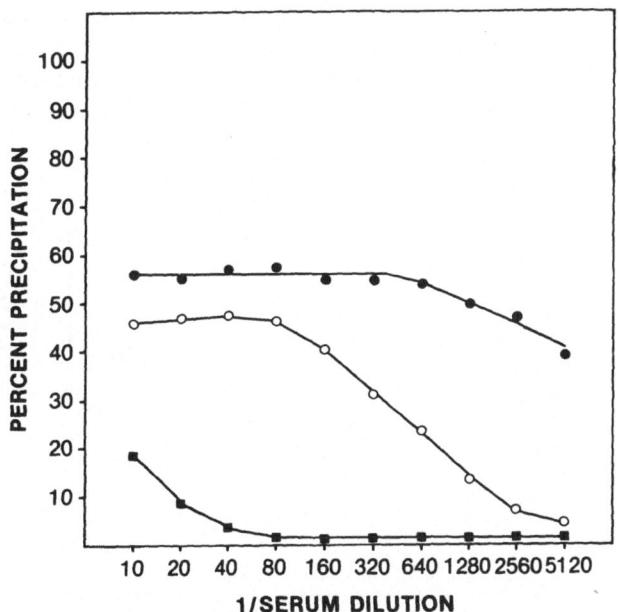

Fig. 5. Titration of $B6C3F_1$ sera against MuLV glycoproteins. Sera from 1.5-year $B6C3F_1$ mice were reacted with ^{125}I-labeled AKR MuLV gp71 (o) or ^{125}I-labeled Rauscher MuLV gp69/71 (■) in direct radioimmune precipitation assays. For comparison is shown the titration curve of a rabbit antiserum to purified Rauscher MuLV gp71 against labeled AKR MuLV gp71 (●).

the autogenous immune response *in vivo* is more closely related to the AKR MuLV and furthermore emphasizes the serological differences in the glyco- proteins of MuLV (Ihle *et al.*, 1976*b*).

An understanding of the function of the immune response is also dependent on knowing the relative contributions of each of the immunological reactions. Since a comparison of titers by direct titration of each purified protein is not possible, an indirect method has to be used. Briefly, autogenous immune sera were reacted with disrupted virions at various concentrations. The amount of each antigen precipitated was determined from SDS polyacrylamide gel electro- phoresis profiles. The results of these determinations are shown in Fig. 6. The titer of this sera is predominantly against gp71, lower against p15(E), and rela- tively weak against gp43. These data provide a relative measure of the specific antigenic titers and further suggest that the reactions observed are immunologi- cally specific and distinct.

The results described above were obtained with normal sera from B6C3F$_1$ mice. However, the antigenic specificity of the autogenous immune response appears to be conserved in a variety of other strains of mice. In particular, STU, C57BL/6, C3H, and BALB/c have given comparable results to those obtained with B6C3F$_1$ mice. Similarly, when NIH mice were immunized with a formalin- ized AKR virus vaccine and their immune response was characterized, only

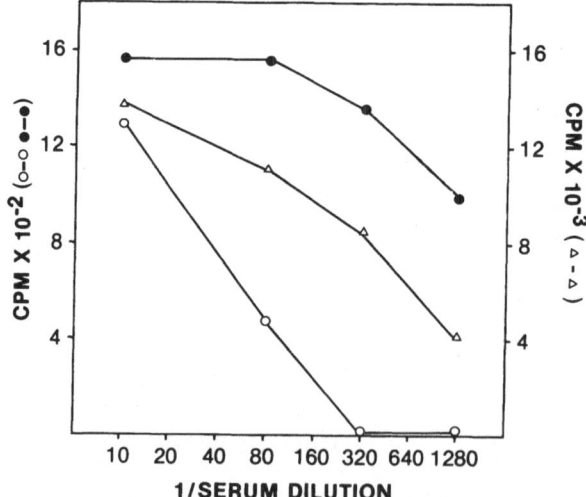

Fig. 6. Titration of B6C3F$_1$ sera against various viral antigens. Sera from 1.5-year B6C3F$_1$ mice were reacted with disrupted labeled ARK MuLV as in Fig. 3 at the dilutions indicated. Immune precipitates were subsequently electrophoresed on SDS polyacrylamide gels and the radioactivity in peaks corre- sponding to gp71 (●), gp43 (○), and p15(E) (△) was determined and plotted here relative to the serum dilution.

reactions with gp71, gp43, and p15(E) were observed (Lee *et al.*, in preparation). Therefore, the recognition of these viral antigens is a consistent feature of the immune response of mice to the expression of endogenous virus or to immunization of mice with this virus.

The antibody specificity of the immune response of B6C3F$_1$ mice to the AKR virus has also been examined (Lee *et al.*, 1974). When 19 S and 7 S immunoglobulins were purified from pooled sera by ammonium sulfate precipitation and chromatography on DEAE-cellulose and G-200 Sephadex, both fractions were found to have precipitating activity against the AKR virus. The results shown in Fig. 7 were obtained when these immunoglobulin fractions were reacted with disrupted virus to determine the antigenic specificity. The 19 S fraction, like the whole serum, specifically precipitated gp71, gp43, and p15. In contrast, the 7 S immunoglobulin fraction precipitated only the p15(E) component. These differences do not appear to be due to quantitative differences in the immunoglobulin fractions because the specific immunoglobulins were quantitated by radial diffusion, and the concentrations used were comparable to

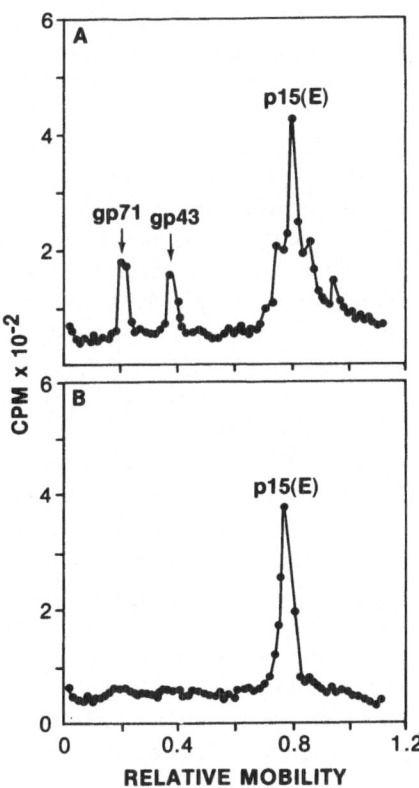

Fig. 7. Immune precipitation of disrupted labeled AKR MuLV by purified immunoglobulin fractions of 1.5-year B6C3F$_1$ sera. Sera were fractionated into the 19 S (A) and 7 S (B) components and reacted with disrupted labeled AKR MuLV and electrophoresed on SDS polyacrylamide gels as in Fig. 3.

those used with whole serum. Furthermore, by radioimmune titration against the intact virus, both fractions had significant titers. This observation suggests that reactivity in general was not lost during purification, although this does not rule out the loss of immunoglobulin reactivity of a specific type. The specificity of the immunoglobulins was also examined with respect to age and was found to be identical in 12-week-, 1.5-year-, and 2.5-year-old mice.

In contrast to the above results when 19 S and 7 S immunoglobulin fractions were titered against purified and iodinated AKR MuLV gp71, both had significant titers. Under the conditions described the 7 S and 19 S titers were approximately 1:160 and 1:40, respectively, relative to initial serum concentrations. The basis for the discrepancy in the apparent immunoglobulin specificity is not known; however, it has been our experience that immune precipitation of disrupted labeled virions can be influenced by many factors and the results must be interpreted with caution. Although the possibility does exist that the 7 S reactivity with the purified protein is a consequence of an alteration of the antigen during purification, this does not appear to be the case. Recent results with a sensitive neutralization assay have demonstrated significant neutralization of AKR MuLV with purified 7 S immunoglubulins, which can be abrogated with purified AKR MuLV gp71 (J.N. Ihle and B. Lazar, in preparation). These results further suggest that 7 S immunoglobulins can interact with gp71 on the virion surface and effect neutralization. Interestingly, in this assay, although 19 S immunoglobulins reacted to a limited extent with AKR MuLV gp71, they did not mediate neutralization. Because of these results we presently feel that both 19 S and 7 S reactivity against the viral antigens gp71 and p15(E) exist.

The significance of the immunological specificities in terms of the viral antigens recognized is not known. In other virus systems, however, distinct differences have been observed between IgM and IgG responses to viral antigens. Schmidt et al. (1968) have shown that 19 S antibodies to Coxsackie virus reacted in a type-specific manner with the major virion antigens, whereas 7 S antibodies reacted in a group-specific manner. Similar results have been obtained for a myxovirus (Heffner and Schluderberg, 1967), although the type specificity of 19 S has not been observed in other systems (Webster, 1968). In this regard, the 19 S and 7 S response of mice to gp71 appears to be highly type-specific. This has been indicated by the precipitation of iodinated glycoproteins from AKR and Rauscher virus as described below. In addition, the antibody specificity appears to be significant in defining the neutralizing potential of the serum. In general, neutralizing efficiency of antibodies appears to be related to their avidity, which is dependent on the affinity of the combining sites, the number of binding sites, and other confirmational characteristics of the antigen, antibody, and antigen–antibody complex (Blank et al., 1972). Presumably one or all of these characteristics are responsible for the 7 S response to AKR virus gp71 to preferentially mediate neutralization of virus infectivity.

IV. VIRUS SPECIFICITY

A number of biologically and serologically distinct murine leukemia viruses have been identified. Thus it becomes necessary to determine to which virus or group of viruses the autogenous immune response is directed. The ability of autogenous immune sera to cross-react among a number of these viruses has been examined (Lee and Ihle, 1975). Typical results are shown in Fig. 8. When sera from normal 1.5-year-old B6C3F$_1$ mice are reacted with [^{3}H] leucine-labeled Friend, Rauscher, or BALB:virus-2 by immune precipitation, titration curves are observed comparable to those obtained with the AKR virus. These results suggest a broad cross-reactivity of autogenous immune sera in terms of the viruses examined. In contrast, these same sera have no reactivity against C-type viruses isolated from other species, including the rat leukemia virus or RD-114 virus.

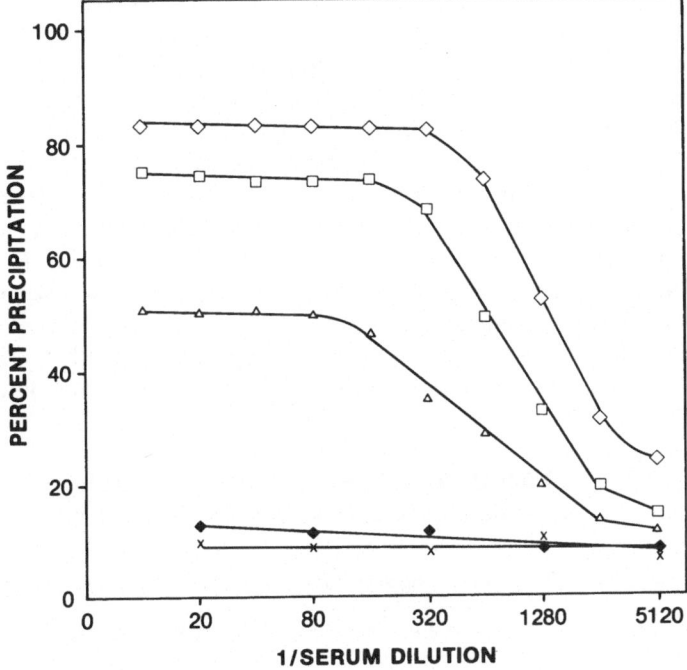

Fig. 8. Reactivity of B6C3F$_1$ sera with various C-type viruses. Sera from 1.5-year B6C3F$_1$ mice were titered against [^{3}H] leucine-labeled Friend (□), Rauscher (◊), BALB:virus-2 (△), RD-114 (♦), or rat leukemia (×) viruses.

The antigenic and immunoglobulin specificities of B6C3F$_1$ sera have also been examined against these various viruses (Lee and Ihle, 1975). Using disrupted [^{3}H] leucine-labeled BALB:virus-2, Rasucher, or Moloney virus, these sera reacted with gp71, gp43, and p15(E) as detected by SDS polyacrylamide gel electrophoresis of the immune precipitates. Comparable amounts of each protein were precipitated from the various viruses at high serum concentrations with the exception of p15(E) from Balb:virus-2. The virion component appears to be quantitatively reduced in the virion relative to the other major components. Similar to the results obtained with the AKR virus, autogenous immune sera had 19 S reactivities against gp71, gp43, and p15(E) and 7 S specificity for the p15 (E) component. These results suggested that at high serum concentrations the various leukemia virus isolates have common antigenic determinants that are recognized by these natural immune sera in an immunologically specific manner. However, as discussed above, direct radioimmunoassays with the purified gp71 from Rauscher and AKR virus demonstrated a strong preference of autogenous immune sera for the glycoprotein from AKR MuLV.

The above results demonstrate a commonality of the natural immune response to all C-type viruses, but fail to distinguish between possible weak cross-reactivity and/or similar but distinct immunological responses. These questions have been approached by using a series of competition and absorption experiments to better define the specificity in terms of virus type. The results of some of these experiments are summarized in Table II. When limiting dilutions of B6C3F$_1$ sera are reacted with [^{3}H] leucine-labeled virus in the presence of increasing amounts of unlabeled virus, antibody precipitation of the labeled virus is progressively competed for by the unlabeled virus. Clearly, this competition is measuring the predominant immunological reactivity, presumably to gp71 as indicated above. Given this limitation, this assay can provide a measure of the specificity of the natural immune response.

Table II shows the micrograms of competing virus required to effect 20% competition of the various labeled viruses. In the homologous reactions, gener-

Table II. Type Specificity of B6C3F$_1$ Serum: Competition Radioimmune Assays with Intact Virions

Competition against	Competing virus (μg of virus required for 20% competition)			
	Rauscher	Friend	AKR	BALB:virus-2
Friend	1.56	1.56	6.25	>200
AKR	100	>200	0.39	200
BALB:virus-2	>200	>200	45	0.78

ally 0.2–1.5 µg of virus is required for 20% competition. These numbers may vary slightly because of such parameters as specific activity of the radioactive virus, serum concentrations used, or the integrity and purity of the competing virus. When B6C3F$_1$ sera are reacted with [^{3}H] Friend virus, then Friend, Rauscher, and AKR viruses can significantly inhibit at relatively low virus concentrations. In contrast, only the AKR virus can compete significantly for precipitation of labeled AKR virus. Lastly, only BALB:virus-2 competes significantly for precipitation of labeled BALB:virus-2, although AKR at a hundredfold higher levels can compete. The results with BALB:virus-2 precipitation, however, must be considered tentative since this virus is replicating in a heterologous cell, the unique cellular, but not viral, antigens of which could contribute to these results. Nevertheless, the inability of BALB:virus-2 to compete does demonstrate that it does not carry antigens common to the ecotropic viruses. The sum of these results suggests that natural antibodies exist in B6C3F$_1$ that are clearly directed against the AKR ecotropic virus. This antibody population can cross-react with Friend and Rauscher type viruses, but is not specifically directed against this group of viruses. Furthermore, the basis of this cross-reactivity is not primarily through the glycoproteins, as indicated by the results of direct radioimmunoassays, but rather appears to be primarily via the antibodies directed against p15(E) (Ihle *et al.*, 1976*b*). The results also suggest that specific antibodies may exist directed against the xenotropic virus which may or may not cross-react with the ecotropic virus. This antibody population, however, does not appear to be able to cross-react with the Friend or Rauscher virus. These conclusions are further supported by absorption experiments summarized in Table III. Compatible with the above results, absorption of B6C3F$_1$ serum with Rauscher or Friend virus completely removes precipitating antibodies for

Table III. Type Specificity of B6C3F$_1$ Serum: Absorption Experiments

Serum titered against	Titer of virus: absorbed serum by radioimmunoassay				
	BALB:virus-2	AKR	Rauscher	Friend	–
AKR	1:1280[a]	1:80	1:1280	1:1280	1:1280
Friend	1:640	1:80	1:80	1:80	1:640
BALB:virus-2	1:40	1:80	1:80	1:80	1:80

[a]Sera were absorbed with 1 mg of the respective virus 45 min at 37°C and 45 min at 4°C. The virus was subsequently pelleted by centrifugation (106,000*g*, 30 min) and the absorbed sera were assayed by radioimmune precipitation assays against the respective [^{3}H] leucine-labeled virus.

Friend virus but not for BALB:virus-2 or AKR. In contrast, absorption with AKR virus completely removes the activity against Friend, Rauscher, or AKR virus, but not against BALB:virus-2. These results strongly suggest that, in this strain of mice, specific antibodies exist for the ecotropic viruses. Obviously, with this knowledge, one can begin to look at virus expression in the host as manifested by the autogenous immune response to distinct endogenous viruses.

V. AUTOGENOUS HUMORAL RESPONSE TO VIRUS-INDUCED CELL-SURFACE ANTIGENS

The preceding results have demonstrated significant natural immunological responses to virion envelope antigens. Of particular significance to the general area of leukemia-specific tumor immunology is the relationship of these antibodies to tumor-specific cell-surface antigens. Although the virion-specific envelope antigens have been extensively characterized biochemically, distinct virus-specific proteins unique to or shared with the cell surface have not been thoroughly examined. In contrast, the majority of the cell-surface antigens have been defined by complex heterologous antisera with unknown specificities. We have approached these questions by examining the distribution of known virion envelope proteins on the cell surface using the techniques of immunoelectron microscopy and employing monospecific heterologous antisera. The results of some of these experiments are summarized in Table IV.

These results demonstrate that, in terms of the virion envelope proteins recognized by autogenous immune sera, only gp71 is consistently observed on the cell surface using a variety of leukemia cell lines. Curiously, however, autogenous immune sera, which have specificity for gp71, fail to react with the

Table IV. Activity of Rabbit Immune Sera Against Murine Leukemia Cell Lines[a]

Serum	EδG2		K-36		EL-4		FLC-745	
	VISA	VEA	VISA	VEA	VISA	VEA	VISA	VEA
Anti-gp71	+++	+++	+++	+++	+++	+++	+++	+++
Anti-p30	+++	−	−	−	−	−	−	−
Anti-p15	−	+++	−	+++	−	+++	−	+++
B6C3F$_1$	−	+++	−	+++	ND		ND	

[a]Immunoferritin labeling of leukemia cell lines. Triple plus signs indicate an average of six to eight ferritin-positive sites/cell perimeter scored on more than 75% positive virions. A minus sign indicates less than two ferritin-labeled sites/cell perimeter or less than 10% positive virions. ND, Not determined. Immunological labeling was with unfixed cells.

cell surface, although they consistently react with the virion surface. This observation suggests that the antigenic specificity of this sera is perhaps unique and restricted in the antigenic determinants recognized. This hypothesis is supported by the observation that heterologous antisera to gp71 have a significantly lower titer against the cell surface than against the virion as detected by immunoelectron microscopy. The relative relationship of the titers of interspecies versus group-specific reactivities suggests that, on the cell surface, the group or interspecies type of antigenic determinants are predominantly expressed. This is compatible with the observation that natural immune sera do not have group or interspecies reactivity against gp71. These points need to be examined further by appropriate absorption and competition experiments. They do emphasize, however, the necessity to approach these questions with well-defined reagents and techniques.

Hanna *et al.* (1975), using a complement-dependent cytotoxicity assay, have previously attempted to correlate the immunological specificity of autogenous immune sera with anticellular (cytotoxic) antibodies. These studies have demonstrated that although these sera react with the virion surface by a number of criteria, they do not have significant cytotoxicity to various virus-replicating and/or -transformed cells. These results may be due to quantitative problems which include either the levels of cytotoxicity relative to the sensitivity of the assay or the level of virus replication of the cells, since autogenous immune sera would be reactive only at sites of budding virions. That the latter possibility contributes significantly has been shown recently by Nowinski *et al.* (1975), who detected natural cytotoxicity, but only with *in vitro* tumor cell lines replicating *abnormally high* levels of virus. This observation further suggests that reactivity is limited to virus budding sites and abundant targets will cause irreparable damage and cytotoxicity (Nowinski, personal communication). The quantitative difference in budding C-type virus in *in vitro* and *in vivo* target cells is an important consideration in using antibody-mediated cytotoxicity assays for determination of coexisting natural antivirus-induced cell-surface or viral-envelope antigens. Disregard of this point (Martin and Martin, 1975) may lend itself to misinterpretation of the functional basis of naturally occurring antibody to virus-associated antigens. Thus the significance of this *in vitro* cytotoxicity is not easily correlated with *in vivo* regulation of virus-transformed cells.

The ability of autogenous immune sera to neutralize various C-type viruses has also been examined (Lee *et al.*, 1974; Hanna *et al.*, 1975; Aaronson and Stephenson, 1974). These results demonstrated weak neutralization of AKR virus, no neutralization of BALB:virus-7 and extremely high levels of inactivation against the xenotropic BALB:virus-2 or the NZB xenotropic virus. Although these data were interpreted to suggest that the antibody reactivity detected in RIP assays was primarily directed against xenotropic virus and was only cross-reactive with AKR virus (Aaronson and Stephenson, 1974), subsequent experiments have clearly demonstrated that the inactivation of xenotropic virus is not antibody-mediated and a serum's ability to inactivate xenotropic virus is not correlated with the presence or absence of antibody detectable in the RIP assay (Levy *et al.*, 1975). However, the significance of this activity to *in vivo* regulation of virus expression has always been in question since these viruses fail to replicate in mouse cells *in vitro*.

The inability to detect neutralization of ecotropic viruses in previous studies, however, appears to be due to technical problems. In particular, C-type viruses are generally extremely labile and, in standard pools of 18-hr-harvested, frozen virus preparations, ratios of non-infectious to infectious particles of 1000–10,000:1 are not uncommon (R. Tennant, personal communication). Clearly, such large excesses of noninfectious particles can compete for binding of potentially neutralizing antibody and minimize the sensitivity of the assays. To circumvent this problem we examined the ability of natural immune sera to neutralize AKR virus infectivity using 2–3 hr-harvested, unfrozen supernatants from producer cultures as a source of infectious virus. As illustrated in Table V, under these conditions naturally immune sera have significant and consistent neutralizing activity against AKR MuLV. The ability of various sera to neutralize AKR MuLV, unlike the ability to inactivate xenotropic virus, is directly correlated with the ability to detect antibodies in the RIP assay. The specificity of this neutralization is also shown in Table V and demonstrates that although natural immune sera can neutralize either N- or B-tropic endogenous viruses they do not neutralize Friend virus. This result is consistent with the above observations that natural immune sera react type-specifically with the major glycoprotein, which is the only viral antigen known to mediate complement-independent

Table V. Neutralization of MuLV Infectivity by Natural Immune Sera[a]

| Serum | RIP titer | Virus | Surviving faction Vn/Vo: serum dilution | | | | |
			1:20	1:40	1:80	1:160	1:320
BALB/c	0	AKR	0.92	0.96	–	–	–
129/J	0	AKR	0.96	0.74	–	–	–
C3H/Anf	1:640	AKR	0.01	0.20	0.48	0.87	0.71
(B6C3)F$_1$	1:1280	AKR	0.01	0.22	0.33	0.74	0.93
(B6C3)F$_1$	0	AKR	0.95	0.91	1.02	0.86	1.23
(B6C3)F$_1$	1:1280	B-tropic	0.1	0.45	0.72	0.86	0.92
(B6C3)F$_1$	1:1280	Friend	0.90	0.94	0.91	0.94	0.98

[a]Neutralization assays were performed with 2–3 hr-harvested, unfrozen virus preparations. Sera were incubated in 0.2 ml with virus at 37° for 60 min, the virus-serum mixture was diluted, and residual virus was detected in S+L-mouse cells (FG-10) as focus-forming units. All sera were heat-inactivated at 56° for 20 min prior to use.

neutralization. Subsequent experiments (J.N. Ihle and B. Lazar, in preparation) have further demonstrated that this neutralization is mediated primarily by 7 S immunoglobulins and can be abrogated by the addition of purified gp71 to the serum at levels that do not cause virus interference. These results, taken together, suggest that *in vivo* this immune response is capable of influencing virus burden by restricting virus infectivity. Clearly, however, the ability of this type of regulation to influence pathogenesis is highly dependent upon other genetic parameters of virus expression and infectivity which strongly influence the total virus burden.

VI. DISCUSSION

The concept that oncogenic viruses such as the murine leukemia viruses can exist as integrated, genetically stable components of the cellular genome has been of profound significance in viral oncology. However, with the emergence of this concept, considerable speculation has arisen bestowing these viral "genes" with unique properties such as a role in differentiation and immunological tolerance. The most important conclusion from the experiments described in this chapter is that mice are not immunologically tolerant to the expression of endogenous C-type viruses but rather maintain a state of immunological surveillance. These observations suggest that, although these viruses are endogenous and vertically transmitted, the host recognizes them as infectious agents, which, in turn, negates the concept of endogenous being "self" in either an immunological or a functional sense. Nevertheless, because of the intimate relationship of the host to the virus some degree of symbiosis may have evolved, but this must clearly be independent of complete infectious virus expression.

The lack of immunological tolerance provides both a basis for immunological regulation of virus expression and control of pathogenesis. Although the role of this natural immune response is not presently well understood, the techniques now exist to critically evaluate this question. The possibility of a relationship between the *Rgv-1* locus and immune regulation is particularly significant and warrants examination. This correlation, if it exists, will provide a relative measure of the efficacy of natural immunological recognition and a basis to assess potential contributions of active immunization.

The role of an immune response would, in part, be to regulate virus burden by restricting virus infection. The significance of reinfection by the virus in pathogenesis has been amply demonstrated for the ecotropic viruses by the *Fv-1* system (Rowe, 1972), where a decrease in tumor incidence can be directly related to decreases in virus burden by restriction of virus replication. These experiments also suggest that immune regulation of virus-mediated pathogenesis could be expected to contribute significantly only in a relatively restricted set of circumstances of "intermediate" levels of virus expression, its influence being modified by other genetic factors involved with expression and infectivity.

The existence of an autogenous immune response to endogenous virus expression of endogenous viruses and virus-mediated antigens. Furthermore, the immunization. In particular, once natural antibodies exist, can the response be modified by immunization? The results to date suggest that the antigenic specificities [i.e., gp71, gp43, and p15(E)] of the natural immune response are conserved, but that antibody type and titer can be changed. However, the significance of these modifications to spontaneous neoplasia has yet to be assessed. A second question of interest is to determine whether immunization prior to the expression of the endogenous virus and the development of a natural immune response alters the pattern of the natural immune response. In particular, could an immunological approach be developed so that qualitative or quantitative changes in the natural immunity were made which would limit early virus replication, and thus subsequent virus burden, and ultimately the incidence of spontaneous neoplasia? One possibility is that maternal influence on virus expression may be due to maternal antibody. Experiments are currently in progress to assess these questions and should indicate the efficacy of immunization in this model system.

The natural immune response can also be used as a sensitive marker for the expression of endogenous viruses and virus-mediated antigens. Furthermore, the type specificity of the immune response, particularly with respect to gp71, allows one to distinguish the particular virus being expressed. These techniques should therefore allow the examination of the influence of a variety of chemical and environmental factors on the expression of viruses *in vivo*. In particular, such experiments should allow an examination of the role of virus activation in radiation-induced leukemogenesis. In addition, it is hoped that this type of analysis can be used to study the factors that control the spontaneous expression of viruses *in vivo*.

Our results have clearly demonstrated that the immune response in a variety of strains of mice is directed against the AKR type of MuLV. In contrast, we have never detected an immune response primarily directed against the Rauscher or Friend gp71 or MuLV, although such an immune response can be experimentally induced by infection or immunization. These results, as well as hybridization data, suggest that these viruses are not entirely endogenous to mice but leave unresolved their origin. These observations suggest that extreme caution should be used in using reagents, particularly gp71, from these viruses to assess endogenous MuLV expression. In this regard, preliminary experiments using homologous competition assays with the AKR MuLV gp71 have failed to detect the widespread noncoordinate expression of "viral glycoprotein" in thymocytes, etc., previously detected with interspecies competition assays using Rauscher gp69/71.

The correlation of the expression of endogenous viruses and the development of an immune response in the murine systems needs to be assessed in other species to determine its general usefulness for detecting virus expression which otherwise requires elaborate techniques and is prone to false negatives. Recently we have found (Ihle *et al.*, 1976*a*) that the techniques used here for C-type viruses are also applicable for B-type viruses in mice and demonstrate distinctly different patterns of immune responses. Similarly, natural antibodies have been detected in baboons with specificity for the endogenous C-type virus of this species, which suggests the general applicability of these techniques for endogenous viruses. Ultimately it is hoped that these techniques will have similar use in humans where complete, infectious virus expression might be a rare event.

ACKNOWLEDGMENTS

This research was sponsored by the National Cancer Institute under Contract No. N01-CO-25423 with Litton Bionetics, Inc.

VII. REFERENCES

Aaronson, S. A., and Stephenson, J. R., 1974, Widespread natural occurrence of high titered neutralizing antibodies to a specific class of endogenous murine type-C virus, *Proc. Natl. Acad. Sci. U.S.A.* **71**:1957.

Aaronson, S. A., Todaro, G. J., and E. M. Scolnick, 1971, Induction of murine C-type viruses from clonal lines of virus-free BALB/3T3 cells, *Science* **174**:157.

Batzing, B. L., Yurconic, M., Jr., and Hanna, M. G., Jr., 1974, Autogenous immunity to endogenous RNA tumor virus: Chronic humoral immune response to virus envelope antigens in B6C3F₁ mice, *J. Natl. Cancer Inst.* **52**:117.

Blank, S. E., Leslie, G. A., and Clem, L. W., 1972, Antibody affinity and valence in viral neutralization, *J. Immunol.* **108**:665.

Breese, S. S., Jr., Stone, S. S., DeBoer, C. J., and Hess, W. R., 1967, Electron microscopy of the interaction of African Swine Fever virus with ferritin-conjugated antibody, *Virology* **31**:508.

Callahan, R., Benveniste, R. E., Lieber, M. M., and Todaro, G. J., 1974, Nucleic acid homology of murine type-C viral genes, *J. Virol.* **14**:1394.

Callahan, R., Lieber, M. M., and Todaro, G. J., 1975, Nucleic acid homology of murine xenotropic type-C viruses, *J. Virol.* **15**:1378.

Chattopadhyay, S. K., Rowe, W. P., Teich, N. M., and Lowry, D. R., 1975, Definitive evidence that the murine C-type virus inducing locus AKV-1 is viral genetic material, *Proc. Natl. Acad. Sci. U.S.A.* **72**:906.

Clapp, N. K., and Yuhas, J. M., 1973, Suggested correlation between radiation-induced immunosuppression and radiogenic leukemia in mice, *J. Natl. Cancer Inst.* **51**:1211.

DeBoer, C. J., Hess, W. R., and Dardiri, A. H., 1969, Studies to determine the presence of neutralizing antibody in sera and kidneys from swine recovered from African swine fever, *Arch. Gesamte Virusforsch.* **27**:44.

Gerloff, R. K., Hoyer, B. H., and McLaren, L. C., 1962, Precipitation of radiolabeled polio virus with specific antibody antiglobulins, *J. Immunol.* **89**:559.

Grant, J. P., Bigner, D. D., Fischinger, P. J., and Bolognesi, D. P., 1974, Expression of murine leukemia virus structural antigens on the surface of chemically-induced murine sarcomas, *Proc. Natl. Acad. Sci. U.S.A.* **71**:5037.

Gross, L., 1951, Pathogeneic properties and vertical transmission of the mouse leukemia agent, *Proc. Soc. Exp. Med.* **78**:342.

Hanna, M. G., Jr., Tennant, R. W., Yuhas, J. M., Clapp, N. K., Batzing, B., and Snodgrass, M., 1973, Autogenous immunity to endogenous RNA tumor virus in mice with a low natural incidence of lymphoma, *Cancer Res.* **32**:2226.

Hanna, M. G., Jr., Ihle, J. N., Batzing, B. L., Tennant, R. W., and Schenley, C. K., 1975, Assessment of reactivities of natural antibodies to endogenous RNA tumor virus envelope antigens and virus-induced cell surface antigens, *Cancer Res.* **35**:164.

Heffner, R. R., Jr., and Schluderberg, A., 1967, Specificity of the primary and secondary antibody responses to myxoviruses, *J. Immunol.* **99**:668.

Hirsch, M. E., Kelly, A. P., Proffitt, M. R., and Black, P. H., 1975, Cell-mediated immunity to antigens associated with endogenous murine C-type leukemia viruses, *Science* **187**:959.

Hollis, V. W., Jr., Aoki, T., Barrera, O., Oldstone, M. B. A., and Dixon, F. J., 1974, Detection of naturally occurring antibodies to RNA-dependent DNA polymerase of murine leukemia virus in kidney eluates of AKR mice, *J. Virol.* **13**:448.

Huebner, R. J., and Todaro, G. J., 1969, Oncogenes of RNA tumor viruses as determinants of cancer, *Proc. Natl. Acad. Sci. U.S.A.* **64**:1087.

Huebner, R. J., Sarma, P. S., Kelloff, G. J., Gliden, R. V., Meier, H., Meyers, D. D., and Peters, R. L., 1971, Immunological tolerance to RNA tumor virus genome expression: Significance of tolerance and prenatal expression in embryogenesis and tumorigenesis, *Ann. N.Y. Acad. Sci.* **181**:246.

Ihle, J. N., Yurconic, M., Jr., and Hanna, M. G., Jr., 1973, Autogenous immunity to endogenous RNA tumor virus: Radioimmune precipitation assay of mouse serum antibody levels, *J. Exp. Med.* **138**:194.

Ihle, J. N., Hanna, M. G., Jr., Roberson, L. E., and Kenney, F. T., 1974, Autogenous immunity to endogenous RNA tumor virus: Identification of antibody reactivity to select viral antigens, *J. Exp. Med.* **136**:1568.

Ihle, J. N., Denny, T., and Bolognesi, D. P., 1975a, Purification and serological characterization of the major envelope glycoprotein from AKR murine leukemia virus and its reactivity with autogenous immune sera from mice, *J. Virol.* **17**:727.

Ihle, J. N., Hanna, M. G., Jr., Schäfer, W., Hunsmann, G., Bolognesi, D. P., and Hüper, G., 1975b, Polypeptides of mammalian oncornaviruses III. Localization of p15 and reactivity with natural antibody, *Virology* **63**:60.

Ihle, J. N., Arthur, L. O., and Fine, D. L., 1976a, Autogenous immunity to mouse mammary tumor virus in mouse strains of high and low mammary tumor incidence, *Cancer Res.* **36**:2840.

Ihle, J. N., Domotor, J. J., Jr., and Bengali, K. M., 1976b, Characterization of the type and group specificities of the immune response in mice to murine leukemia viruses, *J. Virol.* **18**:124.

Ikeda, H., Hardy, W., Jr., Tress, E., and Fleissner, E., 1975, Chromatographic separation and antigenic analysis of proteins of the oncornaviruses. I. Identification of a new murine viral protein, p15(E), *J. Virol.* **16**:53.

Lee, J. C., and Ihle, J. N., 1975, Autogenous immunity to endogenous RNA tumor virus:

Reactivity of natural immune sera to antigenic determinants of several biologically distinct murine leukemia viruses, *J. Natl. Cancer Inst.* **55**:831.

Lee, J. C., Hanna, M. G., Jr., Ihle, J. N., and Aaronson, S. A., 1974, Autogenous immunity to endogenous RNA tumor virus: Differential reactivities of IgM and IgG to virus envelope antigens, *J. Virol.* **14**:773.

Levy, J. A., 1973, Xenotropic viruses: Murine leukemia viruses associated with NIH Swiss, NZB and other mouse strains, *Science* **182**:1151.

Levy, J. A., Ihle, J. N., Oleszko, O., and Barnes, R. D., 1975, Virus-specific neutralization by a soluble non-immunoglobulin factor found naturally in normal mouse sera, *Proc. Natl. Acad. Sci. U.S.A.* **72**:5071.

Lilly, F., 1966, The inheritance of susceptibility to the Gross leukemia virus in mice, *Genetics* **53**:529.

Lilly, F., 1972, Mouse leukemia: A model of a multiple-gene disease, *J. Natl. Cancer Inst.* **49**:927.

Lilly, F., and Pincus, T., 1973, Genetic control of murine viral leukemogenesis advances, *Cancer Res.* **17**:231.

Lilly, F., Duran-Reynals, M. L., and Rowe, W. P., 1975, Correlation of early murine leukemia virus titer and H-2 type with spontaneous leukemia in mice of the BALB/c X AKR cross: A genetic analysis, *J. Exp. Med.* **141**:882.

Martin, S. E., and Martin, W. J., 1975, Naturally occurring cytotoxic tumor reactive antibodies directed against type C viral envelope antigens, *Nature (London)* **256**:498.

Meier, H., Taylor, B. A., Cherry, M., and Huebner, R. T., 1973, Host-gene control of type-C RNA tumor virus expression and tumorigenesis in inbred mice, *Proc. Natl. Acad. Sci. U.S.A.* **70**:1450.

Mellors, R. C., Aoki, T., and Huebner, R. J., 1969, Further implications of murine leukemia-like virus in the disorders of NZB mice, *J. Exp. Med.* **129**:1045.

Mellors, R. C., Shirai, T., Aoki, T., Huebner, R. J., and Krawczynski, K., 1971, Wild-type Gross leukemia virus and the pathogenesis of the glomerulonephritis of New Zealand mice, *J. Exp. Med.* **133**:113.

Nowinski, R. C., and Kaehler, S. L., 1974, Antibody to leukemia virus: Widespread occurrence in inbred mice, *Science* **185**:869.

Nowinski, R. C., and Klein, P. A., 1975, Anomalous reactions of mouse allo antisera with cultured tumor cells. II. Cytotoxicity is caused by antibodies to leukemia viruses, *J. Immunol.* **115**:1261.

Nowinski, R. C., Fleissner, E., Sarkar, N. H., and Aoki, T., 1972, Chromatographic separation and antigenic analysis of proteins of the oncornaviruses. II. Mammalian leukemia-sarcoma viruses, *J. Virol.* **9**:354.

Old, L. J., Boyse, E. A., Oettgen, H. F., 1968. Serologic approaches to the study of cancer in animals and man, *Cancer Res.* **28**:1288.

Oldstone, M. B. A., Aoki, T., and Dixon, F. J., 1972, The antibody response of mice to murine leukemia virus in spontaneous infection: Absence of classical immunologic tolerance, *Proc. Natl. Acad. Sci. U.S.A.* **69**:134.

Peters, R. L., Hartley, J. W., Spahn, G. J., Rabstein, L. S., Whitmire, C. E., Turner, H. C., and Huebner, R. J., 1972, Prevalence of the group-specific (gs) antigen and infectious virus expressions of murine C-type RNA viruses during the life span of BALB/cCR mice, *Int. J. Cancer* **10**:283.

Pincus, T., Hartley, J. W., and Rowe, W. P., 1971, A major genetic locus affecting resistance to infection with murine leukemia viruses. I. Tissue culture studies of naturally occurring viruses, *J. Exp. Med.* **133**:1219.

Rowe, W. P., 1972, Studies of genetic transmission of murine leukemia virus by AKR mice. I. Crosses with $Fv-1^n$ strains of mice, *J. Exp. Med.* **136**:1272.

Rowe, W. P., and Pincus, T., 1972, Quantitative studies of naturally occurring murine leukemia virus infection of AKR mice, *J. Exp. Med.* **135**:429.

Rowe, W. P., Hartley, J. W., Lander, M. R., Pugh, W. E., and Teich, N., 1971, Noninfectious AKR mouse embryo cell lines in which each cell has the capacity to be activated to produce infectious murine leukemia virus, *Virology* **46**:866.

Schäfer, W., Hunsmann, G., Moennig, V., DeNoronha, F., Bolognesi, D. P., Green, R. W., and Hüper, G., 1975, Polypeptides of mammalian oncornaviruses II. Characterization of a murine leukemia virus polypeptide (p15) bearing interspecies reactivity, *Virology* **63**:48.

Schmidt, N. J., Lennette, E. H., and Dennis, J., 1968, Characterization of antibodies produced in natural and experimental coxsackie virus infections, *J. Immunol.* **100**:99.

Steeves, R. A., Strand, M., and August, J. T., 1974, Structural proteins of mammalian oncogenic RNA viruses: Murine leukemia virus neutralization of antisera prepared against purified envelope glycoprotein, *J. Virol.* **14**:187.

Stephenson, J. R., Aaronson, S. A., Arnstein, P., Huebner, R. J., and Tronick, S. R., 1974, Demonstration of two immunologically distinct xenotropic type-C RNA viruses of mouse cells, *Virology* **61**:56.

Strand, M., Wilsnack, R., and August, J. T., 1974, Structural proteins of mammalian oncogenic RNA viruses: Immunological characterization of p15 polypeptide of Rauscher murine virus, *J. Virol.* **14**:1575.

Tennant, R. W., Schlufer, B., Yang, W. K., and Brown, A., 1974, Reciprocal inhibition of mouse leukemia virus infection by *Fv-1* allele cell extracts, *Proc. Natl. Acad. Sci. U.S.A.* **71**:4241.

Webster, R. G., 1968, The immune response to influenza virus. III. Changes in the avidity and specificity of early IgM and IgG antibodies, *Immunology* **14**:29.

Witte, O. N., Weissman, I. L., and Kaplan, H. S., 1973, Structural characteristics of some murine RNA tumor viruses studied by lactoperoxidase iodination, *Proc. Natl. Acad. Sci. U.S.A.* **70**:36.

Chapter 6

Biological and Structural Pleomorphism of the Oncornavirus Envelope Glycoprotein, gp70

Bert C. Del Villano, Stephen J. Kennel, and Richard A. Lerner

Department of Immunopathology
Scripps Clinic and Research Foundation
La Jolla, California 92037

I. INTRODUCTION*

It has been postulated that oncornaviruses play a role in development and differentiation, and that neoplasia is an unforunate consequence of an otherwise important symbiosis (Huebner and Todaro, 1969; Huebner *et al.*, 1970). These concepts are attractive on a theoretical basis, but remained unproved. Nevertheless, the relationship between viral gene expression and normal host-cell functions has been studied in some detail, especially in the case of the interactions between the oncornaviruses and lymphoid cells of the mouse (Tooze, 1973; Gross, 1970). Conceptually, one of the major advances in understanding this relationship has been the demonstration that a protein related to the major envelope glycoprotein of the MuLV gp70 can be a component of normal cells, even in the absence of detectable virus (Del Villano *et al.*, 1975; Tung *et al.*,

This is publication number 1040 from the Department of Immunopathology, Scripps Clinic and Research Foundation, La Jolla, California 92037. This research was supported by grants from the National Cancer Institute, Contract No. NO1CP43375, Grant No. AI-07007; National Foundation, March of Dimes, Contract No. NF1-274; Council for Tobacco Research, Grant No. 766-B; Basil O'Connor Starter Research Grant from the National Foundation; American Cancer Society Grant No. IM-55; and National Science Foundation Grant No.)4B1367-000. R. A. L. is the recipient of USPHS Career Development Award AI-46372.

*Abbreviations: MuLV, murine leukemia virus; SLV, Scripps leukemia virus; SDS PAGE, sodium dodecylsulfate–polyacrylamide gel electrophoresis; MW app., apparent molecular weight; FMR, Friend-Moloney-Rauscher; G, Gross.

1975; Kennel and Feldman, 1976). In this chapter, we review our data which led to this conclusion.

II. MuLV gp70 IS A SURFACE COMPONENT OF VIRUS PARTICLES

In order to identify and characterize molecules which have virus-related antigenic determinants, we applied a system of surface radioiodination using lactoperoxidase, immune precipitation, and analysis by SDS polyacrylamide gel electrophoresis which had been used successfully for the study of cell-surface immunoglobulins (Kennel and Lerner, 1973). The details of surface radioiodination, sample preparation, immune precipitation, and gel electrophoresis have been described previously and will not be emphasized here (Kennel *et al.*, 1973; Del Villano *et al.*, 1975).

Our studies of virus-related antigens began with an analysis of the structure of Scripps leukemia virus (SLV). This virus is a Friend-Moloney-Rauscher (FMR) virus isolated from SCRF 60 A, a lymphoblastoid cell line derived from an NZB mouse (Lerner *et al.*, 1972). *In vitro* labeling of SLV with [^{3}H] glucosamine or with [^{14}C] amino acids indicated that SLV was structurally similar to other murine leukemia virus (MuLV), (Kennel *et al.*, 1973) having major structural components gp70, gp45, p30, and several smaller proteins. Proteins carrying viral antigens could also be identified in radioiodinated virus preparations by indirect immune precipitation, and subsequent sodium dodecylsulfate–polyacrylamide gel electrophoresis (SDS PAGE). For this and most of the other experiments to be described below, we used rat anti-MuLV sera which were prepared by immunization of rats with syngeneic MuLV-induced tumors. Such sera have been widely used by others for the typing of viruses and cell-surface antigens (Old *et al.*, 1965; Aoki *et al.*, 1970, 1972; Aoki and Old, 1966). Since these sera were prepared by syngeneic immunization, they are uniquely suited to studies of viral and cell-surface antigens because they do not have antibodies against fetal calf serum (and other proteins) which are found in most purified virus preparations used for immunization. The immunological reactivity of one such rat anti-MuLV is shown in Fig. 1. NP$_{40}$-disrupted MuLV was radioiodinated and then reacted with rat anti-MuLV. Proteins which react with the rat antibodies were analyzed by SDS PAGE. Three major classes of viral proteins react with the rat antisera: gp70, gp45, and p30. We have used several different rat anti-MuLV sera and have found very similar patterns of reactivity. As a rule, these sera have little reactivity against the lower molecular weight MuLV proteins (i.e., p17, 15, 12, and 10). Further, we showed that the reactivity of these sera with [^{14}C] amino acid- or [^{3}H] glucosamine-labeled virus was similar to that of the radioiodinated preparations, and that the radioiodinated proteins which we detected were not from fetal calf serum (Kennel *et al.*, 1973). We labeled purified virus prepara-

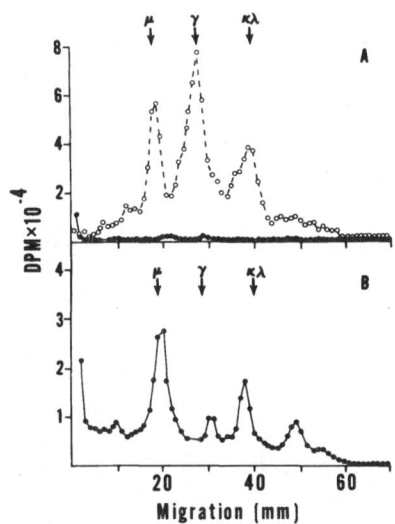

Fig. 1. SDS PAGE of immune precipitates of radioiodinated SLV proteins. SLV was disrupted with NP_{40}, then radioiodinated. Indirect immune precipitates were formed using either rat anti-MuLV (A) or normal rat serum (B) as the primary antibody and then by adding rabbit anti-rat IgG. After extensive washing, samples were disassociated in 8 M urea, 1% SDS, 2% β-mercaptoethanol for electrophoresis. $\circ$, [^{125}I] SLV; $\bullet$, [^{131}I] μ, γ, $\kappa\lambda$ molecular size markers.

tions with "solid-state" lactoperoxidase (David, 1972) either before or after disruption of the virus with a nonionic detergent (Kennel *et al.*, 1973). In the detergent-disrupted virus preparation, all of the viral proteins were labeled essentially in proportion to their mass, whereas in the undisrupted virus preparations, gp70 was selectively labeled (compared to p30). This experiment indicates that the tyrosines of gp70 are more readily iodinated than are those of p30, and also suggests that gp70 is a surface component of the virion. Next, [^{14}C] amino acid-labeled virus was reacted with rat anti-MuLV before or after disruption with Tween 80. The amount of each viral protein in the resulting immune precipitates was determined from SDS PAGE of the precipitates. We found that the ratio of p30 to gp70 in immune precipitates of disrupted virus preparations was three- to fivefold lower than that of undisrupted virus preparations. This experiment indicates that antibodies react with gp70 on the surface of an intact virus particle, and as a result of this reaction the other viral proteins are also precipitated. Thus from the availability of gp70 to labeling with "solid-state" lactoperoxidase and from the availability of gp70 to react with antibody, we can conclude that gp70 is a component of the surface of virus particles. Other experiments (Witte *et al.*, 1973; Steeves *et al.*, 1974; McLellan and August, 1975) also show that gp70 is a surface component of MuLV.

III. MuLV gp70 IS A SURFACE COMPONENT OF INFECTED CELLS

Our initial characterization of MuLV cell-surface antigens was done with SCRF 60 A cells. These lymphoblastoid cells may be described as T cells since they have θ antigen, and do not have surface immunoglobulin. They produce large amounts of MuLV, and by immunofluorescence a MuLV-related cell-surface antigen was detected (Lerner *et al.*, 1972).

To determine which of the viral proteins on the cell surface accounted for this immunofluorescence, we used lactoperoxidase to selectively radioiodinate the surface of SCRF 60 A cells. An extract of the labeled was reacted with rat anti-MuLV and the labeled proteins characterized by SDS PAGE. As shown in Fig. 2, MuLV gp70 was the major component recognized. In similar experiments, gp70 reacted with rat anti-MuLV sera prepared against FMR and Gross (G) type viruses, and with a wide variety of rabbit, guinea pig, and goat antisera prepared by immunization with several MuLVs or with purified MuLV gp70 (Kennel *et al.*, 1973; Del Villano and Lerner, 1975).

Since SCRF 60 A cells produce large amounts of MuLV, the issue of whether the gp70 of these cells was cellular or viral (or both) had to be considered. For example, one possibility is that all of the gp70 observed in these studies was the result of labeling of mature virus particles which had readsorbed to the cells. To determine whether gp70 could be a component of the membrane of infected cells, without being associated with virus particles, we studied the distribution of gp70 by immunoelectron microscopy (Kennel, 1975). As shown in Fig. 3, rat anti-MuLV sera reacted with antigens on virus particles and on cell membranes where virus is not present. In parallel studies, using lactoperoxidase cell-surface labeling, immune precipitation, and SDS gel electrophoresis, it was shown that the rat anti-MuLV was operationally monospecific for gp70. This indicates that gp70 may be a component of the cell membrane, even in areas in

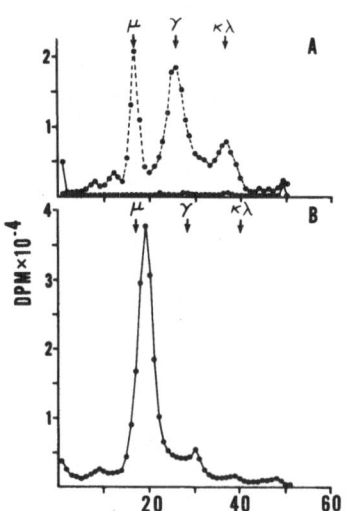

Fig. 2. SDS PAGE of immune precipitates of radioiodinated SCRF 60 A cell-surface proteins. SCRF 60 A cells were "surface-radioiodinated" by the lactoperoxidase procedure and extracted as described by Kennel *et al.* (1973). Indirect immune precipitates were done as in Fig. 1. (A) Primary serum, rat anti-MuLV. (B) Primary serum, normal rat. ○, [^{125}I] SCRF 60 A; ●, [^{131}I] μ, γ, $\kappa\lambda$ molecular size markers.

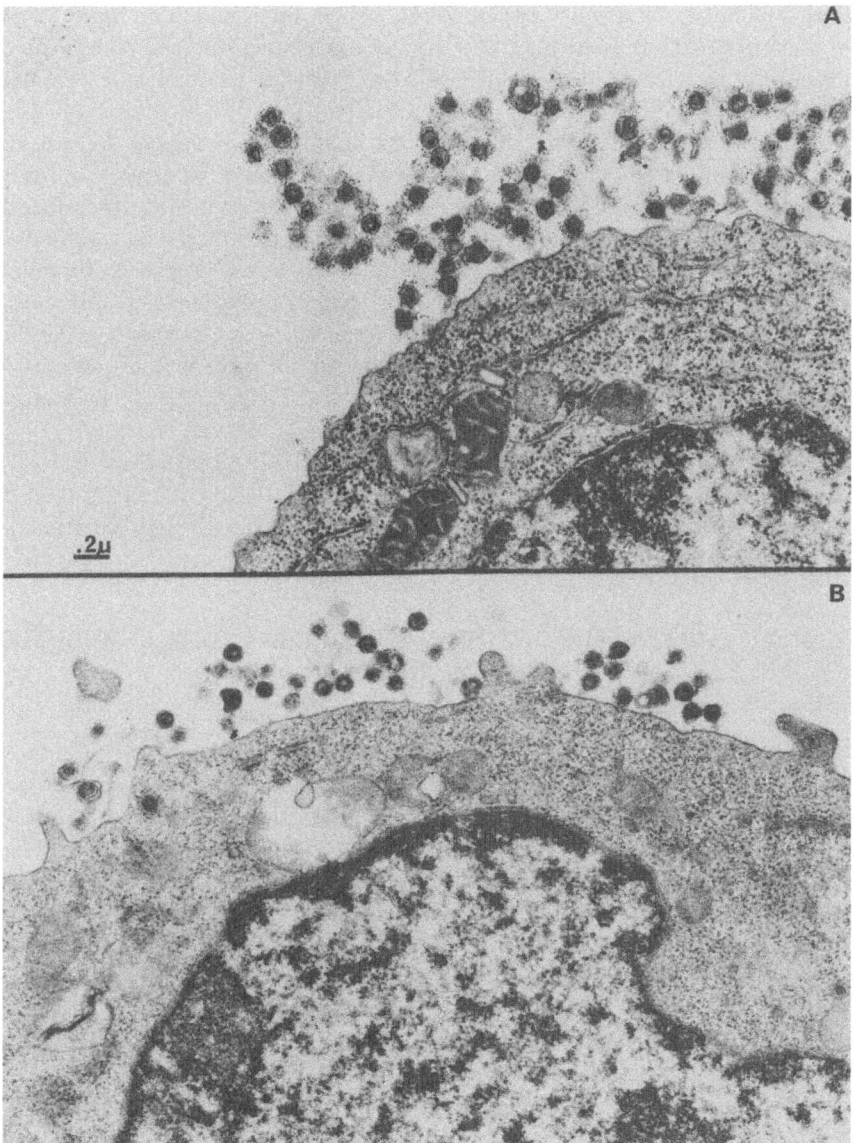

Fig. 3. Immunoelectron microscopy of SCRF 60 A cells using ferritin antibody system. SCRF 60 A cells were fixed with gluteraldehyde and then incubated with rat anti-MuLV (A) or with normal rat serum (B) as described by Kennel (1975). After washing the cells, ferritin-conjugated rabbit anti-rat Ig was added to each. After further incubation and washing, cells were fixed in preparation for electron microscopy. Panel A shows that gp70 is found on the surface of virus particles and on the surface of cells where virus is not apparent. No specific staining is seen in Panel B.

which budding virus was not apparent. As will be discussed later in more detail, we also showed that gp70 may also be a component of the cell membrane of murine thymocytes in the absence of virus particles (Kennel and Feldman, 1975).

In the case of viruses which mature by budding from the cell surface, the distinction between viral and cell-surface antigens becomes somewhat arbitrary, since at some times viral components must also be components of the surface of infected cells. Considering the interactions between infected cells and antibodies, the distinction between "cellular" and "viral" is therefore probably of minimal importance. However, this distinction is of greater importance to our understanding the interactions between infected cells and oncornaviruses, especially when considering the presence of gp70 on the surface of cells following certain pathways of differentiation (Stockert *et al.*, 1971; Tung *et al.*, 1975; Obata *et al.*, 1975; Del Villano *et al.*, 1975).

In summary, the studies of SCRF 60 A cells showed that MuLV gp70 is a component of the surface of virus particles, and is also found in the cell membrane of infected cells, even in regions where there are no virus particles.

IV. MuLV gp70 IS A COMPONENT OF THE SURFACE OF MuLV-INDUCED LYMPHOMAS

The expression of MuLV-related cell-surface antigens on MuLV-induced lymphomas was studied using lactoperoxidase surface labeling, indirect immune precipitation using rat anti-MuLV, and SDS PAGE, just as described above for infected tissue culture cells (Del Villano *et al.*, 1975). As summarized in Table I, 78% of the lymphomas in this series had detectable gp70, and may also have gp45 and p30; we did not identify surface associated gp45 or p30 on any tumor which did not have gp70. In Fig. 4, analysis of four representative MuLV-induced lymphomas are shown. Considerable variation in the relative amounts of the various MuLV surface antigens was observed in different tumors and different organs, but since the techniques used in this study were not quantitative, the significance of this observation is not known.

One of the major points of this study of the virus-related antigens of MuLV-induced lymphomas was the observation that gp70 may be structurally pleomorphic. An example of this pleomorphism is shown in Fig. 5. In this case, lymphoma cells from the thymus and spleen of a single BALB/c mouse that had been neonatally injected with SLV were radioiodinated, then analyzed by indirect immune precipitation with rat anti-MuLV, and then by SDS PAGE. The MW app. of gp70 of the thymus cells was 75,000 and that of the spleen cells was 69,000. Such subtle differences were recognized since we include internal marker proteins in each analytical gel, allowing reliable comparison between

Table I. Classification of MuLV-Related Lymphoma Cell-Surface Antigen[a]

	MuLV component			Positive tissues	Percent
Class	gp70	gp45	p30		
1	+	+	+	2	4
2	+	+	−	10	18
3	+	−	+	2	4
4	+	−	−	29	51
5	−	+	+	0	0
6	−	+	−	0	0
7	−	−	+	0	0
8	−	−	−	14	24

[a]Cells from 57 tissues of mice with MuLV-induced lymphomas were surface-radioiodinated using lactoperoxidase and then analyzed for three classes of MuLV-related antigens by indirect immune precipitation with rat anti-MuLV, followed by SDS PAGE. Tissues were described as positive if a peak, at least twice that observed in trapping controls, was present at the appropriate position.

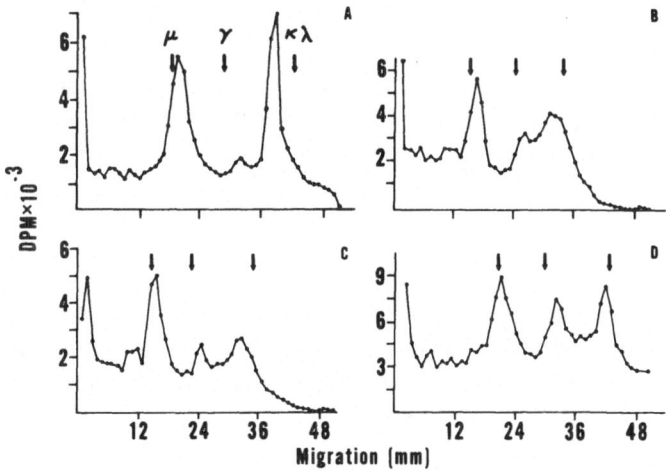

Fig. 4. SDS PAGE of immune precipitates of radioiodinated lymphoma cell-surface proteins. Cell suspensions were obtained from thymic lymphomas of mice which had been injected with MuLV (Scripps). These cells were then "surface-radioiodinated" using lactoperoxidase and analyzed by indirect immune precipitation. In this figure, only specific precipitates formed with rat anti-MuLV are shown, and the positions of the ^{131}I marker proteins formed with rat anti-MuLV are shown, and the positions of the ^{131}I marker proteins are indicated by arrows. Lymphoma cells were as follows: (A) NZB, gp70[+], gp45[−], p30[+]; (B) NZW, gp70[+], gp45[−], p30[−]; (C) C57BL/6, gp70[+], gp45[+], p30[−]; (D) (NZB × NZW)F$_1$, gp70[+], gp45[+], p30[+]. These data indicate the variability of the amount of virus-related antigens among different cell preparations.

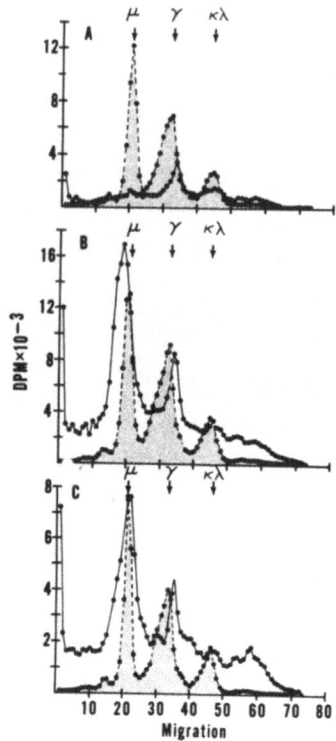

Fig. 5. SDS PAGE of immune precipitates of radio-iodinated lymphoma cell-surface proteins from an MuLV (Scripps) infected BALB/c mouse. (A) ^{125}I-labeled thymus cell-surface proteins which had been reacted with normal rat serum. (B) ^{125}I-labeled thymus cell-surface proteins which had been reacted with rat anti-MuLV serum. (C) ^{125}I-labeled spleen cell-surface proteins which had been reacted with rat anti-MuLV. Both spleen and thymus are gp70$^+$, gp45$^+$, and p30$^+$. However, the electrophoretic mobility of the gp70 from the thymus is signficantly lower than that of the gp70 from the spleen. ○, ^{125}I; ●, [^{131}I]μ, γ, $\kappa\lambda$ molecular size markers, also indicated by shading.

samples. Nevertheless, we confirmed this difference in MW app. by electrophoresis in SDS polyacrylamide gradient slab gels as well as in two different buffer systems (Del Villano *et al.*, 1975). The biochemical basis for the observed variation of MW app. is not known.

V. MuLV gp70 MAY BE EXPRESSED IN NORMAL CELLS

We have studied the expression of MuLV gp70 in normal mouse tissues by a variety of techniques, including cell-surface radioiodination analysis, competition radioimmune assay, and immunofluorescence. Each of these methods contributes unique information so that by analysis using all three methods a comprehensive description of the biology of gp70 may be obtained (Lerner *et al.*, 1975). Briefly, these studies showed that gp70 was found in most mouse tissues and that certain cell types, especially lymphoid and secretory epithelial cells, had very high concentrations of gp70. Although the details of gp70 expression in various mouse strains are beyond the scope of this chapter, the expression of gp70 on the surface of some normal cells will be considered here. Cells obtained from bone marrow, thymus, and sperm cells were studied by lactoperoxidase cell-surface labeling, indirect immune precipitation, and SDS PAGE. As shown in Fig. 6, gp70 was readily detected on the surface of these three cell types from NZB mice. Interestingly, there were marked differences in the electrophoretic mobilities of the gp70 from these organs, compared with the mobility of the μ-chain marker protein. Estimates of the MW app. of these glycoproteins are bone marrow cells 77,000, thymocytes 70,000, and sperm 67,000. Variations in the MW app. of gp70 from these cells were observed in five murine strains and are summarized in Table II (Del Villano, in preparation). Relatively large amounts of gp70 were observed associated with the surface of cells from those mice which are positive for the G_{IX} differentiation antigen. Little or no gp70 was found associated with the surface of these cells in the G_{IX}^- strains. Experiments are currently in progress to identify the biochemical basis for the structural pleomorphism of gp70 from various tissues. It is possible that such variation is the result of cell-specific glycosyltransferases, as has been

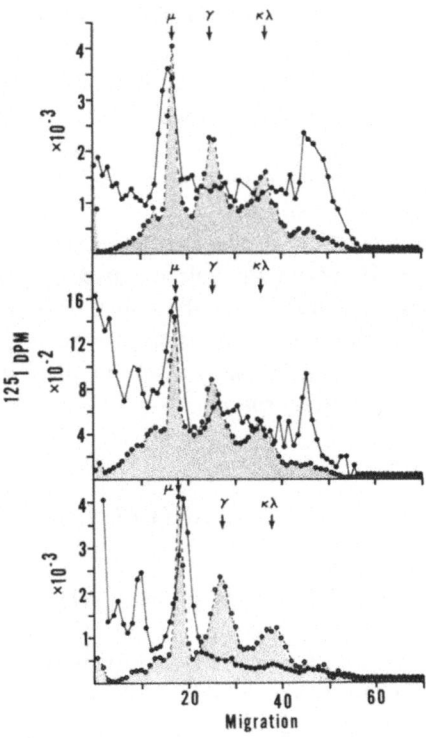

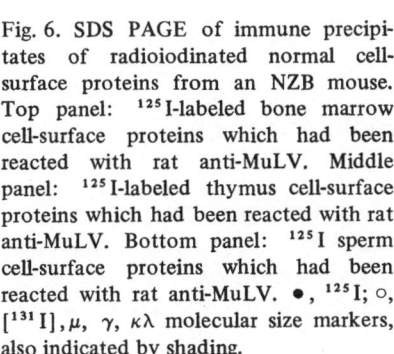

Fig. 6. SDS PAGE of immune precipitates of radioiodinated normal cell-surface proteins from an NZB mouse. Top panel: ^{125}I-labeled bone marrow cell-surface proteins which had been reacted with rat anti-MuLV. Middle panel: ^{125}I-labeled thymus cell-surface proteins which had been reacted with rat anti-MuLV. Bottom panel: [125]I sperm cell-surface proteins which had been reacted with rat anti-MuLV. ●, ^{125}I; ○, [^{131}I], μ, γ, $\kappa\lambda$ molecular size markers, also indicated by shading.

Table II. Relative Electrophoretic
Mobility of gp70 Isolated from Mouse Tissues

	Cell type (MW app. $\times 10^{-3}$)[a]		
Strain	Bone marrow	Thymus	Sperm
NZB	77	70	67
NZW	74	69	67
(NZB $\times$ NXW)F$_1$	74	70	67
129	74	69	67
AKR	72	70	67
BALB/c	$-^b$	$-$	$-$
129 G$_{IX}^-$	$-$	$-$	$-$

[a]Bone marrow, thymus, and sperm cells were isolated from seven different murine strains. Cell-surface antigens were characterized by lactoperoxidase cell-surface radioiodination, indirect immune precipitation [with rat anti-MuLV and with rabbit anti-gp70 (Friend)], and SDS PAGE. MW app. was estimated by comparison with the mobility of $[^{131}I]\mu, \gamma, \kappa\lambda$ marker proteins run in the same gels.
[b]A dash indicates that labeled-cell surface gp70 was not detected in these preparations.

described in other systems (Grimes and Burge, 1971). However, it is also possible that there are significant differences in the primary amino acid structure of these gp70 molecules, since multiple oncornavirus genomes may be integrated into the mouse genome (Lowry *et al.*, 1974).

The presence of gp70 on sperm cells is of particular interest. Boyse has observed that the G$_{IX}$ differentiation antigen may also be expressed on sperm cells. However, the role of gp70 in the biology of the sperm cell is unknown. Since it is likely that the MuLV envelope glycoprotein, gp70, plays a role in the adsorption and penetration of viruses into infected cells, it is also possible that the sperm gp70 plays a role in the "adsorption" and "penetration" phases of fertilization by sperm.

VI. HOST FUNCTIONS AND VIRAL GENES

It is clear that proteins related to oncornavirus gene products can be considered components of normal cells. This may be one of the best examples in higher eukaryotes of symbiosis between endogenous viruses and the host organism. In the case of MuLV gp70, we have described both biological and structural pleomorphism: first, biological pleomorphism in that this molecule may be a component of viruses, normal and malignant cells; and, second, structural pleomorphism in that the relative size of gp70 from different mouse tissues is characteristic of the tissue of origin.

However, a basic question remains unanswered. Are the variants of gp70 transcripts from a single gene, which are modified after synthesis as by glycosylation, or are the proteins products of two or more closely related genes, and have a different primary sequence? The answer to this question is of fundamental importance, both to our understanding of viral leukemogenesis and to our understanding of the "normal" symbiotic relationship between oncornaviruses and their host. In the case of the virus-induced lymphoma, such as that described here, postranscriptional modification of a cell-surface molecule could be a means by which lymphoma cells avoid immune destruction. On the other hand, if the primary structure of the gp70 variants were different, the possibility that two viruses are involved in the leukemias could be considered. These viruses might be present in the infecting inoculum, or might be "activated" during the process of leukemogenesis.

Similarly, in the case of the structural pleomorphism of gp70 in tissues from normal mice, the implications for our understanding of regulation of normal host-cell functions are equally fundamental. That is, if a single molecule is modified in a unique and characteristic manner in different tissues, then we can consider whether this modification is important in differentiation or other cell to cell interactions. However, the possibility that the variant molecules are transcripts from different gene raises intriguing questions about the control of integrated viral genes during differentiation and evolution.

Regardless of the genetic basis for synthesis of variant gp70 molecules, it is interesting to consider their relationship in terms of "molecular mimicry." When considered in the context of stable polymorphisms, "molecular mimicry" between host antigens and viral polypeptides has been considered to take on unique significance. It has been argued (Bodmer, 1972) that the infectious potential of a virus is increased by mimicking a host polypeptide because, in this way, immune response may be evaded or a better fit between the virus surface and a cell receptor may be achieved. Thus the evolutionary advantage of polymorphism in cell-surface polypeptides would be to decrease the rate of virus adaptation. In other words, the pressure of the virus evolving toward the host drives the host to evolve away from the virus. But such arguments may not hold for oncornaviruses which may be important and perhaps necessary symbionts. The suggestion that oncornaviruses are important to the host seems reasonable since potentially oncogenic sequences have persisted in the genome and one needs to explain their selective advantage. In the case of important symbionts, the selective advantage would be toward convergence of structure. Also, "host" proteins coded for by viral genes might show precocious fitness because their extrachromosomal potential allows an evolutionary history distinct from the remainder of the chromosome. Thus apparent mimicry of host proteins by viral polypeptides may be of quite different evolutionary significance, depending on whether symbionts or pathogens are being observed. From a practical point of view, virological mimicking of a host protein may strongly influence the effectiveness of the immune response in elimination of a virus or a tumor.

On the other hand, one can also consider the possibility that integrated viral genes offer little evolutionary advantage to the host, and that by chromosomal rearrangements certain viral genes have become associated with regions of the host chromosome which are involved in certain differentiation pathways. Of course, it is impossible to determine the course or the "will" of integrated viral genes through the evolution of the mouse, and therefore until biological functions can be found for molecules such as gp70, which can be either viral or cellular, we can only speculate about their evolutionary role.

ACKNOWLEDGMENTS

The authors wish to thank Dr. Dani Bolognesi of Duke University Medical Center, Durham, North Carolina, for rabbit anti-gp70 sera and Ms. Barbara Nave for her excellent technical assistance.

VII. REFERENCES

Aoki, T., and Old, L. J., 1966, Occurrence of natural antibody to the G (Gross) leukemia antigen in mice, *Cancer Res.* **26**:1415.

Aoki, T., Boyse, E. A., Old, L. J., de Harven, E., Hammerling, U., and Wood, H. A., 1970, G (Gross) and H-2 cell surface antigens: Location on Gross leukemia cells by electron microscopy with visually labeled antibody, *Proc. Natl. Acad. Sci. U.S.A.* **65**:569.

Aoki, T., Herberman, R. B., Johnson, P. A., Liu, M., and Sturm, M. M., 1972, Wild-type Gross leukemia virus: Classification of soluble antigens (GSA), *J. Virol.* **10**:1208.

Bodmer, W. F., 1972, Evolutionary significance of the HL-A system, *Nature (London)* **237**:139.

David, G. S., 1972, Solid state lactoperoxidase: A highly stable enzyme for simple, gentle iodination of proteins, *Biochem. Biophys. Res. Commun.* **48**:464.

Del Villano, B. C., and Lerner, R. A., 1975, Relationship between the oncornavirus gene product, gp70, and a major protein secretion of the mouse genital tract, *Nature (London)* **259**:497.

Del Villano, B. C., Nave, B., Croker, B. P., Lerner, R. A., and Dixon, F. J., 1975, The oncornavirus glycoprotein gp69/71: A constituent of the surface of normal and malignant thymocytes, *J. Exp. Med.* **141**:172.

Grimes, W. J., and Burge, B. W., 1971, Modification of Sindbis virus glycoprotein by host specified glycosyl transferases, *J. Virol.* **7**:309.

Gross, L., 1970, *Oncogenic Viruses,* 2nd ed., Pergamon Press, New York.

Herberman, R. B., 1972, Serologic analysis of cell surface antigens of tumors induced by murine leukemia viruses, *J. Natl. Cancer Inst.* **48:**265.

Huebner, R. J., and Todaro, G. J., 1969, Oncogenes of RNA tumor viruses as determinants of cancer, *Proc. Natl. Acad. Sci. U.S.A.* **64:**1087.

Huebner, R. J., Kelloff, G. J., Sarna, P. S., Lane, W. T., Turner, A. C., Gilden, R. V., Oroszlan, S., Merer, H., Myers, D. B., and Peters, R. L., 1970, Group specific antigen expression during embryogenesis of the genome of the C-type RNA tumor virus: Implications for ontogenesis and oncognesis, *Proc. Natl. Acad. Sci. U.S.A.* **67:**366.

Kennel, S. J., 1975, Isolation and characterization of virus specific cell surface antigens, in: *Symposium on Cellular Membranes and Tumor Cell Behavior,* University of Texas Press, Houston.

Kennel, S. J., and Feldman, J. D., 1976, Distribution of viral glycoprotein gp 69/71 on cell surfaces of producer and non-producer cells, *Cancer Res.* **30:**200.

Kennel, S. J., and Lerner, R. A., 1973, Isolation and characterization of membrane bound immunoglobulin from cultured human diploid lymphocytes, *J. Mol. Biol.* **76:**485.

Kennel, S. J., Del Villano, B. C., Levy, R. L., and Lerner, R. A., 1973, Properties of an oncornavirus glycoprotein: Evidence for its presence on the surface of virions and infected cells, *Virology* **55:**464.

Lerner, R. A., Jensen, F., Kennel, S. J., Dixon, F. J., Des Roches, G., and Francke, U., 1972, Karyotypic, virologic, and immunologic analyses of two continuous lymphocyte lines established from New Zealand Black mice: Possible relationship of lymphocyte mosaicism to autoimmunity, *Proc. Natl. Acad. Sci. U.S.A.* **69:**2965.

Lerner, R. A., Wilson, C. W., Del Villano, B. C., McConahey, P. J., and Dixon, F. J., 1976, Endogenous oncornaviral gene expression in adult and fetal mice: Quantitative, histologic, and physiologic studies of the major viral glycoprotein, gp70, *J. Exp. Med.* **143:**151.

Lowry, D. R., Chattopadhyay, S. K., Teich, N. M., Rowe, W. P., and Levine, A. S., 1974, AKR murine leukemia virus genome: Frequency of sequences of DNA of high-, low-, and non-virus yielding mouse strains, *Proc. Natl. Acad. Sci. U.S.A.* **71:**3555.

McLellan, W., and August, J. T., 1976, External labeling of envelope glycoproteins of Rauscher murine leukemia virus, *Proc. Natl. Acad. Sci. U.S.A.* (in press).

Obata, Y., Ikeda, H., Stockert, E., and Boyse, E. A., 1975, Relation of the G_{IX} antigen of thymocytes to envelope glycoprotein of murine leukemia virus. *J. Exp. Med.* **141:**188.

Old, L. J., Boyse, E. A., and Stockert, E., 1965, The G (Gross) leukemia antigen, *Cancer Res.* **25:**813.

Steeves, R. A., Strand, M., and August, J. T., 1974, Structural proteins of mammalian oncogenic RNA viruses: Murine leukemia virus neutralization by antisera prepared against purified envelope glycoprotein, *J. Virol.* **14:**187.

Stockert, E., Old, L. J., and Boyse, E. A., 1971, The G_{IX} system: A cell surface allo-antigen associated with murine leukemia virus: Implications regarding chromosomal integration of the viral genome, *J. Exp. Med.* **133:**1334.

Tooze, J., 1973, *The Molecular Biology of Tumour Viruses,* Cold Spring Harbor Laboratory, Cold Spring Harbor, N.Y.

Tung, J. S., Vitetta, E. S., Fleissner, E., and Boyse, E. A., 1975, Biochemical evidence linking the G_{IX} thymocyte surface antigen to the gp 69/71 envelope glycoprotein of murine leukemia virus, *J. Exp. Med.* **141:**198.

Witte, O. N., Weissman, I. L., and Kaplan, H. S., 1973, Structural characteristics of some murine RNA tumor viruses studied by lactoperoxidase iodination, *Proc. Natl. Acad. Sci. U.S.A.* **70:**36.

Chapter 7

Autoimmunity, Oncornaviruses, and Lymphomagenesis

Martin S. Hirsch, Max R. Proffitt, and Paul H. Black

Infectious Disease Unit
Massachusetts General Hospital and Department of Medicine
Harvard Medical School
Boston, Massachusetts 02114

I. INTRODUCTION

C-type oncornaviruses have been associated with a variety of disease states in experimental animals (Hirsch and Black, 1974; Dixon *et al.*, 1974; Levy, 1974; Todaro and Huebner, 1972). Much attention has been directed toward evaluating their role in lymphoproliferative disorders; recently, they have also been considered to play important roles in the induction of, or maintenance of, autoimmune diseases (Hirsch and Proffitt, 1975; Levy, 1974; Dixon *et al.*, 1974). C-type viral genetic information may be acquired through horizontal infection either by experimental injection or by natural transmission of infectious virus; such genetic information may also be vertically transmitted through germ cells from parent to offspring, and may be in the form of integrated proviral DNA (Hirsch and Black, 1974; Todaro and Huebner, 1972; Temin, 1972).

This chapter will attempt to cover two distinct but related areas. We will discuss studies on the immunological activation of endogenous C-type oncornaviruses following skin graft rejection reactions and graft-versus-host reactions. A second area we will discuss is the immunopathogenesis of virus-induced murine lymphomas, which may be a consequence of disseminated autoimmune lymphoproliferation. The potential relationships of these processes to human diseases will also be considered.

II. IMMUNOLOGICAL ACTIVATION OF C-TYPE VIRUSES

A. Skin Graft Rejection Reactions

Kidney transplantation in man has been a major advance in the therapy of chronic renal disease. It has also opened a Pandora's box of viral infections in transplant recipients (Anderson and Spencer, 1969; Coleman *et al.*, 1973; Lopez *et al.*, 1974; Spencer and Anderson, 1970; Strauch *et al.*, 1974). Within the first few months following grafting, nearly all patients will show evidence of infection with one or another of the following agents: cytomegalovirus (CMV), herpes simplex virus (HSV), varicella-zoster virus (VZV), Epstein-Barr virus (EBV), wart virus, or BK papovavirus. Most of these infections are a result of the activation of latent viruses. Renal transplant recipients also have an extraordinarily high incidence of lymphoreticular neoplasms that may or may not be virus induced (Hoover and Fraumeni, 1973; Penn and Starzl, 1972). Although primate C-type viruses have now been isolated from patients with malignancies (Gallagher and Gallo, 1975), their role in human cancer remains conjectural. Studies on the frequency of C-type virus expression in human renal transplant recipients have not yet been reported. However, we have been investigating a murine skin graft model in an effort to determine some of the factors that control immunological activation of endogenous C-type viruses in a situation analogous to human organ transplantation.

Six-week-old BALB/c (H-2^d) male mice were grafted with skin from other A/J (H-2^a) or DBA/2 (H-2^d) male donors; some of the recipients were treated with immunosuppressive drugs to prolong graft survival, whereas others were not. Control groups included BALB/c mice treated with immunosuppressants alone, or left untreated. Transplanted mice were monitored daily for graft rejection. After varying periods up to 4 weeks following grafting, mice were killed, and the following parameters were evaluated on individual mice:

1. Spleen weight and morphology.
2. Lymph node morphology.
3. Virus assays of spleen and, in many cases, thymus, skin graft site, tail, and regional nodes draining the graft.

Summarized data from several studies (Hirsch *et al.*, 1973; Hirsch *et al.*, 1975a) are shown in Tables I and II. The general series of events following skin transplantation in the mouse appears well established. In transplant recipients, C-type viruses are first detected in regional lymph nodes and spleens between 7 and 14 days after grafting; these viruses may be either xenotropic or ecotropic. Thereafter, they appear to reach highest titers in spleens of heavily immunosuppressed mice which maintain their grafts for prolonged periods; either high-dose

Table I. Activation of Ecotropic C-type
Viruses Following Skin Grafting of
BALB/c (H-2^d) Mice

Skin donor	ALS	Incidence of virus positivity	Percent positive
A/J total (H-2^a)	+	34/63	54
Graft retained	+	19/27	70
Graft rejected	+	15/36	42
DBA/2 total (H-2^d)	+	9/13	69
Graft retained	+	4/4	100
Graft rejected	+	5/9	55
A/J or DBA/2 total	+	43/76[a]	57
Graft retained	+	23/31[b]	74
Graft rejected	+	20/45	44
A/J	−	1/10	10
DBA/2	−	0/9	0
No graft	+	8/22	36
No graft	−	2/17	12

[a] $p < 0.001$ compared with control group receiving neither graft nor ALS (x^2).
[b] $p < 0.02$ compared with A/J + DBA/2 graft-rejected group (x^2).

antilymphocyte serum (ALS) or high-dose cyclophosphamide is satisfactory for this purpose. Viruses are not detected in thymuses, in tails, or at skin graft sites in tested graft-recipient mice. Virus activation is usually associated with gross splenomegaly and splenic histological changes consisting of germinal center formation, diffuse hyperplasia of reticulum cells, depletion of periarteriolar lymphocytes, and hyperplasia of red pulp hematopoietic elements. Activated ecotropic viruses may be oncogenic for newborn NIH-Swiss mice, inducing thymic lymphomas within 3–6 months following injection. Whether these viruses induce tumors in the graft recipients themselves, if immunosuppression is maintained for months to years, has not yet been established.

The mechanisms involved in virus activation following skin transplantation remain obscure. It is not even clear whether we are dealing with induction of virus by derepression of genetic material from within cells, or whether we are amplifying infectious virus already present but below threshold levels of detection. Several observations suggest that the former is a more likely possibility. Various groups have now demonstrated that stimulation of lymphocyte blastogenesis by histocompatibility-associated antigens in mixed lymphocyte reactions (MLR) or by certain mitogens can lead to the *in vitro* induction of C-type virus (Hirsch *et al.*, 1972; Greenberger *et al.*, 1975; Moroni *et al.*, 1975; Sherr *et al.*,

Table II. Activation of Xenotropic and Ecotropic Viruses Following Skin Grafting and Various Immunosuppressive Regimens

Group	Number of mice	Skin graft[a]	Suppressive treatment	Skin graft MST ± SE (days)	Mean spleen weight ± SE (g)	Number of virus-positive mice			
						Ecotropic only	Xenotropic only	Ecotropic + xenotropic	Total
A	15	+	None	14.8 ± 2.1	0.157 ± 0.013	2	0	0	2(13%)
B	20	+	ALS	28	0.232 ± 0.016[b]	4	5	4	13(65%)[c]
C	13	+	High-dose cyclophosphamide	20.8 ± 5.8	0.209 ± 0.018[a]	6	1	2	9(69%)[c]
D	16	+	Low-dose cyclophosphamide	16.0 ± 5.8	0.189 ± 0.020	0	0	0	0(0%)
E	14	+	High-dose cortisone	15.9 ± 4.1	0.086 ± 0.007[b]	0	1	0	1(7%)
F	18	+	Low-dose cortisone	15.1 ± 1.8	0.127 ± 0.004[d]	0	1	0	1(7%)
G	15	−	High-dose cyclophosphamide	—	0.118 ± 0.010	0	0	0	0(0%)
H	15	−	None	—	0.124 ± 0.012	0	0	0	0(0%)

[a] BALB/c mice grafted with DBA/2 skin.
[b] $p < 0.01$ compared with group A (t test).
[c] $p < 0.01$ compared with group A (x^2).
[d] $p < 0.05$ compared with group A (t test).

1974), indicating that virus can be induced from lymphocytes by direct stimulation. In addition, our studies indicate that treatment of BALB/c mice with cyclophosphamide alone does not result in virus activation, whereas in combination with skin grafting it does (Hirsch *et al.*, 1975a). If virus detection were merely a result of virus amplification, immunosuppression secondary to cyclophosphamide alone should accomplish this goal. ALS alone does increase the incidence of virus-positive animals, although not to the levels observed when it is combined with skin transplantation. However, ALS is a potent antigen in itself, as well as an immunosuppressant, and chronic ALS treatment results in marked germinal center proliferation and plasma cell hyperplasia in lymph nodes and spleens (Lance, 1968).

The accumulated data suggest the following sequence of events in murine skin transplant recipients. Placement of histoincompatible grafts results in a vigorous immune response in regional nodes and spleens. Certain lymphocyte populations undergo blastogenesis, and during this process C-type viruses become activated within this responding population. In the presence of immunosuppression, these viruses may replicate within other dividing target cells and are not eliminated by host defense mechanisms. The subsequent events that may culminate in lymphomagenesis will be discussed in a later section.

Viruses other than C-type oncornaviruses may become activated by similar immunological mechanisms. Murine cytomegaloviruses have been activated by skin transplantation and allogeneic blood transfusion *in vivo* (Wu *et al.*, 1975; Cheung *et al.*, 1975) and by histocompatibility reactions and certain mitogens *in vitro* (Olding *et al.*, 1975). It is likely that the described pheomena will subsequently be extended to still other viruses and to other species.

B. Graft-Versus-Host Reactions

Several human disorders are characterized by chronic reactivity against self antigens. Some of them, e.g., Sjögren's syndrome and systemic lupus erythematosus, appear to be complicated by an increased incidence of lymphomas, particularly reticulum cell sarcomas or immunoblastic lymphomas (Anderson and Talal, 1972; Canoso and Cohen, 1975). One murine model which parallels these human disorders is the graft-versus-host reaction (GVHR), wherein parental lymphoid cells are injected into F_1 recipients. Antigens from the opposite parent are recognized as foreign by the donor lymphocytes and a chronic rejection reaction ensues. Depending on the strains employed, and the age of the recipients, a variety of immunopathological disorders may develop (Elkins, 1971). In one combination, where BALB/c splenocytes are injected into (BALB/c × A/J)F_1 hybrid mice (hereafter referred to as CAF$_1$), a high incidence of reticulum cell sarcoma develops in recipients (Armstrong *et al.*, 1970).

Several years ago we became interested in evaluating the possibility that C-type oncornaviruses might be activated by GVHR, and might be associated with subsequent lymphomagenesis (Hirsch *et al.*, 1970, 1972). It became readily apparent that ecotropic C-type viruses rapidly appeared in spleens of CAF_1 mice following injection of parental BALB/c spleen cells, whereas uninjected CAF_1 mice and BALB/c donors were generally virus negative by the techniques employed (Table III). In addition, treating donor cells with mitomycin C prevented GVHR, virus activation, and subsequent oncogenesis. These studies were confirmed and extended by Armstrong *et al.* (1973), who made the additional important observation that cell-free extracts from CAF_1 mice undergoing GVHR could induce lymphoreticular tumors in syngeneic neonatal mice. Subsequent studies by others (Sherr *et al.*, 1974) have also indicated that xenotropic C-type viruses may be activated during GVHR in this strain combination, and under certain experimental conditions may be selectively demonstrated. Several additional strain combinations have been tested for ecotropic virus activation during GVHR (Hirsch *et al.*, 1972; Phillips *et al.*, 1975b). The incidence of virus activation is generally higher in those mice with a high incidence of subsequent neoplasia [BALB/c → CAF_1, BALB/c → (BALB/c × C57BL6)F_1] than in those with a low tumor incidence [BALB/c → (C57BL6 × DBA/2)F_1], C57BL6 → [(C57BL6 × C57BL10)F_1], although there are exceptions to this rule (Phillips *et al.*, 1975b).

Analysis of the source and mechanism of virus activation is complicated by the nature of the GVHR, which involves a major early response by parental cells followed by an extensive proliferation of F_1 cells (Elkins, 1971). In the strain combination we have studied, most of the tumors that develop are of F_1 origin (Gleichmann *et al.*, 1975). However, as in the previously discussed skin graft response and MLR, the major initial responding cell, i.e, the BALB/c splenocyte, is the likely source of the activated virus (André-Schwartz *et al.*, 1973). Since

Table III. Incidence of Spleens Positive for Ecotropic C-type Viruses in Mice with and without Graft-Versus-Host Reactions (GVHR)[a]

Strains	Number	Number virus positive	Percent positive
CAF_1 ← BALB/c	52	47	90
CAF_1 uninjected	51	6	12
BALB/c uninjected	25	1	4
A/J uninjected	14	0	0

[a]Assay employed for C-type viruses was the XC mixed culture cytopathogenicity assay.

treatment of GVHR cells *in vitro* with anti-θ serum and complement eliminates their capacity to release ecotropic C-type viruses, it appears that BALB/c T cells are likely the initial source of virus production (Phillips *et al.*, 1975*b*). Certain immune responses are depressed in CAF_1 mice undergoing GVHR (Solnik *et al.*, 1973; Phillips *et al.*, 1975*a*), although it is not yet established whether these mice are hyporesponsive to their own activated viruses. Normal CAF_1 mice, like other strains of mice, can respond immunologically to their own endogenous C-type viruses (Hirsch *et al.*, 1975*b*), and it is likely that GVHR-associated hyporesponsiveness to viral antigens contributes to virus replication and subsequent lymphomagenesis. It is of interest that morphological changes in spleens of GVHR animals are very similar to those observed in skin graft recipients undergoing immunosuppression, a situation also characterized by C-type virus activation. In both models, virus replication is accompanied by depletion of periarteriolar lymphocytes and hyperplasia of reticulum cells.

A reasonable interpretation of the events observed in CAF_1 mice undergoing GVHR is the following. As in the skin graft model, BALB/c lymphoid cells when exposed to A/J antigens in CAF_1 mice undergo blastogenesis with subsequent activation of C-type viruses. In the face of GVHR-associated immunosuppression and in the presence of a large number of proliferating CAF_1 lymphoreticular cells, virus replication occurs in these F_1 cells. If these target cells are sufficiently altered, neoplastic lymphoproliferation can develop. In other strains where virus activation is more tightly restricted, where immunosuppression is less marked, or where the appropriate proliferating target cells are not available, lymphomas would not develop. It is also possible that immune-complex glomerulonephritis seen in certain GVHR combinations may, in part, be due to activation of xenotropic C-type viruses that are not lymphomagenic, but rather provide a large source of antigen for immune-complex formation. Xenotropic viruses appear to play this role in certain mouse strains with a high spontaneous rate of glomerulonephritis, e.g., the (NZB × NZW)F_1 hybrid strain (Levy, 1974).

C-type oncornavirus information can also be activated from murine lymphocytes *in vitro* by establishment of certain culture conditions (Lonai *et al.*, 1974), by MLR (Hirsch *et al.*, 1972; Sherr *et al.*, 1974), by halogenated pyrimidines (Phillips *et al.*, 1975*b*), and by certain mitogens such as lipopolysaccharide or concanavalin-A (Greenberger *et al.*, 1975; Moroni *et al.*, 1975). Mitogens and nucleoside derivatives may have additive or synergistic effects on virus activation (Moroni *et al.*, 1975). Different mechanisms are probably involved in these various forms of virus activation. Lymphoblastic proliferation alone is not sufficient for virus activation, since other mitogens and antigens, e.g., phytohemagglutinin and sheep erythrocyte stroma, induce marked blastogenesis, but not virus activation (Phillips *et al.*, 1975*b*; Hirsch *et al.*, 1972; Greenberger *et al.*, 1975). Although it is possible that subtle differences in the way lymphocytes respond to different stimuli may influence virus activation, it is more likely that stimulation of certain specific lymphocyte subpopulations is necessary for efficient virus activation.

The possible mechanisms by which C-type oncornaviruses induce lymphoreticular neoplasms will be discussed in the following section.

III. VIRUS-INDUCED AUTOIMMUNITY AND LYMPHOMAGENESIS

Another murine model we have been studying closely links autoimmunity and lymphomas to C-type murine oncornaviruses (Proffitt *et al.*, 1975a,b), and may provide a clearer understanding of the pathogenesis of at least some lymphoproliferative diseases. Mice infected as neonates with murine leukemia virus of the Moloney strain (MuLV-M carriers) develop disseminated lymphomas of thymic origin and die within approximately 4–6 months. Prior to the appearance of lymphomas, a severe, premature, bilateral but asynchronous involution of the thymus occurs. This is accompanied by pronounced intrathymic cell destruction and proliferation of lymphoblastic cells. Eventually, the thymus enlarges with malignant lymphoblasts which subsequently spread to peripheral lymphoid tissues and other organs (Siegler, 1968; Metcalf, 1966). Similar events occur spontaneously in AKR mice that are naturally infected with endogenous MuLV of the Gross strain (MuLV-G) (Siegler, 1968).

In order to study the relationship of the immune response to the pathogenesis of lymphoma, a colony of C3H/He mice carrying MuLV-M was established by injecting newborns with MuLV-M during the first 24 hr after birth. These mice reached breeding age and bore at least one litter before the onset of lymphoma. All subsequent generations transmitted the virus to their offspring. The incidence of lymphoma in mice from this colony is 90–100% by approximately 6 months. Employing an *in vitro* microcytotoxicity assay, we have shown that thymocytes from these carrier mice cause a dramatic reduction of normal syngeneic target cells (fibroblasts) long before premature thymic involution or overt lymphoma is apparent (Proffitt *et al.*, 1975a). In contrast, thymocytes from C3H/He mice carrying the lactic dehydrogenase virus (LDV carriers) or the lymphocytic choriomeningitis virus (LCMV carriers) since birth do not cause reduction of the same target cells (Proffitt *et al.*, 1976). Infection of the syngeneic C3H/HE target cells with MuLV-M spares them from reduction by MuLV-M carrier thymocytes (Proffitt *et al.*, 1975a). Similarly, infection of the target cells with MuLV-G causes them to be spared; however, LCMV does not have a comparable effect (Proffitt *et al.*, 1976). Normal C3H thymocytes, on the other hand, often enhance the growth of normal, noninfected target cells and usually have little significant effect on target cells infected with MuLV-M.

Occasionally a normal mouse exhibits modest thymic reactivity against MuLV-infected target cells; this may reflect a low-level, naturally occurring cell-mediated immunity to endogenous MuLV similar to that evident in CAF_1 mice (Hirsch et al., 1975b).

These data, summarized in Table IV, indicate that MuLV-M-infected thymocytes may have their normal capacity to recognize "self" antigen altered such that a normal antigen(s) is recognized as foreign, whereas MuLV-associated antigens are now viewed as "self." The failure of LCMV, an RNA virus which, like MuLV, replicates by budding from cell membranes, to confer protection on the cells infected by it indicates that the phenomenon is specific. The mechanisms involved in these interactions are presently unclear. It is possible that MuLV-M alters the behavior of thymocytes by altering the genetic machinery of these cells. Alternatively, oncornaviruses may provide bridges between viral receptors on cells of different types allowing closer contact between lymphocytes and target cells and thereby expression of potentially autoimmune reactivity. Preliminary evidence suggests that such "virus-bridging" may be important in these cytotoxic reactions.

Table V provides a summary of the salient characteristics of the autoreactive MuLV-M carrier thymocytes. They are lymphoid in morphology and must be viable to mediate target-cell reduction. They occur in a nonadherent, light buoyant density fraction on Ficoll-Hypaque gradients; in the presence of complement, they are lysed by anti-θ-C3H and anti-H-2^k sera, but not by anti-mouse IgG. They are infected with MuLV as indicated by their sensitivity to antisera directed against MuLV-associated antigens. Their resistance to in vivo treatment

Table IV. Summary of Cytotoxic Reactivity in Vitro

	Target cells[a]			
Effector cells	Uninfected	MuLV-M infected	MuLV-G infected	LCMV infected
Thymocyte–normal	−	±	±	−
Thymocyte–MuLV-M-carrier	+	−	−	+
Lymphoma–in situ	+	−	NT[b]	NT
Lymphoma–transplantable	+	−	NT	NT
Peripheral lymphocyte (early)	−	+	NT	NT
Peripheral lymphocyte (late)	+	−	NT	NT
Thymocyte–LCMV-carrier	−	−	NT	−
Thymocyte–LDV-carrier	−	−	NT	NT

[a]C3H/HeJ embryo cells either uninfected or infected with Moloney (MuLV-M) or Gross (MuLV-G) leukemia virus or with lymphocytic choriomeningitis virus (LCMV).
[b]Not tested.

Table V. Characteristics of Autoreactive
MuLV-M-Carrier Thymocytes

Cell type		Sensitivity to treatment with	
Lymphoid morphology	Yes	Anti-θ-C3H	Yes
Nonadherent	Yes	Anti-mouse IgG	No
Cortisone resistant	Yes	Anti-H-2^k	Yes
MuLV infected	Yes		

with hydrocortisone helps to classify them as functionally-mature immunocytes (Proffitt *et al.,* 1975*b*).

Specificity studies using syngeneic, allogeneic, and xenogeneic target cells have shown that thymocytes from MuLV-M carriers are reactive against cells of all mouse strains so far tested except for AKR (Table VI). When xenogeneic cells were used as targets, there was very slight reactivity against monkey cells, but this was of borderline significance. However, there was no reduction of human, rat, or hamster cells. In fact, there was marked growth enhancement of the latter two cell types even though syngeneic target cells were dramatically reduced in the same experiments. It remains to be determined whether the reactivity by MuLV-M carrier thymocytes is monoclonal and directed against one antigen common to all mouse strains, or whether there is restricted reactivity directed against a variety of murine but not xenogeneic antigens. The lack of reactivity against AKR cells may simply reflect sparing due to the presence of endogenous MuLV-G similar to that seen when C3H cells were infected exogeneously with MuLV-G.

Additional studies have shown that the aggressive behavior of MuLV-M carrier thymocytes may be an integral part of the pathogenesis of lymphoma in these mice. Lymphoma cells, prepared from thymic tumors arising *in situ* or after their multiple subcutaneous transplantation into normal young adult mice, significantly reduced noninfected but spared MuLV-M infected target cells. This suggests that the tumors themselves may be composed of autoreactive cells. That interpretation is further supported by the fact that spleen and lymph node lymphocytes from seven out of ten young, preleukemic carrier mice (8–10 weeks old) caused significant reduction of MuLV-M-infected target cells (Table VII). However, lymphocytes from older preleukemic carriers (16–17 weeks old) taken at about the time lymphoma disseminates from the thymus reacted in a manner similar to thymocytes from preleukemic carriers; i.e., they significantly reduced noninfected target cells, but spared infected target cells.

We have proposed a possible mechanism to explain the linkage of virus infection to autoreactivity and malignant lymphoma. This is depicted diagram-

Table VI. Percent Reduction of Syngeneic, Allogeneic, and Xenogeneic Target Cells by Thymocytes from Normal or MuLV-M-Carrier C3H/He Mice[a]

		Target cells							
		Mouse				Human	Monkey	Rat	Hamster
Experiment No.	Thymocytes	C3H/He	BALB/c	C57BL/6	AKR				
74-5-28A	Normal	-73^b	17^c					-56^b	
	Carrier	32^b	20^b					-23^b	
74-6-3B	Normal	-59^b	6				0	-40^b	-47^b
	Carrier	32^b	37^b				5	-67^b	-33^b
74-7-9A	Normal	-20^b		16		8	5		-5
	Carrier	65^b		32^b		4	15^b		-40^b
74-7-23C	Normal	8			1				
	Carrier	32^b			-17^c				
74-10-12B	Normal	-20^c			-1				
	Carrier	69^b			-3				

[a]Percent reduction relative to target cells grown in culture medium alone. Negative percentages of reduction indicate enhancement of target cell growth.
[b]$p < 0.01$ (Student's t test).
[c]$0.05 > p > 0.01$ (Student's t test).

matically in Fig. 1. Infection by MuLV of a thymic subpopulation with potential antiself reactivity (Cohen and Wekerle, 1973; Howe, 1973; von Boehmer, 1973) might activate and/or fix this function during subsequent differentiation of those cells. Thus a population(s) or clone(s) of mature, virus-infected, auto-aggressive cells would arise. These cells could, in turn, interact with uninfected lymphocytes including those with antiviral reactivity. A "civil war" might then ensue, the outcome of which would determine the subsequent course of lympho-ma development. If antiviral T cells were able to keep the autoaggressive cells in check, lymphoma development would be curtailed or prevented. If, on the other hand, normal immunocompetent cells, including those involved in antiviral and/or antitumor immune surveillance, were destroyed, the autoaggressive cells would be free to replicate, leading to disseminated lymphoma. This "civil war" may well account for much of the cellular destruction associated with premature thymic involution and lymphomagenesis in MuLV-M-infected mice. This may, in turn, be at least partially responsible for the diminished numbers of positive T cells and for the generally immunodepressed state in MuLV-M carriers (Proffitt *et al.*, unpublished observations).

It is also possible that in MuLV-M carriers, virus-infected clones with reactivities against other, not necessarily autoantigenic, specificities might arise and proliferate, resulting in a variety of immunopathological manifestations. Thus an assortment of aberrant immune responses might be expected during the course of lymphoma development.

Table VII. Cell-Mediated Reactivity by
Peripheral Lymphocytes from MuLV-M
Carrier Mice of Different Ages Against
Syngeneic Target Cells Infected
or Not Infected with MuLV-M

	Number of mice having demonstrable, significant reactivity[a]	
Target cells	Preleukemic carriers (young)[b]	Preleukemic carriers (older)[c]
Infected	7/10	3/11
Noninfected	1/10	8/11

[a]Significant cytotoxicity ($p < 0.05$, Student's t test) compared with the effect of lymphocytes from normal mice of the same age.
[b]8–10 weeks old.
[c]Older than 16 weeks.

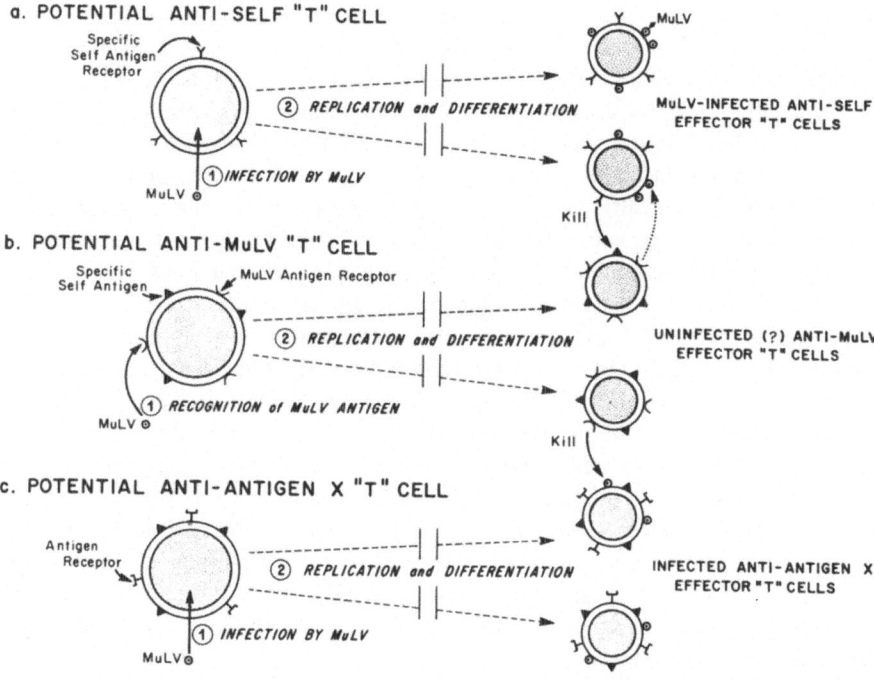

Fig. 1. Hypothetical model of intrathymic cellular interactions in mice infected with MuLV-M. Represented are antigen-reactive thymocytes with varied capabilities to respond to different antigens. Thymocyte (a) has potential reactivity against certain specific self-antigens; ordinarily, this self-reactivity is unexpressed. Upon infection by MuLV, cell (a) might be stimulated to divide and express its autoreactive potential. Other thymic cells have different reactive potentials: cell (b) against MuLV-M-associated antigens and cell (c) against a hypothetical antigen X. Upon recognition of MuLV-associated antigens, cell (b) would divide and proliferate into a clone able to react against MuLV-infected cells. If antiself cells were to destroy anti-MuLV cells, the infected clones of antiself cells would selectively replicate; if anti-MuLV cells were to destroy infected antiself cells, the infection and autoaggressive reactivity would be contained. Cell (c) also might be infected by MuLV, resulting in the expansion of cell clones with varied immunological capabilities (e.g., reactivity against certain other nonself antigens). Figure reprinted from the *International Journal of Cancer* 15:230, 1975, with the permission of the International Union Against Cancer, Geneva, Switzerland.

IV. DISCUSSION

The two phenomena we have described, immunological activation of MuLV and leukemia virus-induced autoreactivity, may be bound by a common thread. In both types of responses, the organ most intensely involved in localized immune reactions is also the organ that first becomes neoplastic; thus the thymus is the primary site of virus replication, autoreactivity, and lymphoma development following MuLV-M infection, whereas the spleen is the primary site for virus activation, replication, and lymphoma development following the GVH reaction. Perhaps similar events develop in both models, triggered in one case by exogenous MuLV infection and in the other by immune activation of endogenous MuLV. Once initiated, the sequence might involve the appearance of virus-induced autoaggressive T cells capable of eliminating host lymphocytes active in immune surveillance. This is supported by several lines of evidence, including diminished numbers of identifiable θ-positive thymus cells in carrier mice and B cells in GVH animals prior to appearance of lymphomas, and hyporesponsiveness to a variety of antigens and mitogens in both models prior to the appearance of lymphomas (Solnik *et al.,* 1973; Proffitt *et al.,* unpublished). The combined effects of proliferation of aggressor cells and alteration of immune surveillance could lead to the unrestricted replication and dissemination of those cells, culminating in frank lymphoma in carriers or GVH mice. Although the histological, virological, and immunological data are compatible with such a theory, alternative explanations are also possible. For example, elimination of suppressor T cells (Gershwin and Steinberg, 1973) either by direct virus effects or by autoimmune destruction could further potentiate the proliferation of autoimmune lymphoid populations.

Analogous mechanisms can be proposed to explain the relationship of viruses, autoimmune responses, and lymphomas in several animal models (East, 1970; Porter, 1971; Cox and Keast, 1973; Walters *et al.,* 1973; Levy, 1974; Hirsch and Proffitt, 1975). In one of the most studied of these models, the NZB mouse, it is increasingly apparent that an endogenous xenotropic MuLV is intimately related to an array of immunopathological phenomena seen in these mice and perhaps to their high incidence of lymphoma as well (Levy, 1974). Like MuLV-M carriers, NZB mice show evidence of intrathymic cellular destruction (DeVries and Hijmans, 1967) associated with a sharp decline in functionally normal peripheral T cells with age (Talal and Steinberg, 1974). Interestingly, the lymphocytes from aging NZB mice are cytotoxic for normal NZB fibroblasts *in vitro* (Stiller *et al.,* 1973). This may reflect a spontaneous virus-induced "civil war" like that which we have described in MuLV-M carriers. A similar mechanism may further account for the intrathymic cellular destruction and thymic atrophy seen in cats infected with feline leukemia virus (Essex, 1975), and may operate in other murine leukemias as well. Sklar and Rowe (unpublished) have found that following infection of mice with Abelson leukemia virus (MuLV-A), a virus that induces B-cell lymphomas, there is an analogous selective autoimmune cytotoxicity.

A variety of human disorders may also be tied by a similar thread. Sjögren's syndrome (SS) and systemic lupus erythematosus (SLE) share many features with the murine models we have discussed. Patients with either disorder have been reported to show cell-mediated and humoral hyperreactivity to autoantigens (Bloch *et al.*, 1965; Berry *et al.*, 1972; Abe *et al.*, 1973; Tannenbaum and Schur, 1974), and depression of certain T-cell-mediated immune responses (Sucia-Foca *et al.*, 1974; Tannenbaum and Schur, 1974; Leventhal *et al.*, 1967). Sjögren's syndrome patients display an increased incidence of lymphoreticular hyperplasia often progressing to immunoblastic sarcoma (Anderson and Talal, 1972; Lukes and Collins, 1974); the frequency of malignancy, often of lymphoreticular elements, may also be increased in SLE patients (Canoso and Cohen, 1975). Evidence of increased expression of primate C-type viruses in SLE has come from immunochemical, immunofluorescent, and ultrastructural studies (Strand and August, 1974; Lewis *et al.*, 1974; Dixon, 1974); although the evidence for viral participation in SS is still weak (Cremer *et al.*, 1974), many observers have found ultrastructural evidence of particles resembling viruses in SS tissues (Grimley *et al.*, 1973; Györkey *et al.*, 1972) and newer techniques to look for C-type viruses have yet to be employed in this disorder. In both SS and SLE, the activation of endogenous C-type viruses or the acquisition of exogenous viruses may lead to a selective proliferation of virus-altered B or T cells expressing autoimmune responses. If held partially in check by suppressor T cells or by a competent immune surveillance mechanism, these events may lead to recurrent or persistent autoimmune phenomena; if ineffectively controlled, lymphoid hyperplasia advancing to B- or T-cell immunoblastic lymphomas may result.

Myasthenia gravis is another human disorder characterized by autoimmunity occasionally progressing to lymphoma; as in the murine MuLV-M carrier, a major target organ is the thymus (Abdou *et al.*, 1974; Castleman, 1966; Goldstein and Schlesinger, 1975). In mixed leukocyte reactions, thymic cells from myasthenia patients may stimulate peripheral lymphocytes and *vice versa* (Abdou *et al.*, 1974). Such patients may show histological evidence of thymitis (Goldstein and Schlesinger, 1975) and 10% develop thymomas (Castleman, 1966). Although a viral relationship to myasthenia gravis has not been demonstrated, a persistent virus infection within the thymus is possible and should be further explored.

Finally, mention should again be made of the human organ transplant recipient, extraordinarily susceptible to the activation of latent viruses and to the development of lymphoreticular neoplasms. Many questions regarding these patients are of great interest, and should be answered in the next few years. Among them are the following: Are C-type oncornaviruses activated following human organ transplantation? Are viruses (oncorna, herpes, papova, or other) important in the development of lymphomas in these patients, and if so, by what mechanisms? Can the incidence of lymphomas be reduced by diminishing viral expression with agents such as interferon? Answers to these questions may provide a better understanding of the complex interrelationships among viruses, immunopathology, and cancer in man.

V. SUMMARY

The interactions between aberrant immune responses and C-type oncorna-viruses in mice are complex. These viruses may be activated during certain immune responses, e.g., histocompatibility reactions, in the face of chronic immunosuppression. Oncornaviruses, themselves, may induce autoaggressive cell-mediated responses in certain lymphoid subpopulations, and these auto-immune reactions may be important in subsequent lymphomagenesis.

Parallel events may occur in other animal models, e.g., the NZB mouse, and in certain human disorders, e.g., Sjögren's syndrome, systemic lupus erythemato-sus, and myasthenia gravis.

ACKNOWLEDGMENTS

Work from our laboratory described in this chapter was supported by PHS Grants CA16177-01 and CA12464-05 and Contrast NIH-N01-CP-43222 of the Virus Cancer Program of the National Cancer Institute. Max R. Proffitt is a Special Fellow of the Leukemia Society of America.

VI. REFERENCES

Abdou, N. I., Lisak, R. P., Zweiman, B., Abrahamsohn, I., and Penn, A. S., 1974, The thymus in myasthenia gravis: Evidence for altered cell populations, *N. Engl. J. Med.* **291**:1271.

Abe, T., Hara, M., Yamesaki, K., and Homma, M., 1973, Cell mediated immune response in systemic lupus erythematosus: *In vitro* cellular response to native DNA by macrophage inhibitory test, *Arthritis Rheum.* **16**:688.

Anderson, H. K., and Spencer, E. S., 1969, Cytomegalovirus infection among renal allograft recipients, *Acta Med. Scand.* **186**:7.

Anderson, L. G., and Talal, N., 1972, The spectrum of benign to malignant lymphoprolifera-tion in Sjögren's syndrome, *Clin. Exp. Immunol.* **10**:199.

André-Schwartz, J., Schwartz, R. S., Hirsch, M. S., Phillips, S. M., and Black, P. H., 1973, Activation of leukemia viruses by graft-versus-host and mixed-lymphocyte culture reactions: Electron microscopic evidence of C-type particles, *J. Natl. Cancer Inst.* **51**:507.

Armstrong, M. Y. K., Gleichmann, E., Gleichmann, H., Beldotti, L., André-Schwartz, J., and Schwartz, R. S., 1970, Chronic allogeneic disease. II. Development of lymphomas, *J. Exp. Med.* **132**:417.

Armstrong, M. Y. K., Ruddle, N. H., Lipman, M. B., and Richards, F. F., 1973, Tumor induction by immunologically activated murine leukemia viruses, *J. Exp. Med.* **137**:1163.

Berry, H., Bacon, P. A., and Davis, J. D., 1972, Cell mediated immunity in Sjögren's syndrome, *Ann. Rheum. Dis.* 31:298.

Bloch, K. J., Buchanan, W. W., Wohl, M. J., and Bunim, J. J., 1965, Sjögren's syndrome: A clinical, pathological and serological study of sixty-two cases, *Medicine (Baltimore)* 44:187.

Boehmer, H. von, 1973, Direct cell contact is required in the syngeneic mixed lymphocyte reaction, *Eur. J. Immunol.* 3:109.

Canoso, J. J., and Cohen, A. S., 1975, Malignancy in a series of 70 patients with systemic lupus erythematosus, *Arthritis Rheum.* 17:383.

Castleman, B., 1966, The pathology of the thymus gland in myasthenia gravis, *Ann. N.Y. Acad. Sci.* 135:496.

Cheung, K., Smith, H. M., and Lang, D. J., 1975, The transmission of cytomegalovirus (CMV) in blood transfusion: A murine model, *Pediatr. Res.* 9:339 (abst.).

Cohen, I. R., and Wekerle, H., 1973, Regulation of autosensitization. The immune activation and specific inhibition of self-recognizing thymus-derived lymphocytes, *J. Exp. Med.* 137:224.

Coleman, D. V., Gardner, S. D., and Field, A. M., 1973, Human polyomavirus infection in renal allograft recipients, *Br. Med. J.* 3:371.

Cox, K. O., and Keast, D., 1973, Rauscher virus infection, erythrocyte clearance studies, and autoimmune phenomena, *J. Natl. Cancer Inst.* 50:941.

Cremer, N. E., Daniels, T. E., Oshiro, L. S., Marcus, F., Claypool, R., Sylvester, R. A., and Talal, N., 1974, Immunological and virological studies of cultured labial biopsy cells from patients with Sjögren's syndrome, *Clin. Exp. Immunol.* 18:213.

DeVries, M. J., and Hijmans, W., 1967, Pathological changes of thymic epithelial cells and autoimmune disease in NZB, NZW, and (NZB X NZW)F$_1$ mice, *Immunology* 12:179.

Dixon, F., as quoted in 1974 *Lancet* editorial, 2:1302.

Dixon, F., Croker, B., Del Villano, B., Jensen, F., and Lerner, R., 1974, Oncornavirus infection and "auto" immune complex disease of mice, *Prog. Immunol. II* 5:49.

Elkins, W. L., 1971, Cellular immunology and the pathogenesis of graft versus host reactions, *Prog. Allergy* 15:78.

East, J., 1970, Immunopathology and neoplasms in New Zealand black (NZB) and SJL/J mice, *Prog. Exp. Tumor Res.* 13:84.

Essex, M., 1975, Horizontally and vertically transmitted oncornaviruses of cats, *Adv. Cancer Res.* 21:175.

Gallagher, R. E., and Gallo, R. C., 1975, Type C RNA tumor virus isolated from cultured human acute myelogenous leukemia cells, *Science* 187:350.

Gershwin, M. E., and Steinberg, A. D., 1973, Loss of suppressor function as a cause of lymphoid malignancy, *Lancet* 2:1174.

Gleichmann, E., Gleichmann, H., Schwartz, R. S., Weinblatt, A., and Armstrong, M. Y. K., 1975, Immunologic induction of malignant lymphoma: Identification of donor and host tumors in the graft-versus-host model, *J. Natl. Cancer Inst.* 54:107.

Goldstein, G., and Schlesinger, D. M., 1975, Thymopoietin and myasthenia gravis: neostigmine-responsive neuromuscular block produced in mice by a synthetic peptide fragment of thymopoietin, *Lancet* 2:25.

Greenberger, J. S., Phillips, S. M., Stephenson, J. R., and Aaronson, S. A., 1975, Induction of mouse type-C RNA virus by lipopolysaccharide, *J. Immunol.* 115:317.

Grimley, P. M., Decker, J. L., Michelitch, H. J., and Frantz, M. M., 1973, Abnormal structures in circulating lymphocytes from patients with systemic lupus erythematosus and related disease, *Arthritis Rheum.* 16:313.

Györkey, F., Sinkovics, J. G., Min, K. W., and Györkey, P., 1972, A morphological study on the occurrence and distribution of structures resembling viral nucleocapsids in collagen disease, *Am. J. Med.* **53**:148.

Hirsch, M. S., and Black, P. H., 1974, Activation of mammalian leukemia viruses, *Adv. Virus Res.* **19**:265.

Hirsch, M. S., and Proffitt, M. R., 1975, Autoimmunity in viral infections, in: *Viral Immunology and Immunopathology* (A. L. Notkins, ed.), pp. 419–434, Academic Press, New York.

Hirsch, M. S., Black, P. H., Tracy, G. S., Leibowitz, S., and Schwartz, R. S., 1970, Leukemia virus activation in chronic allogeneic disease, *Proc. Natl. Acad. Sci. U.S.A.* **67**:1914.

Hirsch, M. S., Phillips, S. M., Solnik, C., Black, P. H., Schwartz, R. S., and Carpenter, C. B., 1972, Activation of leukemia viruses by graft-versus-host and mixed lymphocyte reactions *in vitro, Proc. Natl. Acad. Sci. U.S.A.* **5**:1069.

Hirsch, M. S., Ellis, D. A., Black, P. H., Monaco, A. P., and Wood, M. L., 1973, Leukemia virus activation during homograft rejection, *Science* **180**:500.

Hirsch, M. S., Ellis, D. A., Kelly, A. P., Proffitt, M. R., Black, P. H., Monaco, A. P., and Wood, M. L., 1975a, Activation of C-type viruses during skin graft rejection in the mouse. Interrelationships between immunostimulation and immunosuppression, *Int. J. Cancer* **15**:493.

Hirsch, M. S., Kelly, A. P., Proffitt, M. R., and Black, P. H., 1975b, Cell-mediated immunity to antigens associated with endogenous murine C-type viruses, *Science* **187**:959.

Hoover, R., and Fraumeni, J. F., Jr., 1973, Risk of cancer in renal transplant recipients, *Lancet* **2**:55.

Howe, M. L., 1973, Isogenic lymphocyte interaction: responsiveness of murine thymocytes to self antigens, *J. Immunol.* **110**:1090.

Lance, E. M., 1968, The effects of chronic ALS administration in mice, *Adv. Transplant.* **8**:107.

Leventhal, B. G., Waldorf, D. S., and Talal, N., 1967, Impaired lymphocyte transformation and delayed hypersensitivity in Sjögren's syndrome, *J. Clin. Invest.* **46**:1338.

Levy, J. A., 1974, Autoimmunity and neoplasia. The possible role of C-type viruses, *Am. J. Clin. Pathol.* **62**:258.

Lewis, R. M., Tannenberg, W., Smith, C., and Schwartz, R. S., 1974, C-type viruses in systemic lupus erythematosus, *Nature (London)* **252**:78.

Lonai, P., Declève, A., and Kaplan, H. S., 1974. Spontaneous induction of endogenous murine leukemia virus-related antigen expression during short-term *in vitro* incubation of mouse lymphocytes, *Proc. Natl. Acad. Sci. U.S.A.* **71**:2008.

Lopez, C., Simmons, R. L., Mauer, S. M., Najarian, J. S., and Good, R. A., 1974, Association of renal allograft rejection with virus infections, *Am. J. Med.* **56**:280.

Lukes, R. J., and Collins, R. D., 1974, Immunologic characterization of human malignant lymphomas, *Cancer* **34**:1488.

Metcalf, D., 1966, *The Thymus,* pp. 100–117, Springer-Verlag, New York.

Moroni, C., Schumann, G., Robert-Guroff, M., Suter, E. R., and Martin, D., 1975, Induction of endogenous murine C-type virus in spleen cell cultures treated with mitogens and 5-bromo-2'-deoxyuridine, *Proc. Natl. Acad. Sci. U.S.A.* **72**:535.

Olding, L. B., Jensen, F. C., and Oldstone, M. B. A., 1975, Pathogenesis of cytomegalovirus infection. I. Activation of virus from bone marrow-derived lymphocytes by in vitro allogeneic reaction, *J. Exp. Med.* **141**:561.

Penn, I., and Starzl, T. E., 1972, Malignant tumors arising de novo in immunosuppressed organ transplant recipients, *Transplantation* **14**:407.

Phillips, S. M., Gleichmann, H., Hirsch, M. S., Black, P. H., Merrill, J. P., Schwartz, R. S., and Carpenter, C. B., 1975a, Cellular immunity in the mouse. IV. Altered thymic-dependent lymphocyte reactivity in chronic graft vs host reaction and leukemia virus activation, *Cell. Immunol.* 15:152.

Phillips, S. M., Hirsch, M. S., André-Schwartz, J., Solnik, C., Black, P. H., Schwartz, R. S., Merrill, J. P., and Carpenter, C. B., 1975*b*, Cellular immunity in the mouse. V. Further studies on leukemia virus activation in allogeneic reactions of mice: stimulatory parameters, *Cell. Immuno.* 15:169.

Porter, D. D., 1971, A quantitative review of the slow virus landscape, *Prog. Exp. Tumor Res.* 13:339.

Proffitt, M. R., Hirsch, M. S., Gheridian, B., McKenzie, I. F. C., and Black, P. H., 1975*a*, Immunological mechanisms in the pathogenesis of virus-induced murine leukemia. I. Autoreactivity, *Int. J. Cancer* 15:221.

Proffitt, M. R., Hirsch, M. S., McKenzie, I. F. C., Gheridian, B., and Black, P. H., 1975*b*, Immunological mechanisms in the pathogenesis of virus-induced murine leukemia. II. Characterization of autoreactive thymocytes. *Int. J. Cancer* 15:230.

Proffitt, M. R., Hirsch, M. S., Ellis, D. A., Gheridian, B., and Black, P. H., 1976, Immunologic mechanisms in the pathogenesis of virus-induced murine leukemia. III. Target cell specificity of autoreactive thymocytes, *J. Immunol.* 117:11.

Sherr, C. J., Lieber, M. M., and Todaro, G. J., 1974, Mixed splenocyte cultures and graft versus host reactions selectively induce an "S-tropic" murine type-C virus, *Cell* 1:55.

Siegler, R., 1968, Pathology of murine leukemias, in: *Experimental Leukemia* (M. Rich, ed.), pp. 51–95, Appleton-Century-Crofts, New York.

Solnik, C., Gleichmann, H., Kavanah, M., and Schwartz, R. S., 1973, Immunosuppression and malignant lymphomas in graft versus host reactions, *Cancer Res.* 33:2068.

Spencer, E. S., and Anderson, H. K., 1970, Clinically evident, non-terminal infections with herpesviruses and the wart virus in immunosuppressed renal allograft recipients, *Br. Med. J.* 3:251.

Stiller, C. R., Russell, A. S., McConnachie, P., Dossetor, J. B., and Diener, E., 1973, Cell-mediated autoimmunity in NZB mice, *Clin. Exp. Immunol.* 15:445.

Strand, M., and August, J. T., 1974, Type-C RNA virus gene expression in human tissue, *J. Virol.* 14:1584.

Strauch, B., Siegel, N., Andrews, L., and Miller, G., 1974, Oropharyngeal excretion of Epstein-Barr virus by renal transplant recipients and other patients treated with immunosuppressive drugs, *Lancet* 1:234.

Suciu-Foca, N., Buda, J. A., Thiem, T., and Reemtsma, K., 1974, Impaired responsiveness of lymphocytes in patients with systemic lupus erythematosus, *Clin. Exp. Immunol.* 18:295.

Talal, N., and Steinberg, A. D., 1974, The pathogenesis of autoimmunity in New Zealand black mice, *Curr. Top. Microbiol. Immunol.* 64:79.

Tannenbaum, H., and Schur, P. H., 1974, The role of lymphocytes in rheumatic diseases, *J. Rheumatol.* 1:4.

Temin, H. M., 1972, the RNA tumor viruses-background and foreground, *Proc. Natl. Acad. Sci. U.S.A.* 69:1016.

Todaro, G. J., and Huebner, R. J., 1972, The viral oncogene hypothesis: new evidence, *Proc. Natl. Acad. Sci. U.S.A.* 69:1009.

Walters, M. L., Stanley, N. F., Dawkins, R. L., and Alpers, M. P., 1973, Immunological assessment of mice with chronic jaundice and runting induced by reovirus 3, *Br. J. Exp. Pathol.* 54:329.

Wu, B. C., Dowling, J. N., Armstrong, J. A., and Ho, M., 1975. Enhancement of mouse cytomegalovirus infection during host-versus-graft reaction, *Science* 190:56.

Chapter 8

Natural Immunity to Murine Mammary Tumor Viruses

P. Bentvelzen and P. C. Creemers

Radiobiological Institute TNO
Rijswijk, The Netherlands

I. HISTORICAL REVIEW

The best-known route of transmission of the mouse mammary tumor virus (MTV) is via the milk (Bittner, 1936). In inbred mouse strains selected for a high incidence of mammary carcinoma, a milkborne tumor-inciting agent has been passed for numerous generations. Disregarding the occasional loss of virus from such high-cancer strains (Andervont and Dunn, 1962), the perpetuation of the virus and the disease for so many years has been regarded as indicative for true viral tolerance of high-cancer-strain mice. The immunogenicity of MTV to its natural host was very much in doubt (Bittner, 1962; Squartini, 1966; Andrewes and Pereira, 1967), while its antigenicity to other species was clearly demonstrated at an early stage of mammary tumor virus research (Andervont and Bryan, 1944; Green *et al.*, 1946; Bittner and Imagawa, 1955).

However, Andervont (1945) and Bentvelzen (1968*b*) observed that infected females of resistant low-mammary cancer strain mice could passively immunize their otherwise susceptible hybrid offspring against MTV. Blair (1968) reported the induction of neutralizing antibodies to the virus in mice. Several investigators succeeded in the induction of mouse antibodies that can precipitate either complete virions (Blair *et al.*, 1966; Hilgers *et al.*, 1971) or various soluble viral antigens in the double immunodiffusion test (Nowinski *et al.*, 1967; Fink *et al.*, 1968; Bentvelzen *et al.*, 1970*a*; Hilgers *et al.*, 1971).

Mammary tumors from high-cancer strains can evoke strong transplantation immunity in syngeneic mice which do not carry the milkborne viral agent (Weiss *et al.*, 1966). A similar immunity could be evoked with formalinized viral preparations (Burton *et al.*, 1969), indicating that probably transplantation immunity is directed against a viral coat protein deposited on the tumor cell surface. However, mice which are neonatally infected with the virus via the mother's milk cannot become immunized against a cross-reactive mammary-tumor transplantation antigen (Morton, 1965, 1969; Weiss *et al.*, 1966) but only against weak antigens unique to each tumor (Vaage, 1968a,b; Morton *et al.*, 1969). This has been interpreted as a tolerance of the infected mice to the virus.

Blair *et al.* (1966) and Hilgers *et al.* (1971) found that neonatally infected C3H mice upon immunization produce viral antibodies. Tumor-bearing mice of this strain contain precipitating antibodies to MTV in their serum (Bentvelzen *et al.*, 1970a; Müller *et al.*, 1971). True tolerance to the virus does not seem to exist at the humoral level. It remains to be established to which viral antigens the antibody reactivity is directed.

An important question is whether these antibodies exert an influence on tumor growth. The enhancing role of serum factors from immunized animals on the growth of transplanted tumors has been clearly established (Attia and Weiss, 1966; Müller, 1967; Dezfulian *et al.*, 1968). Immunization with mammary tumor tissue or virus and complete Freund's adjuvant may lead to the accelerated appearance of "spontaneous" tumors in neonatally infected mice (Hirsch and Iversen, 1961; Bentvelzen *et al.*, 1970a), suggesting the role of enhancing antibodies. A very interesting observation by Stolfi *et al.* (1975) is that serum from tumor-bearing mice at high dilutions has a cytotoxic activity to tumor cells in the presence of complement. The failure to lyse tumor cells at low dilutions, as we also repeatedly observed, has been ascribed to the presence of an inhibitor.

Yunis *et al.* (1969) noticed that injection of spleen cells from adult C3H mice into neonatally thymectomized mice caused a significant inhibition of "spontaneous" mammary carcinogenesis, while spleen cells from syngeneic but "virus-free" C3Hf mice had no such an effect. It is not clear whether this adoptive transfer of immunity can be ascribed to antibody-synthesizing cells that cause neutralization of the virus which is introduced during the nursing period. It must be mentioned here that the length of the period of nursing by infected females is critical for the tumor incidence (Andervont and McEleney, 1939; Andervont, 1949; Bentvelzen, 1968a,b). Another explanation for the results obtained by Yunis *et al.* (1969) is the transfer of cellular immunity directed against virus-producing cells.

Utilizing the colony-inhibition test, Heppner (1969) found that mammary-tumor-bearing mice have lymphocytes that can arrest the growth of mammary tumor cells. However, there was little evidence that this cellular reactivity was directed against viral antigens. This led to the concept of partial tolerance to the virus, i.e., cellular unresponsiveness to virus-coded cell-surface antigens, in contrast to the humoral response to virions (Blair, 1971). In the latter case, it was assumed that upon immunization tolerance was "broken" more readily at the humoral level. Van der Gugten and Bentvelzen (1969) assumed that some form of immunity to the virus existed at both levels in neonatally infected mice. They termed it "underground immunity."

By means of the, in our opinion, somehow unreliable microcytotoxicity test, Blair and Lane (1974a,b) and Blair et $al.$ (1974) observed cytotoxic cellular activity of spleen cells from neonatally infected BALB/c mice toward virus-induced mammary tumor cells. In view of the cross-reactivity, this cytotoxic activity seems to be virus related. This cell-mediated form of immunity would develop as early as three weeks of age (Blair and Lane, 1975). Mice with small tumors also would have cytotoxic cells in their spleens, but such cells could not be detected in mice with large tumors. Incubation of the target cells with serum from infected mice partially blocked the cytotoxic activity. Time-course studies seemed to indicate two separate events: an early-appearing cytostasis, which could not be blocked by serum factors, and later cell destruction, which could be abrogated by preincubation of the target cells with serum from BALB/cfC3H mice. It was suggested by Blair and Lane (1975) that two different spleen cell populations would be involved in the separate events. By treatment of spleen cells with anti-θ serum, the later-appearing cell destruction was abolished, which might indicate that T cells were involved. The early-appearing cytostasis could be blocked by treatment of spleen cells with heat-aggregated human γ-globulin, indicating that a different cell population could be held responsible for this phenomenon (Lane et $al.$, 1975).

Uninfected BALB/c mice would also have spleen cells that are cytotoxic to virally induced mammary tumor cells when they are over 14 weeks of age (Blair and Lane, 1974a). It was thought to be due to horizontal transmission of MTV in the mouse colony (Blair and Lane, 1974b), but this is difficult to deduce from experimental groups with only one mouse. The reactivity of the BALB/c cells could not be blocked by preincubation of the tumor cells with serum from BALB/cfC3H mice (Blair and Lane, 1975). The cytotoxic action of normal BALB/c spleen cells did not seem to be caused by T cells (Lane et $al.$, 1975).

An extensive study of cellular immunity to MTV in BALB/cfC3H mice has been undertaken in our laboratory, involving more than one technique and larger groups of mice than in the aforementioned studies of Blair. It is our experience that the microcytotoxicity test is technically cumbersome and not very reliable (see also Howell et $al.$, 1974). We also utilized the leukocyte adherence inhibition test (Halliday and Miller, 1972) using peritoneal exudate cells and the leukocyte stimulation test, in which the [^{14}C] thymidine uptake by lymphocytes in the presence of purified disrupted MTV is taken as an indication for cellular reactivity to the virus. The results of this investigation will be detailed elsewhere (P. C. Creemers, manuscript in preparation), but the outcome of the two latter tests is that only when BALB/cfC3H mice have medium-sized tumors do they display strong cellular activity against the virus.

For the standard mammary tumor virus (MTV-S), besides the milkborne and erratic male transmission, no other modes of transmission seem to exist (for a review, see Mühlbock and Bentvelzen, 1968). However, in the GR mouse strain a virulent, somewhat different MTV-strain is vertically transmitted by the gametes produced by either sex (Mühlbock and Bentvelzen, 1968). Extensive genetic analysis (Bentvelzen, 1968a; Bentvelzen and Daams, 1969; Bentvelzen et al., 1970b; Bentvelzen, 1972a) led to the hypothesis that this virus was transmitted as a genetic factor of the host.

Retrospectively, the gamete-borne transmission of the low-oncogenic strain of MTV in C3Hf as noticed by Pitelka et al. (1964) had to be explained on the same basis. It was also realized that low-cancer-strain mice would carry a germinal provirus of MTV in their cellular genome (Bentvelzen, 1968a; Bentvelzen and Daams, 1969). Molecular hybridization experiments have confirmed the correctness of this view (Varmus et al., 1972).

The GR mouse strain, which is exceptional in many respects, is the best releaser of MTV (Haaijman and Brinkhof, unpublished results). There was little evidence for an immunological responsiveness to its endogenous MTV-P (Bentvelzen et al., 1970b; Hilgers et al., 1971; Bentvelzen, 1974). However, immunization of GR mice with the antigenically different MTV-S leads to a significant delay in tumor development (Van der Gugten and Bentvelzen, 1969; Bentvelzen et al., 1970a), the production of precipitating antibodies to either MTV (Hilgers et al., 1971; Bentvelzen, 1972b), and considerable cellular immunity to the virus as estimated by various techniques (P. C. Creemers, unpublished results). It was assumed that such manipulations led to a break in tolerance to the endogenous MTV. Noteworthy is that hyperimmunization with MTV-S caused an accelerated appearance of mammary tumors in GR mice (Bentvelzen, 1972b).

II. IMMUNOFLUORESCENCE STUDIES ON THE PRESENCE OF ANTIBODIES TO MTV IN MOUSE SERA

By means of the indirect immunofluorescence technique on mammary tumor slices, Müller and Zotter (1973) claimed to have found antibodies to MTV in neonatally infected mice. As no rigid tests of specificity had been performed by these authors, an additional study in our laboratory (reported in the following section) has been carried out in order to assess the validity of these claims.

For the first series of experiments, acetone-fixed slides of cultures grown in Leighton tubes were used (Dulbecco's medium plus 10% fetal calf serum in the presence of 10% CO_2 in humidified air). Two kinds of mammary tumor cultures were used: one derived from primary GR mouse strain tumors, harboring MTV-P, and the other from tumors induced in BALB/c mice by the endogenous MTV-O (see Hageman *et al.*, 1972). Secondary BALB/c embryonic fibroblast cultures, whether infected or not with Rauscher leukemia virus (RLV), were used as controls. The slides were incubated in a humidified chamber at 37°C for either 45 min or 16 hr with various dilutions of mouse serum, beginning at tenfold. After repeated washing, the slides were incubated with a fluorescein isothiocyanate-conjugated (FITC) goat anti-mouse IgG serum (Nordic, Tilburg, The Netherlands) at a twentyfold dilution for 45 min. This antiserum has been tested for specificity in immunoelectrophoresis and in every immunofluorescence experiment for aspecific reactions with any tissue culture. No aspecificity was found.

The slides were embedded in Elvanol and kept at −28°C until examined. They were viewed under a Leitz Orthoplan microscope with the Ploemopak 2.1, with the two filter systems for FITC (2X KP 490 nm, 1 nm GG 455 nm, TK 510 nm—interference dividing plate—and K 515 nm + SAL 525 nm as barrier filters). With this excellent optical system, no counterstain of the cultures is needed.

From the results shown in Table I, it can be concluded that the reaction proved to be specific for MTV. Usually no reaction was observed with any serum when the slides were incubated for only 45 min. It must be mentioned here that rigid criteria had to be met before fluorescence was called positive. It is obvious that when the slides were incubated for 16 hr all mice with known MTV-expression proved to have antibodies in their serum which reacted with an intracytoplasmic viral antigen. The virus specificity was further demonstrated when incubation of the mouse sera with purified MTV-S (0.01 mg/0.1 ml serum) overnight at 4°C led to a complete abrogation of the reaction. Mice without known MTV expression had no detectable antibodies by this technique, but possibly more sensitive techniques such as the radioimmunoassay might pick them up.

In addition, some immunofluorescence studies were performed with living cells in order to detect MTV-associated membrane antigens. Undiluted mouse sera were used, since dilution led rapidly to the disappearance of positive fluorescence. From the results shown in Table II it is obvious that tumor-bearing mice have antibodies in their serum which give a broad cross-reactive membrane fluorescence with GR mammary tumor cells producing MTV-P. It is quite remarkable that mice with large tumors have no detectable antibodies in this test. Surprisingly, mice which were infected with MTV-S instead of the endogenous MTV-O had a much stronger reaction. Absorption of the sera with purified MTV did not lead to complete abrogation of the reaction in contrast to the cytoplasmic immunofluorescence. It has been theorized that the p28 protein of MTV (an internal core protein in the virion) would accumulate in the cytoplasm and that gp 52 (the spike protein) would be deposited at the cell

Table I. Immunofluorescence Reactions of Mouse Sera with an MTV-Associated Cytoplasmic Antigen

Mouse strain	Age (months)	MTV-expression	Number of sera	Endpoint titers[a] (geometric mean) on cultures of			
				MTV-O	MTV-P	BALB/c-EF	BALB/c-EF + RLV
C57BL	3	−	4	0–0	0–0	0–0	0–0
BALB/c	4	−	10	0–0	0–0	0–0	0–0
BALB/cfC3H	2	+	4	0–17	0–10	0–0	0–0
BALB/cfC3H	6–8	+ (tumor)	15	18–92	0–52	0–0	0–0
BALB/c-MTV-O	6–8	+ (tumor)	12	23–64	8–60	0–0	0–0
GR	2	+	4	0–15	0–20	0–0	0–0
GR	6	+ (tumor)	10	14–184	10–104	0–0	0–0

[a]First number 45 min incubation, second 16 hr.

Table II. MTV-Associated Membrane Fluorescence
with Sera from Tumor-Bearing BALB/c Mice

| | | Fluorescence on cultures of | | | |
| | | GR tumors | | BALB/c-EF | |
Virus strain	Tumor weight (g)	45 min	16 hr	45 min	16 hr
MTV-O	2.0	−	+	−	−
	3.2	−	+	−	−
	4.0	−	±	−	−
MTV-S	0.7	−	−	−	−
	1.3	±	+	−	−
	1.8	++	++	−	−
	2.3	++	++	−	−
	5.0	−	−	−	−

surface. The failure to completely absorb out the reactivity toward tumor membranes after incubation with an excess of MTV might indicate that a nonvirion but MTV-associated antigen is present at the cell surface. More extensive investigations are needed in this respect.

There is a lack of correlation when mouse sera are tested for both intracytoplasmic and membrane fluorescence. This might indicate that antibodies to different viral or virus-associated antigens are involved. Investigations utilizing more sensitive immunoassays and purified MTV proteins are in progress to solve this problem.

ACKNOWLEDGMENTS

The work upon which this publication is based was performed pursuant to Contract NIH NO1 CP43328 with the National Cancer Institute, Division of Cancer Cause and Prevention, Viral Oncology, Department of Health, Education, and Welfare, Bethesda, Maryland.

III. REFERENCES

Andervont, H. B., 1945, Susceptibility of young and adult mice to the mammary tumor agent, *J. Natl. Cancer Inst.* 5:397.

Andervont, H. B., 1949, Studies on the disappearance of the mammary tumor agent in mice of strains C3H and C, *J. Natl. Cancer Inst.* 10:201.

Andervont, H. B., and Bryan, W. R., 1944, Properties of the mouse mammary tumor agent, *J. Natl. Cancer Inst.* **5**:143.

Andervont, H. B., and Dunn, T. B., 1962, Studies of the mammary-tumor agent of strain RIII mice, *J. Natl. Cancer Inst.* **28**:159.

Andervont, H. B., and McEleney, A., 1939, Influence of foster-nursing upon the incidence of spontaneous breast cancer in strain C3H mice, *Public Health Rep.* **54**:1597.

Andrewes, C., and Pereira, H. G., 1967, *Viruses of Vertebrates,* p. 139, Ballière, Tindall, and Cassell, London.

Attia, M. A., and Weiss, D. W., 1966, Immunology of spontaneous mammary carcinomas in mice. V. Acquired tumor resistance and enhancement in strain A mice infected with mammary tumor virus, *Cancer Res.* **26**:1787.

Bentvelzen, P., 1968a, *Genetical Control of the Vertical Transmission of the Mühlbock Mammary Tumour Virus in the GR Mouse Strain,* Hollandia, Amsterdam.

Bentvelzen, P., 1968b, Resistance to small amounts of Bittner mammary tumor virus in offspring of female mice with the virus, *J. Natl. Cancer Inst.* **41**:757.

Bentvelzen, P., 1972a, Hereditary infections with mammary tumor viruses in mice, in: *RNA Viruses and Host Genome in Oncogenesis* (P. Emmelot and P. Bentvelsen, eds.), p. 309, North-Holland, Amsterdam.

Bentvelzen, P., 1972b, Attempts to immunize GR mice against tumour development, in: *Fundamental Research on Mammary Tumours* (J. Mouriquand, ed.), p. 129, INSERM, Paris.

Bentvelzen, P., 1974, Host–virus interactions in murine mammary carcinogenesis, *Biochim. Biophys. Acta* **355**:236.

Bentvelzen, P., and Daams, J. H., 1969, Hereditary infections with mammary tumor viruses in mice. *J. Natl. Cancer Inst.* **43**:1025.

Bentvelzen, P., van der Gugten, A., Hilgers, J., and Daams, J. H., 1970a, Breakthrough in tolerance to eggborne mammary tumor viruses, in: *Immunity and Tolerance in Oncogenesis* (L. Severi, ed.), p. 525, IVth Perugia Quadriennial International Conference, Perugia, Italy.

Bentvelzen, P., Daams, J. H., Hageman, P., and Calafat, J., 1970b, Genetic transmission of viruses that incite mammary tumor in mice, *Proc. Natl. Acad. Sci. U.S.A.* **67**:377.

Bittner, J. J., 1936, Some possible effects of nursing on the mammary gland tumor incidence in mice, *Science* **84**:162.

Bittner, J. J., 1962, Biologic assay and serial passage of the mouse mammary tumor agent in mammary tumors from mothers and their hybrid progeny, in: *CIBA Foundation Symposium: Tumor Viruses of Murine Origin,* p. 55, Little, Brown, Boston.

Bittner, J. J., and Imagawa, D. T., 1955, Effect of the source of the mouse mammary tumor agent (MTA) upon neutralization of the agent with antisera, *Cancer Res.* **15**:464.

Blair, P. B., 1968, Immunology of the mouse mammary tumor virus (MTV): Neutralization of MTV by mouse antiserum, *Cancer Res.* **28**:148.

Blair, P. B., 1971, Immunological aspects of the relationship between host and oncogenic virus in the mouse mammary tumor system, *Isr. J. Med. Sci.* **7**:161.

Blair, P. B., and Lane, M. A., 1974a, Serum factors in mammary neoplasia: Enhancement and antagonism of spleen cell activity *in vitro* detected by different methods of serum factor assay, *J. Immunol.* **112**:439.

Blair, P. B., and Lane, M. A., 1974b, Immunologic evidence for horizontal transmission of MTV, *J. Immunol.* **113**:1446.

Blair, P. B., and Lane, M. A., 1975, *In vitro* detection of immune responses to MTV-induced mammary tumors: Qualitative differences in response detected by time studies, *J. Immunol.* **114**:17.

Blair, P. B., Lavrin, D. H., Dezfulian, M., and Weiss, D. W., 1966, Immunology of the mouse mammary tumor virus (MTV): Identification *in vitro* of mouse antibodies against MTV, *Cancer Res.* 26:647.

Blair, P. B., Lane, M. A., and Yagi, M. J., 1974, *In vitro* detection of immune responses to MTV induced mammary tumors: Activity of spleen cell preparations from both MTV-free and MTV-infected mice, *J. Immunol.* 112:693.

Burton, D. S., Blair, P. B., and Weiss, D. W., 1969, Protection against mammary tumors in mice by immunization with purified mammary tumor virus preparations, *Cancer Res.* 29:971.

Dezfulian, M., Zee, T., DeOme, K. B., Blair, P. B., and Weiss, D. W., 1968, Role of the mammary tumor virus in the immunogenicity of spontaneous mammary carcinomas of BALB/c mice and in the responsiveness of the hosts, *Cancer Res.* 28:1759.

Fink, M. A., Feller, W. F., and Sibal, L. R., 1968, Methods for detection of antibody to the mammary tumor virus, *J. Natl. Cancer Inst.* 41:1395.

Green, R. G., Moosey, M. M., and Bittner, J. J., 1946, Antigenic character of the cancer milk agent in mice, *Proc. Soc. Exp. Biol. Med.* 61:115.

Gugten, A. van der, and Bentvelzen, P., 1969, Interference between two strains of the mouse mammary tumor virus in the GR mouse strain, *Eur. J. Cancer* 5:361.

Hageman, P. C., Calafat, J., and Daams, J. H., 1972, The mammary tumor viruses, in: *RNA Viruses and Host Genome in Oncogenesis* (P. Emmelot and P. Bentvelzen, eds.), p. 238, North-Holland, Amsterdam.

Halliday, W. J., and Miller, S., 1972, Leukocyte adherence inhibition: A simple test for cell-mediated tumour immunity and serum blocking factors, *Int. J. Cancer* 9:477.

Heppner, G. H., 1969, Studies on serum-mediated inhibition of cellular immunity to spontaneous mouse mammary tumors, *Int. J. Cancer* 4:608.

Hilgers, J., Daams, J. H., and Bentvelzen, P., 1971, The induction of precipitating antibodies to the mammary tumor virus in several inbred mouse strains, *Isr. J. Med. Sci.* 7:154.

Hirsch, H. M., and Iversen, I., 1961, Accelerated development of spontaneous mammary tumors in mice pretreated with mammary tumor tissue and adjuvant, *Cancer Res.* 21:752.

Howell, S. B., Dean, J. H., Esber, E. C., and Law, L. W., 1974, Cell interactions in adoptive immune rejection of a syngeneic tumor, *Int. J. Cancer* 14:662.

Lane, M. A., Roubinian, J., Slomich, M., Trefts, P., and Blair, P. B., 1975, Characterization of cytotoxic effector cells in the mouse mammary tumor system, *J. Immunol.* 114:24.

Morton, D. L., 1965, Acquired immunological tolerance to spontaneous mammary adenocarcinomas following neonatal infection with mammary tumor agent (MTA), *Proc. Am. Assoc. Cancer Res.* 5:46.

Morton, D. L., 1969, Acquired immunological tolerance and carcinogenesis by the mammary tumor virus. I. Influence of neonatal infection with the mammary tumor virus on the growth of spontaneous mammary adenocarcinomas, *J. Natl. Cancer Inst.* 42:311.

Morton, D. L., Miller, G. F., and Wood, D. A., 1969, Demonstration of tumor-specific immunity against antigens unrelated to the mammary tumor virus in spontaneous mammary adenocarcinomas, *J. Natl. Cancer Inst.* 42:289.

Mühlbock, O., and Bentvelzen, P., 1968, The transmission of the mammary tumor viruses, in: *Perspectives in Virology*, Vol. 6 (M. Pollard, ed.), p. 75, Academic Press, New York.

Müller, M., 1967, Immunologic interactions between isologous or F_1 hybrid hosts and spontaneous mammary tumors in CBA/Bln mice, *Cancer Res.* 27:2272.

Müller, M., and Zotter, S., 1973, Mammary tumor virus (MTV) infection of CBA/Bln mice involving production of antibodies to MTV, *J. Natl. Cancer Inst.* 50:713.

Müller, M., Hageman, P. C., and Daams, J. H., 1971, Spontaneous occurrence of precipitating antibodies to the mammary tumor virus in mice, *J. Natl. Cancer Inst.* **47**:801.

Nowinski, R. C., Old, L. J., Moore, D. H., Geering, G., and Boyse, E. A., 1967, A soluble antigen of the mammary tumor virus, *Virology* **31**:1.

Pitelka, D. R., Bern, H. A., Nandi, S., and DeOme, K. B., 1964, On the significance of virus-like particles in mammary tissues of C3Hf mice, *J. Natl. Cancer Inst.* **33**:867.

Squartini, F., 1966, Tumours arising from vertical transmission, in: *Handbook of Experimental Pharmacology XVI/13*, p. 1, Springer-Verlag, Berlin.

Stolfi, R. L., Fugmann, R. A., Stolfi, L. M., and Martin, D. S., 1975, Development and inhibition of cytotoxic antibody against spontaneous murine breast cancer, *J. Immunol.* **114**:1824.

Vaage, J., 1968*a*, Non-cross-reacting resistance to virus induced mouse mammary tumours in virus-infected C3H mice, *Nature (London)* **218**:101.

Vaage, J., 1968*b*, Nonvirus-associated antigens in virus induced mouse mammary tumors, *Cancer Res.* **28**:2477.

Varmus, H. E., Bishop, J. M., Nowinski, R. C., and Sarkar, N. H., 1972, Mammary tumour virus specific nucleotide sequences in DNA of high and low incidence mouse strains, *Nature (London) New Biol.* **238**:189.

Wainberg, M. A., Markson, Y., Weiss, D. W., and Doljanski, F., 1974, Cellular immunity against Rous sarcoma of chickens: Preferential reactivity against autochthonous target cells as determined by lymphocyte adherence and cytotoxicity tests *in vitro*, *Proc. Natl. Acad. Sci. U.S.A.* **71**:3565.

Weiss, D. W., Lavrin, D. H., Dezfulian, M., Vaage, J., and Blair, P. B., 1966, Studies on the immunology of spontaneous mammary carcinomas in mice, in: *Viruses Inducing Cancer—Implications for Therapy* (W. J. Burdette, ed.), p. 138, University of Utah Press, Salt Lake City.

Yunis, E. J., Martinez, C., Smith, J., Stutman, O., and Good, R. A., 1969, Spontaneous mammary adenocarcinoma in mice: Influence of thymectomy and reconstitution with thymus grafts or spleen cells, *Cancer Res.* **29**:174.

Chapter 9

Immunogenicity and MuMTV-like Antigenicity of Human Breast Cancer Tissues

Maurice M. Black

New York Medical College
Flower & Fifth Avenue Hospitals
New York, New York 10029

I. INTRODUCTION

In 1936 Bittner reported that a transmissible factor in murine milk was related to the development of mammary tumors. Since that time, Bittner's milk factor has been shown to be a specific type of RNA virus, and the relationship between this RNA virus and murine mammary carcinogenesis has been extensively documented by biological, ultrastructural, immunological, and biochemical techniques (Moore and Charney, 1975). Despite such compelling observations regarding the viral etiology of murine mammary tumors, parallel studies of human mammary cancers have, until recently, yielded essentially negative data. Viral particles are rarely demonstrable in human mammary tissues, benign or malignant. Nor do temporal or geographic variations in incidence rates of human breast cancer correlate with nursing habits (MacMahon *et al.*, 1970). Nevertheless, within the past several years there have been a number of reports indicating that some human breast tissues may harbor particles and/or RNA components which resemble murine mammary tumor virus (MuMTV) (Spiegelman *et al.*, 1972; Schlom *et al.*, 1972, 1973; Seman and Dmochowski, 1973; Müller and Grossmann, 1972; Müller *et al.*, 1972, 1973; Moore, 1974). While such findings are of interest, it remains to be shown that they are specifically related to the development and/or behavior of human breast cancers.

It should be noted that murine mammary tumor research typically employs highly inbred populations maintained under controlled conditions. Furthermore, murine mammary tumors are characterized by progressive local growths. Metastatic dissemination of murine mammary tumors is usually of limited clinical consequence. In contrast, human breast cancer is a nonrandom event in an outbred population and its clinical course is largely determined by metastatic growth. Moreover, the human disease may exhibit extreme variations in behavior in individual patients. Some breast cancer patients die of rapidly progressive disease within months, while others may remain apparently disease-free for decades before recurrent lethal disease appears. Unfortunately, the use of the singular designation, breast cancer, in contrast to the plural form, breast cancers, is so universal that nonclinical investigators, epidemiologists, biochemists, immunologists, virologists, etc., come to believe that their techniques are being applied to precisely defined homogeneous test materials. Even clinical investigators commonly conduct their studies or apply therapy as if they were dealing with homogeneous populations. It is not surprising that the literature is replete with pointless polemics regarding the results of analytical and therapeutic procedures.

It is not unreasonable to expect that even if MuMTV were biologically significant in some human breast cancers it might not be equally significant in all breast cancers or even in all stages of any breast cancer. It is paradoxical that investigators who would demand detailed information regarding the source and nature of experimental tumor tissues (strain, age, nutrition, breeding status, etc.) will accept for analysis any chunk of human tissue designated as "breast cancer" by a "cooperative" pathologist. While it may be difficult to define human tissues with the same precision as is possible for inbred strains of mice, it is indeed possible to recognize a number of biologically significant variables of structure and stage of development. In fact, such characteristics are more adequately definable in the human than in mice. Moreover, the diverse variations in tumor–host interactions provide natural experiments which would be difficult to duplicate in the laboratory. An awareness of such realities is a prerequisite of a meaningful approach to the general problem of human breast cancer and the particular role of viruses in human mammary carcinogenesis.

The following presentation will demonstrate that clinicopathological individualization of patients and their lesions are of critical importance in investigations of human mammary carcinogenesis and behavior. Such individualization would seem to be particularly pertinent to studies of tumor-specific and viral-associated antigens. It will be shown that structural variables lead to immunological interpretations which can be confirmed by immunological measurements. The latter lead, in turn, to the demonstration of MuMTV-like properties of prognostically significant immunogens of human breast cancer tissues.

II. IMMUNOGENICITY OF HUMAN BREAST CANCER

It is readily demonstrable that the postoperative survival of breast cancer patients is inversely correlated with the extent (stage) of the disease at the time of diagnosis. It is also apparent that postoperative survival is correlated with the degree of histological (Bloom, 1950) or nuclear differentiation (Black and Speer, 1957). The majority of patients having breast cancers with well-differentiated nuclei, nuclear grade III, have prolonged postoperative survivals. In contrast, prolonged postoperative survivals are uncommon among patients having undifferentiated nuclei, nuclear grade I. Nevertheless, appreciable variations in biological behavior remains even among those patients who are grouped according to such "tumor-oriented" variables. Such findings, coupled with uncommon, yet real, instances of spontaneous regressions suggest that host-related variables might influence the biological behavior of breast cancer.

In the 1950s this laboratory initiated an ongoing study of prognostically significant structural characteristics of the lymphoreticuloendothelial (L-RE) system of breast cancer patients (Black *et al.*, 1953). In numerous reports we described distinctive L-RE responses to human breast cancer (Black and Speer, 1958, 1960; Black, 1965, 1970*a,b*; Cutler *et al.*, 1969; Black *et al.*, 1975*b*). Most significantly, distinctive types of L-RE response in the primary tumor and regional lymph nodes were found to be prognostically favorable. Such responses included sinus histiocytosis (SH) in the axillary nodes, diffuse lymphoid cellular infiltrations (LI) among the cancer cells of the primary tumor, and perivenous lymphoid cellular infiltrations (PVI) in the region of the primary tumor. Carefully controlled studies demonstrated that the biological behavior of breast cancer patients could be correlated with the intrinsic aggressive potential of the breast cancer, reflected in the nuclear grade, and tumor-retarding influences of the host, reflected in L-RE responses. Similar observations were also reported by others (Anastassiades and Pryce, 1966; Hamlin, 1968; Silverberg *et al.*, 1970).

The cellular nature of the prognostically significant L-RE responses suggested that they represented an immunological response of the delayed (cellular) type of hypersensitivity (Black and Speer, 1959*b*; Black, 1965; Black, 1973). In short, it appeared that an appreciable proportion of human mammary carcinomas were immunogenic in the host of origin and the biological behavior of breast cancers reflected the immunogenicity of the cancer tissue and the specific hypersensitivity responses of the host. Such evidence of immunogenicity was most regularly demonstrable in the earliest recognizable stage of human breast cancer, viz., *in situ* stage (Black and Chabon, 1969, 1970; Black, 1972; Black *et al.*, 1972*b*). LI and/or PVI responses are associated with approximately 80% of those *in situ* breast cancers which are not accompanied by invasive breast cancer. L-RE responses are also observed in an appreciable proportion of precancerous types of mammary duct atypia (precancerous mastopathy). It thus appears that immunogenicity is an early accompaniment of mammary carcinogenesis. It is noteworthy that lymph nodes draining spontaneous murine mammary tumors also display reactive hyperplasia (Black and Speer, 1959*a*).

Table I demonstrates that L-RE responses are also commonly associated with foci of *in situ* carcinoma in breasts which contain invasive breast cancer.

Table I. Percent LI or PVI Response to
in Situ and Invasive Areas of Breast
Cancers Having Both Types of Lesions

	Total	L-RE +	L-RE −
In situ	230	130 (57)	100
		↓	↓
Invasive	230	↓	↓
	↓	↓	↓
L-RE+	100 (43)	92 (71)	8 (8)

However, the percent L-RE-positive response to the *in situ* foci in such breasts is lower than that against *in situ* breast cancer without invasive breast cancer, *viz.*, 57 and 80%, respectively. Table II also demonstrates that L-RE responsiveness to invasive breast cancer is related to the L-RE responses to the associated *in situ* lesion. In those breasts lacking a response to the *in situ* areas, L-RE responses to the invasive areas are uncommon (8%). In contrast, L-RE responses to the invasive cancer are found in the majority (71%) of those cases having L-RE responses to *in situ* foci. However, the lack of response to the invasive lesions in 30% of those cases having reactivity to their *in situ* foci suggests that some invasive cancer cells lack immunogens which are present in the *in situ* cancer cells in the same breast.

While tumor-specific antigenic changes seem to be regular if not universal accompaniments of the developmental stages of breast cancer, such antigenicity is seen less regularly among invasive breast cancer tissues. It should also be noted that the type of L-RE responses is correlated with the degree of nuclear differentiation of the cancer cells. LI responses are found almost exclusively in association with breast cancers (*in situ* and invasive) which have a low (anaplas-

Table II. Response of Breast Cancer Patients'
Leukocytes to Autologous Breast Cancer Tissues

Target	Stage of disease	Number	MI < 0.80
In situ carcinoma	0	16	11 (70)[a]
In situ carcinoma	I	9	6 (67)
In situ carcinoma	II	6	2 (33)
Invasive carcinoma	I	89	32 (36)
Invasive carcinoma	II	69	19 (28)

[a]Percentages are given in parentheses.

tic) nuclear grade. On the other hand, PVI responses are not preferentially associated with the nuclear grade (Black *et al.*, 1975*b*).

It should be noted that LI and SH responses are more regularly associated with breast cancers in Japanese women than with breast cancers in Western women (Morrison *et al.*, 1973; Friedell *et al.*, 1974). Not only is breast cancer infrequent among Japanese women, but also Japanese breast cancer patients have superior stage and survival characteristics. Thus the structural and biological observations suggest that tumor-specific immunogenic changes influence the course and possibly the development of mammary carcinoma. It follows that analytical studies of tumor immunogenicity should take cognizance of the structural characteristics of tissues to be analyzed. The same caveat seems applicable to attempts to demonstrate virions or their genomic products.

Considered *in toto* the microscopic studies suggest that (1) breast cancer patients vary in regard to biologically significant immunogenicity of their cancer tissue and specific hypersensitivity responses to their cancer tissue; (2) prognostically significant immunogenicity and hypersensitivity are maximally present during the preinvasive stage of the disease; and (3) the progression of the disease is associated with or reflects a loss of immunogenicity and/or specific hypersensitivity.

The clinical implications of the microscopic studies served as a stimulus and a reference for more direct studies of tumor immunogenicity and specific hypersensitivity of breast cancer patients. The following presentation will demonstrate that *in vivo* and *in vitro* measurements of cellular hypersensitivity against breast cancer tissues support the interpretations derived from the microscopic studies. In addition, they suggest a relationship between the immunogens of human breast cancer tissues and specific proteins of MuMTV.

III. IMMUNOLOGICAL MEASUREMENTS

A. Autologous Breast Cancer Tissue

1. Skin Window Testing

Hypersensitivity responses to autologous breast lesions were evaluated by a modification of the Rebuck (1955) skin window (SW) technique. Cryostat sections of autologous breast tissues, benign and malignant, were mounted on coverslips and applied to microabrasions of the skin of the forearm for 28–30 hr. The coverslips were then removed, stained (Wright's), and the nature of the cellular exudate evaluated. Approximately one-third of the breast cancer patients tested against autologous breast cancer tissue showed distinctive types of mononuclear cell exudates which were not seen in response to autologous benign breast tissues. The details of such responses may be found in previous publications (Black and Leis, 1971, 1973). The findings of current interest are (1) a stage-response relationship with maximal responsiveness in patients with noninvasive *in situ* carcinoma > stage I > stage II > stage III, and (2) SW responsiveness to autologous invasive breast cancer tissue was greater in PVI-positive–SH-positive patients and in LI-positive patients (53%) as contrasted with patients lacking such L-RE responses (29%). It should be noted that positive SW responses were found repeatedly in some patients who were clinically free of disease 2–3 years postoperatively. We have also observed changes from positive to negative SW responses preceding and associated with the appearance of recurrent disease. Since the same target tissue was used in such repetitive tests, the change from a positive to negative response must reflect a systemic change, either a loss of specific hypersensitivity and/or blocking factors.

The SW studies support the prior conclusion that L-RE responses to breast cancer tissue reflect prognostically significant immunological responses to immunogens in breast cancer tissues. Positive responses with both techniques are indicative of the presence of immunogenicity and specific hypersensitivity. However, neither procedure provides direct information as to the basis of negative responses, *viz.*, lack of immunogenicity, lack of specific hypersensitivity or the presence of blocking factors. Accordingly, we have utilized an *in vitro* assay of cellular hypersensitivity in an attempt to obtain data bearing on the antigenic properties of breast cancer tissue. The procedure employed was the leukocyte migration technique.

2. Leukocyte Migration Procedure

The essential feature of this procedure is a comparison of the migration in the presence of the putative antigen with that found in the absence of the antigen. The ratio is termed the "migration index" (MI). A MI < 0.80 is commonly considered to indicate a positive response. Other investigations have shown that this procedure is capable of revealing hypersensitivity responses of some breast cancer patients against extracts of autologous and homologous breast cancer tissues (Anderson *et al.*, 1970; Anderson *et al.*, 1972; Blasecki and Tevethia, 1973; Fossati *et al.*, 1972; Herberman, 1973*a,b*; McCoy *et al.*, 1974).

In keeping with our particular interest in the antigenic characteristics of microscopically characterized breast cancer tissues, we utilized cryostat sections as antigenic preparations (Black *et al.*, 1974*a*). The cryostat sections are mounted on circular coverslips which become the roof of a Sykes-Moore chamber. The use of cryostat sections makes it possible to choose several microscopically defined samples of tissue from the same breast—*viz.*, areas of *in situ* carcinoma, invasive cancer, and normotypic benign area—and correlate the *in vitro* measurements with the clinicopathologic characteristics.

Table II presents the responsiveness of breast cancer patients' leukocytes according to the nature of the target and the clinical stage of the disease. It is evident that positive responses (MI < 0.80) were obtained most regularly when the target was autologous *in situ* cancer tissue from stage 0 and stage I cases. In contrast, such responses were least common when the target was invasive breast cancer tissue from stage II breast cancer patients. When the target was invasive breast cancer from patients having metastases to 6+ lymph nodes, only 9 (20%) of 45 patients had MI < 0.80. Thus leukocyte responses, like the L-RE responses, to autologous breast cancer tissues vary with specific characteristics of the target and with the stage of the disease.

Further evidence of the influence of target and host characteristics on responses to autologous breast cancer tissues is presented in Table III. It will be seen that the response of leukocytes to autologous invasive breast cancer tissues, having similar nuclear grades, is correlated with the L-RE responses. Indices < 0.80 were significantly more frequent against L-RE-positive autologous invasive breast cancer tissues (45%) than against L-RE-negative targets (20%). As shown in Table IV, leukocyte preparations which were responsive (MI < 0.80) to autologous L-RE-positive breast cancer tissue were commonly cross-reactive with L-RE-positive homologous breast cancer tissues (72%). In contrast, leukocytes which were nonreactive to L-RE-positive autologous breast cancer tissues were uncommonly responsive to L-RE-positive homologous breast cancer tissues (23%).

It appears from the previous *in vitro* measurements that immunogenic breast cancers from different patients may share antigenic characteristics. Such antigenic similarity between homologous breast cancer tissues is reminiscent of the antigenic similarity found in viral-induced experimental tumors. It thus seemed of interest to investigate the responsiveness of breast cancer patients' leukocytes to preparations of murine mammary tumor virus (MuMTV).

Table III. Response of Breast Cancer Patients' Leukocytes to Autologous Invasive Breast Cancer Tissue Having Similar Nuclear Grades

Breast cancer	MI	
	Number	< 0.80
L-RE-positive	62	28 (45)[a,b]
L-RE-negative	74	15 (20)[a,b]

[a] x^2 with Yates correction: MI < 0.80, $x^2 = 8.55$; $P < 0.01$.
[b] Percentages are given in parentheses.

Table IV. Leukocytes from L-RE-Positive
Breast Cancer Patients: MI Response to
Homologous L-RE-Positive Breast Cancer
Tissues by Response to L-RE-Positive
Autologous Breast Cancer Tissue

	Response to homologous[a]	
Response to autologous	Number of tests	MI < 0.80
MI < 0.80		
Number of patients—10	21	15 (72)[b]
MI 0.80+		
Number of patients—21	43	10 (23)

[a]Note: MI < 0.80 were uncommon when leukocytes from control women were tested against L-RE-positive breast cancer
tissues, *viz.*, 5/122 (4%).
[b]Percentages are given in parentheses.

MI < 0.80 was found in approximately one-third of the tests of breast
cancer patients' leukocytes against MuMTV-containing milk from RIII mice
(Black *et al.*, 1974*b*, 1975*a*). Such responsive leukocyte preparations were
commonly cross-reactive to purified preparations of MuMTV but were nonresponsive to MuMTV-free milk from RIIIf, C57BL, and Swiss mice. In contrast,
leukocyte preparations from control women and women with benign breast
lesions rarely (5%) responded to RIII milk or purified MuMTV preparations.

B. Cross-Reactivity against MuMTV and Immunogenic Breast Cancer

1. Autologous Breast Cancer Tissue

The finding that breast cancer patients' leukocytes may respond to MuMTV
is certainly of interest. By itself, however, its significance in regard to human
mammary carcinogenesis and behavior is problematical. It is thus of interest that
we observed correlations between leukocyte responses to RIII milk and biologically significant features of autologous and homologous breast cancer tissues
(Black *et al.*, 1975*a*). As shown in Table V, the responsiveness of breast cancer
patients' leukocytes to RIII milk is correlated with the degree of nuclear differentiation of the autologous cancer: NG I, 20%; NG II, 28%; NG III, 40%. It is
noteworthy in this connection that molecular hybridization studies indicate that
MuMTV-homologous RNA is preferentially found in human breast cancer tissues
having grade III nuclei (see below).

Table V. Response of Breast Cancer Patients' Leukocytes
to RIII Mouse Milk in Relation to Nuclear Grade (NG) of the
Cancer Tissue and Response to Autologous Breast Cancer
Tissue in Relation to Response to RIII Milk

Nuclear grade	Total	Response to RIII milk	
		RIII-positive Autologous positive	RIII-negative Autologous positive
I	74	15 (20)[a]	59
		11 (73)	11 (19)
II	65	18 (28)	47
		11 (61)	11 (23)
III	35	14 (40)	21
		10 (71)	5 (24)

[a]Percentages are given in parentheses.

Table V also demonstrates that within each NG grouping the leukocyte response to autologous breast cancer tissue is correlated with responsiveness to RIII milk, while Table VI demonstrates that the responsiveness of breast cancer patients' leukocytes to autologous breast cancer tissues is a function of the immunogenic properties of the tissue (L-RE-positive > L-RE-negative) and the responsiveness of the leukocytes to MuMTV-containing RIII milk (RIII-positive > RIII-negative). The maximal responsiveness is found between RIII-positive leukocytes and L-RE-positive autologous targets (84%). These data suggest that breast cancer tissues may differ in their antigenic properties and that biologically significant immunogens are antigenically similar to some component of MuMTV (Black et al., 1975a, 1976).

Further evidence of antigenic similarity between MuMTV and immunogens of human breast cancer is provided in Tabel VII. These data demonstrate that positive SW responses are maximal in those patients whose leukocytes are

Table VI. Percent MI < 0.80 vs.
Autologous Breast Cancer Tissue by L-RE
Status and Leukocyte Response to RIII Milk

RIII	L-RE +	L-RE −	Total
< 0.80	16/19 (84)[a]	15/31 (49)	31/50 (62)
0.80+	10/42 (24)	11/57 (19)	21/99 (21)
Total	26/61 (43)	26/88 (30)	

[a]Percentages are given in parentheses.

Table VII. Percent Positive Skin Window Response
in Relation to L-RE Response, and MI Versus RIII
Milk and Autologous Breast Cancer Tissue

| | L-RE-positive breast cancer patients | | | |
| | Autologous | | | |
RIII	< 0.80	0.80+	?	Total
< 0.80	9/12	2/3	2/2	13/17 (76)[a]
0.80+	2/6	9/24	4/5	15/35 (43)
?	9/20	6/15		
Total	20/38 (53)	17/42 (40)		43/87 (49)

| | L-RE-negative breast cancer patients | | | |
| | Autologous | | | |
RIII	< 0.80	0.80+	?	Total
< 0.80	6/14	4/13	3/5	13/32 (41)
0.80+	3/9	8/39	2/7	13/55 (24)
?	3/6	3/13		
Total	12/29 (41)	15/65 (23)		32/106 (30)

| | Total series | | | |
| | Autologous | | | |
RIII	< 0.80	0.80+	?	Total
< 0.80	15/26 (58)	6/16 (38)	5/7	26/49 (53)
0.80+	5/15 (33)	17/63 (27)	6/12	28/90 (31)
?	12/26	9/28		
Total	32/67 (48)	32/107 (30)		75/193 (39)

[a]Percentages are given in parentheses.

simultaneously responsive (MI < 0.80) to RIII milk and autologous breast cancer tissues. Here too, L-RE-positive targets are "seen" by the leukocytes more consistently than L-RE-negative targets.

2. Homologous Breast Cancer Tissue

As indicated previously, breast cancer patients' leukocytes which are responsive to L-RE-positive autologous breast cancer tissues are commonly cross-reactive to L-RE-positive homologous breast cancer tissues. As shown in Table

VIII, reactivity to homologous breast cancer tissue is also a function of reactivity to RIII milk. Leukocytes which respond to RIII milk and autologous breast cancer tissue are simultaneously cross-reactive to a majority (73%) of L-RE-positive homologous breast cancer tissues. In contrast, leukocytes which are simultaneously nonresponsive to RIII milk and L-RE-positive breast cancer tissues are uncommonly responsive (17%) to L-RE-positive homologous breast cancer tissues. It should be noted, however, that an appreciable minority (43%) of L-RE-positive autologous breast cancers were "seen" by RIII-negative leukocytes (Table VII). A similar level of cross-reactivity was found when autologous-positive, RIII-negative leukocytes were tested against homologous breast cancer tissues. It appears that immunogenic human breast cancer tissues may contain tumor-associated and/or viral-associated antigens or neither. Similar conclusions have been drawn regarding the antigens of murine mammary tumors (Morton *et al.*, 1969; Heppner and Pierce, 1969). It should be noted that the preferential responsiveness to *in situ* as compared with invasive breast cancer tissues is almost

Table VIII. Percent MI < 0.80 Versus
Homologous Breast Cancer Tissue by L-RE Status
and Leukocyte Response to RIII Milk and
Autologous Breast Cancer Tissue

Autologous	L-RE-positive homologous breast cancer tissue		
	RIII < 0.80	RIII 0.80+	Total
< 0.80	46/63 (73)[a]	18/46 (39)	64/109 (59)
0.80+	13/34 (38)	31/181 (17)	44/215 (20)
Total	59/97 (61)	49/227 (22)	108/324 (33)

Autologous	L-RE-negative homologous breast cancer tissue		
	RIII < 0.80	RIII 0.80+	Total
< 0.80	4/11 (36)	4/9	8/20 (40)
0.80+	0/4	3/44 (7)	3/48 (6)
Total	4/15 (27)	7/53 (13)	11/68 (16)

Autologous	Total homologous breast cancer series		
	RIII < 0.80	RIII 0.80+	Total
< 0.80	50/74 (68)	22/55 (40)	72/129 (56)
0.80+	13/38 (34)	34/225 (15)	47/263 (18)
Total	63/112 (56)	56/280 (20)	119/392 (30)

[a]Percentages are given in parentheses.

exclusively demonstrable with RIII-positive leukocyte preparations (Black *et al.*, 1974*b*). The latter observation suggests that MuMTV-like antigenicity is an early accompaniment of mammary carcinogenesis.

IV. PHYSICOCHEMICAL MEASUREMENTS

If some breast cancer tissues contain components which are readily diffusible from cryostat sections and are antigenically similar to components of MuMTV, it should be possible to identify such common components by non-immunological procedures. Accordingly we initiated a study of protein components in eluates of cryostat sections of breast cancer tissues. Parallel eluates were also prepared from cryostat sections of benign breast tissues. The eluates were cleared by centrifugation and Millipore filtration and their protein components were then studied by polyacrylamide gel electrophoresis (PAGE) with and without pretreatment with sodium dodecylsulfate (SDS). Simultaneous comparative studies were also performed on proteins of MuMTV derived from RIII mouse milk. The SDS PAGE procedure provides a display of the protein components according to their molecular weights, while the former procedure separates proteins on the basis of charge as well as size. While a detailed description of methods and results will be reported elsewhere (Black *et al.*, 1975*c*), the salient findings are as follows.

A. SDS PAGE

Figure 1 demonstrates that eluates of human breast cancer tissues may indeed contain proteins which resemble those of MuMTV. Of particular interest is a protein whose molecular weight approximates that of gp52 of MuMTV. Accordingly we have designated it as p50. A p50 component was found in 23 of 32 breast cancer tissues but was lacking in five of five eluates of benign tissues from cancerous breasts and six of six eluates of benign tissues from noncancerous breasts. As shown in Table IX, p50 was found in eight of ten prognostically favorable stage I breast cancers and in six of seven breast cancers having metastases to <4 axillary lymph nodes. In contrast, it was lacking in six of 15 breast cancers having metastases to 4+ lymph nodes.

B. Native Proteins PAGE

When the proteins of breast tissue eluates are separated electrophoretically in 8.5% polyacrylamide gels, they all demonstrate a protein band whose mobility is

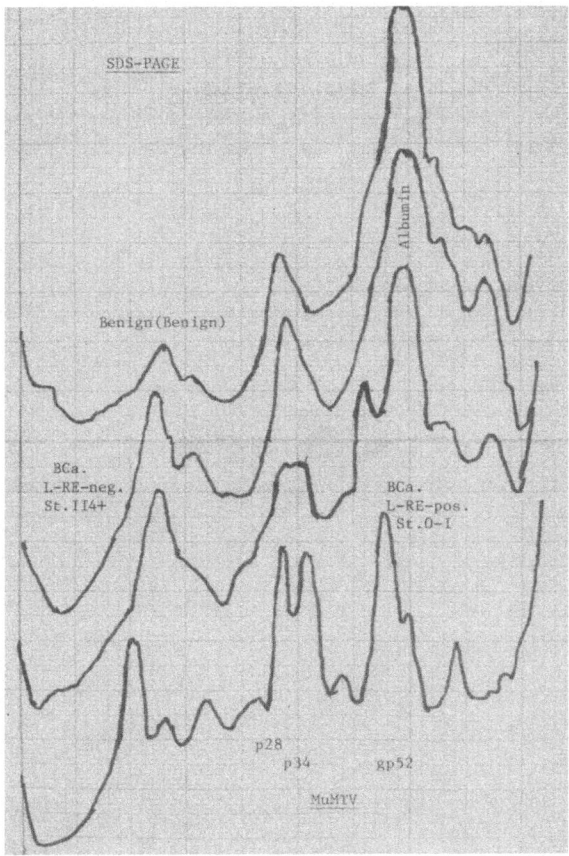

Fig. 1. Densitometer tracings of SDS PAGE of proteins from MuMTV, L-RE-positive stage 0–I, and L-RE-negative stage II4+ human breast cancer tissues and benign tissue of a benign breast. The benign and malignant breast tissues contain proteins which migrate similarly to p28 of MuMTV. The L-RE-positive stage 0–I breast tissue also has components which migrate similarly to p34 and gp52 of MuMTV. These components are lacking in benign breast tissue. The gp52-like component is commonly inconspicuous in L-RE-negative breast cancer tissues.

approximately 0.55 that of serum albumin. This band, designated as B, provides a reference for other bands found in breast tissue eluates. All eluates which in SDS PAGE studies were found to have a well-defined p50 band were found on PAGE studies to contain protein bands which migrated between 0.82 and 0.60 of the B-band migration. Such protein bands were found in only three of the ten eluates of breast cancer tissues which lacked a well-defined p50 band and in none of the eluates of benign tissues.

As shown in Fig. 2, the gp52 protein of MuMTV is separable on 8.5% PAGE into subfractions whose peaks are found at approximately 0.70, 0.75, and 0.80

**Table IX. Stage Distribution of Breast
Cancers According to Presence of
50,000 MW Protein**

Stage	Present	Absent–minimal	Total
I	8	2	10
II < 4	6	1	7
II 4+	9	6	15
Total	23	9	32

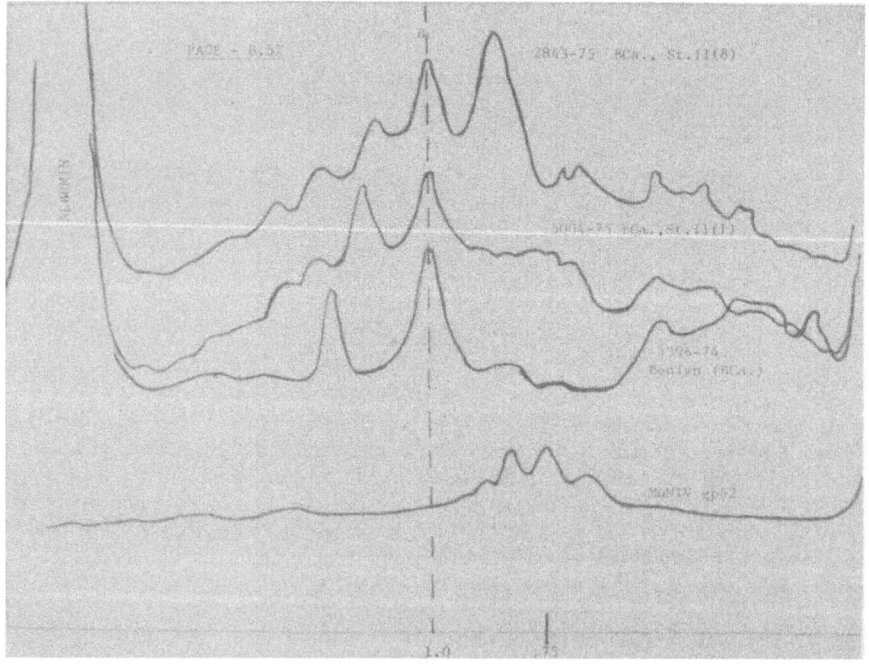

Fig. 2. Densitometer tracings of 8.5% PAGE of proteins from benign and malignant breast tissues and gp52 of MuMTV. The human breast tissues all contain a protein (B) which migrates 0.55 of the albumin. The viral gp52 protein separates into subgroups whose migration peaks are found at approximately 0.70, 0.75, and 0.80 of the B component of human breast tissues. A majority of breast cancer tissues contain proteins which migrate to one or several of these positions. Such protein components are lacking in benign breast tissues from control and cancerous breasts.

of the B-band migration. It appears that the eluate proteins which migrate in the same region are subfractions of the p50 band seen in SDS PAGE preparations. Figure 2 demonstrates that eluates may differ in regard to their p50 subfractions. Some eluates contain a single sharp band while others contain combinations of differently migrating proteins. The 52 breast cancer eluates studied by 8.5% PAGE were separable into four groups according to the migration of their subfractions relative to the B band: *viz.*, eluates having proteins migrating exclusively or predominantly to a position 0.8 that of the B band (p50-0.80), 17 cases; eluates having proteins migrating exclusively to a position 0.75 that of the B band (p50-0.75), six cases; eluates having proteins migrating exclusively to a position 0.70 that of the B band (p50-0.70), one case; eluates having a mixture of p50-0.70, p50-0.75, and/or 0.80 (p50-0.70+), 14 cases; and eluates having minimal amounts of the above components (p50-neg.), 15 cases.

It appears from the data shown in Table X that the protein patterns have biological significance. Of the 17 patients whose eluates had a p50-0.80 pattern, only four had stage I disease, while 11 had stage II 4+ disease. Only six of the 17 cancers were associated with an L-RE response. In contrast, of the 14 patients whose eluate patterns were p50-0.70 or 0.70+ only two had stage II 4+ disease, while nine had stage I disease. Furthermore, eight of the 14 cancers showed positive L-RE responses. Of the 15 cases having p50-negative patterns, ten had stage II 4+ disease and only three showed L-RE responses. The prognostic significance of the p50 protein patterns is also suggested by the data shown in Table XI. Seven of the ten eluates from prognostically favorable L-RE-positive stage I lesions had p50-0.70 proteins. In contrast, only one of 20 eluates from prognostically poor L-RE-negative stage II 4+ lesions had a p50-0.70 protein, seven eluates had a p50-0.80 pattern, while nine had a p50-negative pattern.

It appears that some breast cancer tissues do indeed contain proteins whose physicochemical characteristics are similar to proteins of MuMTV. It also seems that the protein patterns of the breast cancer tissues are prognostically significant. In order to obtain data on the antigenic significance of the protein

Table X. Clinicopathological Characteristics of Breast Cancers in Relation to Their P50 Protein Patterns

p50 pattern	Number	Stage I	Stage II<4	Stage II4+	L-RE-positive
0.80	17	4	2	11 (65)[a]	6 (35)
0.75	6	2	1	3 (50)	2 (33)
0.70, 0.70+	14	9	3	2 (14)	8 (57)
Negative	15	5	—	10 (67)	3 (20)
Total	52	20	6	26	19

[a]Percentages are given in parentheses.

Table XI. p50 Protein Patterns of
Prognostically Favorable and Prognostically
Unfavorable Breast Cancer Tissues

p50 pattern	Stage I, L-RE +	Stage II 4+, L-RE–
0.80	1	7
0.75	1	3
0.70, 0.70+	7	1
Negative	1	9
Total	10	20

patterns, we examined the response of breast cancer patients' leukocytes to cryostat sections of homologous breast cancer tissues according to the protein patterns of the cancer tissues and the leukocyte responses to RIII milk. The leukocyte migration data were obtained from our records of previously performed independent studies.

As shown in Table XII, RIII-positive leukocytes were maximally responsive to breast cancer tissues having a p50-0.70 protein component, *viz.*, 14/27 (52%). However, such leukocytes also responded in five (45%) of 11 tests against p50-negative breast cancer tissues. This latter response is greater than that of RII-positive leukocytes against benign breast tissues from control and cancerous

Table XII. Response of Breast Cancer Patients'
Leukocytes to Homologous Breast Cancer Tissues in
Relation to the p50 Proteins of the Cancer Tissues and
Leukocyte Responsiveness to RIII Mouse Milk

p50 patterns	Leukocyte responses		Total
	RIII-positive	RIII-negative	
0.80			
Mi < 0.80/total	0/6	1/32 (3)[a]	1/38 (3)
Mean ± SE	0.98 ± 0.06	0.97 ± 0.02	
0.75			
MI < 0.80/total	1/12 (8)	3/36 (8)	4/48 (8)
Mean ± SE	0.93 ± 0.03	0.95 ± 0.02	
0.70, 0.70+			
MI < 0.80/total	14/27 (52)	19/59 (32)	33/86 (38)
Mean ± SE	0.82 ± 0.03	0.88 ± 0.02	
Negative			
MI < 0.80/total	5/11 (45)	3/19 (16)	8/30 (27)
Mean ± SE	0.85 ± 0.05	0.91 ± 0.03	

[a]Percentages are given in parentheses.

breasts, *viz.*, 12% of 25 tests. The finding that RIII-positive leukocytes are more responsive to p50-negative breast cancer tissues than to benign breast tissues, which are also p50-negative, suggests that the antigenicity of breast cancer tissue is not exclusively dependent on the presence of the p50-0.70 component. It should be noted, however, that RIII-negative leukocytes responded more regularly to p50-0.70-containing breast cancer tissues (32%) than they did to p50-negative breast cancer tissues (16%). It would seem more than coincidental that p50-0.70 breast cancers are associated with high antigenicity and unusually favorable stage and L-RE characteristics.

In contrast to the leukocyte responses to the p50-0.70 and p50-negative homologous cancer tissues, neither RIII-positive nor RIII-negative leukocytes were appreciably responsive to p50-0.75 and p50-0.80 homologous breast cancers. The striking difference in antigenicity between the p50-0.70 and the latter two subgroups suggest that subtle changes in the protein components may be antigenically significant.

While our data are still limited, they do suggest that the antigenic properties of breast cancer tissues are correlated with protein components which have antigenic and physicochemical similarities to proteins of MuMTV. Moreover, the data of Tables X and XI suggest that the protein components of breast cancer tissues are correlated with the clinical behavior of breast cancer. Similar inferences may be drawn from the data of Hollinshead *et al.* (1974), who used gradient PAGE to separate soluble components of breast cancers, control breast tissues, and benign breast tumors. The pattern of separation of the cancer extracts was demonstrably different from those of the noncancer tissues. The cancer extracts contained a distinct protein component which was lacking in the control extracts. This component corresponds in location to the p50 protein band when our eluates are run in similar gradient gels. When Hollinshead *et al.* (1974) tested various segments of their gels for skin-reactive antigens, they found that region 2b of their cancer extracts (containing the distinctive component) elicited reactivity in breast cancer patients but was negative in patients with other types of cancer. Region 2b of the control tissue extracts produced no response in patients with breast cancer or other types of cancer. These data, coupled with our own, suggest that the distinctive protein component may indeed represent a breast cancer-specific antigen. Hollinshead *et al.* (1974) found that stage I and stage IV breast cancer patients were equally responsive to fraction 2b from breast cancer tissues. They also found that fraction 2a of control and cancer tissues produced skin responses in stage I breast cancer patients but not in stage IV breast cancer patients. Some patients with gynecological cancers other than breast also responded to fraction 2a.

It is evident that much remains to be learned in regard to the antigenic properties of specific components of control and cancer cells. More specifically, there is a need for more precise characterization of MuMTL-like proteins in human cancer tissues and specific cellular hypersensitivity to MuMTV-like antigens. It should be mentioned that despite the physicochemical and antigenic similarities between immunogenic human breast cancer tissues and MuMTV it remains to be proven that a true identity exists. As yet we have been unable to demonstrate that antisera prepared against MuMTV gp52 cross-reacts with eluates of a number of cancerous or benign breast tissues. Nor have we been able to demonstrate cross-reactivity against such eluates in rabbits having delayed hypersensitivity to MuMTV. However, the potency of the antiserum and the responsiveness of the sensitizied rabbits were decidedly lower than that of the *in vitro* responses of breast cancer patients' leukocytes to RIII milk. The point to be emphasized is the need to isolate and characterize the immunogens of breast cancer tissues and compare such purified preparations with specific fractions of MuMTV.

C. Molecular Hybridization

In considering the possible role of MuMTV in human mammary carcinogenesis, it is pertinent to take note of data derived from molecular hybridization studies. Schlom and Spiegelman (1973) reported that RNA derived from a significant proportion of different breast cancers hybridizes with DNA generated by reverse transcriptase activity from MuMTV-RNA templates. On the other hand, Vaidya *et al.* (1974) found that hybridization with RNA from unselected breast cancer tissues was uncommon. Their data suggest that homology between human breast tissue RNA and the MuMTV genome is a nonrandom occurrence. Homologous RNA appears to be preferentially associated with a positive family history and/or the *in situ* phase of the disease. It should be noted that homologous RNA was also found in two of five samples of noncancerous areas of cancerous breasts. Both of the homologous samples were derived from breasts having invasive breast cancers which lacked detectable homologous RNA. Both patients were less than 35 years of age and both had a family history of breast cancer. The nonrandom distribution of hybridizable RNA among breast cancer tissues is also manifest in terms of the NG. None of the seven positive samples was obtained from breast cancers having NG-I (anaplastic). In contrast, 10 of the 16 negative breast cancer RNA preparations were derived from NG-I cancers. The need for correlating analytical findings with clinicopathological characteristics is no less applicable to molecular hybridization than it is to immunological and therapeutic studies.

V. COMMENTS

Data obtained by such diverse techniques as microscopy, *in vivo* and *in vitro* immunological measurements, and physicochemical characterization of breast cancer proteins indicate, separately and collectively, that some breast cancers possess prognostically significant immunogens. Such immunogenicity is most consistently demonstrable during the *in situ* phase of the disease, while progressive disease is associated with, or the result of, diminished immunogenicity and/or specific hypersensitivity. Since breast cancer immunogens exhibit MuMTV-like antigenic and physicochemical properties, it would seem that *in situ* breast cancers would provide a particularly favorable resource for investigating the participation of MuMTV and other candidate viruses in human mammary carcinogenesis.

The common occurrence of shared immunogens among *in situ* breast cancers also offers a potential approach to immunotherapy. Surgical resection of the local lesion would prevent the progression of the disease, yet leave the hypersensitivity intact. Since subsequently developing breast cancers would encounter an already sensitized host, their progression should be impeded. The validity of this expectation is suggested by the finding that breast cancers arising after prior removal of *in situ* carcinomas and precancerous lesions have unusually favorable stage and survival characteristics as compared with breast cancers arising after removal of (1) nonimmunogenic, normotypic lesions, (2) invasive breast cancer, or (3) no prior breast lesion (Black *et al.*, 1972a). These observations suggest that immunogens isolated from *in situ* breast carcinomas might be capable of provoking biologically important specific hypersensitivity against subsequently developing breast carcinomas. If such isolated immunogens are in fact antigenically similar to specific components of MuMTV, the latter might serve as a source of such material. It is pertinent to note that Charney and Moore (1972) and Charney *et al.* (1973) have shown that immunization with formalin-inactivated MuMTV reduces the incidence of mammary tumors in selected strains of mice.

The finding that invasive breast cancers may differ in immunogenicity is also pertinent to attempts at immunotherapy (Black, 1975). It seems unlikely that immunogen-deficient breast cancers would be influenced by attempts to increase nonspecific or even specific hypersensitivity of the host. On the other hand, immunogenic tumors progressing in an immunologically compromised host might be benefited by immunostimulation, particularly if specific hypersensitivity could be increased.

If all human breast cancers were similar in development and biological behavior, it would be reasonable to expect uniformly positive or negative results with diverse investigative techniques, *viz.,* epidemiological, virological, biochemical, immunological, and therapeutic. If, on the other hand, the development and biological behavior of breast cancers were influenced by constellations of exogenous and endogenous factors, it would not be surprising if investigations using unselected targets obtained different answers to the same question. The point to be emphasized is that the more precisely we can characterize the immunogenicity of individual cancers and the specific hypersensitivity responses of individual patients the more valid will be our therapeutic approaches. It appears from the available data that MuMTV-like antigenicity and protein patterns may provide an approach toward the biologically significant characterization of individual cancers. Similarly, immunological responsiveness to MuMTV seems to provide an additional index for classifying the host. It should be noted that the empirical value of such indices is not necessarily dependent on proving the identity of breast cancer immunogens and MuMTV components.

Some additional comments are appropriate concerning some commonly overlooked questions regarding mammary carcinogenesis in both mice and humans. The demonstration that MuMTV satisfies Koch's postulates as the etiological agent of murine breast cancer is not synonymous with an understanding of either the mechanism of carcinogenesis or the unique subcellular characteristics of cancer cells. We are essentially ignorant of the critical events which transform a portion of the normal, virus-producing, murine mammary gland into a malignant neoplasm. The same question is of course applicable to the usually focal area of one of the paired human breasts, or perhaps the question should be stated in a reverse fashion: how does most of the mammary parenchyma avoid malignant transformation despite the presence of all the factors necessary for such a transformation? Another question of almost equal basic significance and certainly of clinical importance is what factors determine whether a particular breast cancer will have prognostically unfavorable grade I nuclei or prognostically favorable grade III nuclei. An allied question is why clinically significant metastases are so uncommon in murine mammary carcinomas. If all human breast cancers had grade III nuclei or the limited metastases of murine mammary cancer, the breast cancer problem would be far less acute.

The previous questions are raised for the purpose of emphasizing that the complexity displayed by human breast cancer demands more than the demonstration that a particular virus is sometimes associated with human breast cancer tissues. It might be most rewarding if such analytical techniques as molecular hybridization (Schlom and Spiegelman, 1973; Varmus *et al.*, 1973) and immunoelectron microscopy (Hoshino and Dmochowski, 1973) were applied to targets selected for their clinicopathological characteristics. A multidisciplined attack on such selected material should significant advance our knowledge of viral participation in the development and behavior of human breast cancer. Equally important, such an approach may yield therapeutic and prophylactic benefits long before all the basic questions are answered.

ACKNOWLEDGMENTS

These studies were supported in large measure by Contracts NO1-CP-33398 within the Special Virus-Cancer Program and NO1-CP-33321 of the Field Studies and Statistics Program, National Cancer Institute, National Institutes of Health, USPHS.

Appreciation is due the following individuals who were associated with the author in various phases of this ongoing study: Mr. Alfred M. Andrade, Thomas H. C. Barclay, M. D., Ada B. Chabon, M. D., Mr. Jesse Charney, Sidney J. Cutler, Sc.D., Dr. Arnold S. Dion, Bejamin F. Hankey, Sc.D., Dan H. Moore, Ph.D., Ms. Bella Shore, Francis D. Speer, M.D., Dr. Akhil B. Vaidya, and Reinhard E. Zachrau, M.D.

VI. REFERENCES

Anastassiades, O. T., and Pryce, D. M., 1966, Immunological significance of morphologic changes in lymph nodes draining breast cancer, *Br. J. Cancer* **20**:239.

Andersen, V., Bjerrum, O., Bendixen, G., Schiødt, T., and Dissing, I., 1970, Effect of autologous mammary tumour extracts on human leukocyte migration *in vitro*, *Int. J. Cancer* **5**:357.

Anderson, R. J., McBride, C. M., and Hersh, E. M., 1972, *In vitro* lymphocyte responses to malignant, benign neoplastic and normal tissue extracts, *Proc. Soc. Exp. Biol. Med.* **140**:465.

Bittner, J. J., 1936, Some possible effects of nursing on the mammary gland tumor incidence in mice (preliminary report), *Science* **84**:162.

Black, M. M., 1965, Reactivity of the lymphoreticuloendothelial system in human cancer, in: *Progress in Clinical Cancer* (I. Ariel, ed.), pp. 26–49, Grune and Stratton, New York.

Black, M. M., 1970a, Lymphoreticuloendothelial reactivity as a component of the tumor–host relationship, in: *Immunity and Tolerance in Oncogenesis* (L. Severi, ed.), pp. 863–876, Division of Cancer Research, Perugia, Italy.

Black, M. M., 1970b, Human breast carcinoma. I. Clinical considerations; II. Research potential, *N.Y. State J. Med.* **70**:863; 962.

Black, M. M., 1972, Cellular and biological manifestations of immunogenicity to precancerous mastopathy, *Natl. Cancer Inst. Monogr.* **35**:73.

Black, M. M., 1973, Human breast cancer: A model for cancer immunology, *Isr. J. Med. Sci.* **9**:284.

Black, M. M., 1975, Cell mediated response in human mammary cancer, in: *Host Defence in Breast Cancer* (B. A. Stoll, ed.), pp. 48–77, William Heinemann Medical Books, London.

Black, M. M., and Chabon, A. B., 1969, *In situ* carcinoma of the breast, in: *Pathology Annual* (S. C. Sommers, ed.), pp. 185–210, Appleton-Century-Crofts, New York.

Black, M. M., and Chabon, A. B., 1970. Incipient carcinoma of the breast: structural characteristics and host reactivity, in: *Immunity and Tolerance in Oncogenesis* (L. Severi, ed.), pp. 923–936, Division of Cancer Research, Perugia, Italy.

Black, M. M., and Leis, H. P., Jr., 1971, Cellular responses to autologous breast cancer tissue: Correlation with stage and lymphoreticuloendothelial reactivity, *Cancer* **28**:263.

Black, M. M., and Leis, H. P., Jr., 1973, Cellular responses to autologous breast cancer tissue: sequential observations, *Cancer* **32**:384.

Black, M. M., and Speer, F. D., 1957, Nuclear structure in cancer tissues, *Surg. Gynecol. Obstet.* **105**:97.

Black, M. M., and Speer, F. D., 1958, Sinus histiocytosis of lymph nodes in cancer, *Surg. Gynecol. Obstet.* **106**:163.

Black, M. M., and Speer, F. D., 1959*a*, Lymph node structure and metallophilia in tumor-bearing mice, *Arch. Pathol.* **67**:58.

Black, M. M., and Speer, F. D., 1959*b*, Immunology of cancer, *Surg. Gynecol. Obstet.* **109**:105.

Black, M. M., and Speer, F. D., 1960, Lymph node reactivity in cancer patients, *Surg. Gynecol. Obstet.* **110**:477.

Black, M. M., Kerpe, S., and Speer, F. D., 1953, Lymph node structure in patients with cancer of the breast, *Am. J. Pathol.* **29**:505.

Black, M. M., Cutler, S. J., and Barclay, T. H. C., 1972*a*, Post biopsy breast carcinoma: A natural experiment in cancer immunology, *Cancer* **29**:61.

Black, M. M., Barclay, T. H. C., Cutler, S. J., Hankey, B. F., and Asire, A. J., 1972*b*, The association of atypical characteristics of benign breast lesions with subsequent risk of breast cancer, *Cancer* **29**:338.

Black, M. M., Leis, H. P., Jr., Shore, B., and Azchrau, R. E., 1974*a*, Cellular hypersensitivity to breast cancer: Assessment by a leukocyte migration procedure, *Cancer* **33**:952.

Black, M. M., Moore, D. H., Shore, B., Zachrau, R. E., and Leis, H. P., Jr., 1974*b*, Effect of murine milk samples and human breast tissues on human leukocyte migration indices, *Cancer Res.* **34**:1054.

Black, M. M., Zachrau, R. E., Shore, B., Moore, D. H., and Leis, H. P., Jr., 1975*a*, Prognostically favorable immunogens of human breast cancer tissue: Antigenic similarity to murine mammary tumor virus, *Cancer* **35**:121.

Black, M. M., Barclay, T. H. C., and Hankey, B. F., 1975*b*, Prognosis in breast cancer utilizing histological characteristics of the primary tumor, *Cancer* **36**:2048.

Black, M. M., Dion, A., Zachrau, R. E., and Shore, B., 1975*c*, Distinctive protein components of human breast cancer tissues: MuMTV-like properties, *Cancer Res.*, in press.

Black, M. M., Zachrau, R. E., Shore, B., and Leis, H. P., Jr., 1976, Biological considerations of tumor-specific and virus-associated antigens of human breast cancers, *Cancer Res.* **36**:769.

Blasecki, J. W., and Tevethia, S. S., 1973, *In vitro* assay of cellular immunity to tumor-specific antigen(s) of virus-induced tumors by macrophage migration inhibition, *J. Immunol.* **110**:590.

Bloom, H. T. G., 1950, Prognosis in carcinoma of the breast, *Br. J. Cancer* **4**:259.

Charney, J., and Moore, D. H., 1972, Immunization studies with mammary tumor virus, *J. Natl. Cancer Inst.* **48**:1125.

Charney, J., Moore, D. H., Holben, J. A., and Cody, C., 1973, Prevention of multiple tumor development in mice by immunization with inactivated mammary tumor virus, in: *Multiple Primary Malignant Tumors* (L. Severi, ed.), pp. 1125–1133, Division of Cancer Research, Perugia, Italy.

Cutler, S. J., Black, M. M., Mork, T., Harvei, S., and Freeman, C., 1969, Further observations on prognostic factors in cancer of the female breast, *Cancer* **24**:653.

Fossati, G., Canevari, S., Della Porta, G., Balzarini, G. P., and Veronesi, M., 1972, Cellular immunity to human breast carcinoma, *Int. J. Cancer* **10**:391.

Friedell, G. H., Soto, E. A., Kumaoka, S., Abe, O., Hayward, J. L., and Bullbrook, R. D., 1974, Sinus histiocytosis in British and Japanese patients with breast cancer, *Lancet* **2**:1228.

Hamlin, I. M. E., 1968, Possible host resistance in carcinoma of the breast: A histological study, *Br. J. Cancer* **22**:383.

Heppner, G. H., and Pierce, G., 1969, *In vitro* demonstration of tumor-specific antigens in spontaneous mammary tumors of mice, *Int. J. Cancer* **4**:212.

Herberman, R. B., 1973a, *In vivo* and *in vitro* assays of cellular immunity to human tumor antigens, *Fed. Proc.* **32**:160.

Herberman, R. B., 1973b, Cellular immunity to human tumor-associated antigens, *Isr. J. Med. Sci.* **9**:300.

Hollinshead, A. C., Jaffurs, W. T., Alpert, L. K., Harris, J. E., and Herberman, R. B., 1974, Isolation and identification of soluble skin-reactive membrane antigens of malignant and normal human breast cells, *Cancer Res.* **34**:2961.

Hoshino, M., and Dmochowski, L., 1973, Electron microscopic study of antigens in cells of mouse mammary tumor cell lines by peroxidase labeled antibodies in sera of mammary tumor-bearing mice and of patients with breast cancer, *Cancer Res.* **33**:2551.

MacMahon, B., Cole, P., Lin, T. M., Lowe, C. R., Mirra, A. P., Ravnihar, B., Salber, E. J., Valaoras, V. G., and Yuasa, S., 1970, Age at first birth and breast cancer risk, *Bull. WHO* **43**:209.

McCoy, J. L., Jerome, L. F., Dean, J. H., Cannon, G. B., Alford, T. C., Doering, T., and Herberman, R. B., 1974, Inhibition of leukocyte migration by tumor-associated antigens in soluble extracts of human breast carcinoma, *J. Natl. Cancer Inst.* **53**:11.

Moore, D. H., 1974, Evidence in favor of the existence of human breast cancer virus, *Cancer Res.* **34**:2322.

Moore, D. H., and Charney, J., 1975, Breast cancer: Etiology and possible prevention, *Am. Scientist* **63**:160.

Morrison, A. S., Black, M. M., Lowe, C. R., MacMahon, B., and Yuasa, S., 1973, Some international differences in histology and survival in breast cancer, *Int. J. Cancer* **11**:261.

Morton, D. L., Miller, G. F., and Wood, D. A., 1969, Demonstration of tumor-specific immunity against antigens unrelated to the mammary tumor virus in spontaneous mammary adenocarcinomas, *J. Natl. Cancer Inst.* **42**:289.

Müller, M., and Grossmann, H., 1972, An antigen in human breast cancer sera related to the murine mammary tumor virus, *Nature London New Biol.* **231**:116.

Müller, M., Zotter, S., Grossmann, H., and Kemmer, C., 1972, Immunological cross reaction between human breast cancer, mastopathy and virus-producing mammary carcinoma of mice, *Arch. Geschwulstforsch.* **40**:285.

Müller, M., Kemmer, C., Zotter, S., Grossmann, H., and Micheel, B., 1973, Cross reaction between human breast cancer, mastopathy and murine mammary carcinoma: localization of the antigen in type A particle virus, *Arch. Geschwulstforsch.* **41**:100.

Rebuck, J. W., 1955, A method of studying leukocytic functions *in vivo, Ann. N.Y. Acad. Sci.* **59**:757.

Schlom, J., and Spiegelman, S., 1973, Evidence for viral involvement in murine and human mammary adenocarcinoma, *Am. J. Clin. Pathol.* **60**:44.

Schlom, J., Spiegelman, S., and Moore, D. H., 1972, Reverse transcriptase and high molecular weight RNA in particles from mouse and human milk, *J. Natl. Cancer Inst.* **48**:1197.

Schlom, J., Michalides, R., Kufe, D., Hehlmann, R., Spiegelman, S., Bentvelzen, P., and Hageman, P., 1973, A comparative study of the biologic and molecular basis of murine mammary carcinoma: A model for human breast cancer, *J. Natl. Cancer Inst.* **51**:541.

Seman, G., and Dmochowski, L., 1973, Electron microscope observation of virus-like particles in comedocarcinoma of the human breast, *Cancer* **32**:148.

Silverberg, S. G., Chitale, A. R., Hind, A. D., Frazier, A. B., and Levitt, S. H., 1970, Sinus histiocytosis and mammary carcinoma: Study of 366 radical mastectomies and a historical review, *Cancer* **26**:1177.

Spiegelman, S., Axel, R., and Schlom, J., 1972, Virus-related RNA in human and mouse mammary tumors, *J. Natl. Cancer Inst.* **48**:1205.

Vaidya, A. B., Black, M. M., Dion, A. S., and Moore, D. H., 1974, Homology between human breast tumor RNA and mouse mammary tumor virus genome, *Nature (London)* **249**:565.

Varmus, H. E., Quintrell, N., Medeiros, E., Bishop, J. M., Nowinski, R. C., and Sarkar, N. H., 1973, Transcription of mouse mammary tumor virus genes in tissues from high and low tumor incidence mouse strains, *J. Mol. Biol.* **79**:663.

Chapter 10

Clinical Implications of Immunity to Oncogenic Viruses

Paul H. Levine

Laboratory of Viral Carcinogenesis
National Institutes of Health
National Cancer Institute
Bethesda, Maryland 20014

I. INTRODUCTION

The evidence pointing to a viral etiology for at least some forms of human cancer, a possibility that has long been considered on the basis of animal studies, has continued to accumulate to such an extent that viral oncologists must now reevaluate their clinical and experimental data in order to consider which specific approaches are now ready for clinical trials. Although ethical restrictions continue to inhibit attempts to prove that specific viruses cause certain human tumors, as outlined by Bryan *et al.* (1967; Bryan, 1962), epidemiological studies have been able to suggest not only which human tumors are most likely to be caused by infectious agents (Burkitt, 1962; Cole *et al.,* 1968; Correa and O'Conor, 1971; Heath and Hasterlik, 1963; Kessler, 1974; Levine, 1974; Levine and Gravell, 1975; Morrow *et al.,* 1971) but some have even suggested the pattern of the agents' transmission (Kessler, 1976; Vianna *et al.,* 1971).

The classical approach to control of virus-induced diseases has been the development of preventive vaccines, and viral oncologists have usually seen as their goal the development of a preventive vaccine which would control leukemia or lymphoma in the same way that vaccines for polio and smallpox have controlled these once awesome threats to mankind. Several factors, however, have required a broader approach to the control of potentially virus-induced human tumors. One of the most important of these factors is the growing effect of conventional therapeutic techniques, particularly chemotherapy, which has led to decreasing mortality in certain tumors that are most likely of viral origin, particularly acute lymphocytic leukemia (ALL) of childhood and Burkitt's lymphoma (BL). It has been estimated, for example, that only two children per 100,000 should now die from ALL (Holland, 1976). Even if a viral vaccine to prevent human leukemia were developed, one would have to think very carefully about the risks involved in inoculating normal individuals with such a vaccine regardless of its efficacy. Studies on prevention of other potentially virus-induced human tumors with high mortality rates should still be pursued, of course; breast cancer, cervical cancer, and nasopharyngeal cancer (NPC) continue to have sufficient impact in high-risk populations to remain as obvious targets. Other means of exploiting the information being obtained by viral immunologists have become increasingly apparent, however, and untapped opportunities in diagnosis and therapy are continually being discovered. It is therefore timely to take another look at the state of the art in the immunology of oncogenic viruses, and to reevaluate which experimental findings appear to have the most immediate relevance to the control of human cancer.

II. ETIOLOGY

Etiology continues to be the area in which immunity to oncogenic viruses plays the most obvious role, since specific control measures cannot be applied until one has the etiological agent well characterized. In this particular aspect of research, perhaps more than any other, a multidisciplinary approach is needed since the tools of the laboratory investigator must be applied to etiological problems in conjunction with epidemiologist's knowledge of the different patterns of viral transmission, as well as the different patterns of disease potentially occurring as a result of the infection. The growing number of model systems has given virologists, immunologists, and epidemiologists many choices for the study of human cancer, particularly in leukemia (Gardner *et al.*, 1976; Gross, 1951; Jarrett *et al.*, 1973), lymphoma (Ablashi and Pearson, 1974; Churchill and Biggs, 1968; Melendez *et al.*, 1968), and breast cancer (Bittner, 1952, 1960; Blair and Lane, 1974; Chopra and Mason, 1970). Therefore, a close comparison of the human and animal diseases is required to enable the selection of the best animal-model system for the specific human disease. General questions that must be answered for each disease include the following:

1. Does the tumor appear to be induced by an environmental factor?
2. Does the pattern of disease suggest a prominent genetic influence?
3. Is there a virus associated with the human tumor that shares any features with the virus(es) causing the apparent homologous animal tumor?

4. Does the host response to the candidate human tumor virus parallel the host response to the known oncogenic virus in a comparable animal system?

More specific immunological approaches to the question of viral etiology depend on the degree of characterization possible for the putative tumor virus-associated antigens involved. Different approaches can be applied to systems where the investigator is clearly dealing with a human virus as with the Epstein-Barr virus (EBV), herpes simplex type II (HSV-2), or the papovaviruses (Padgett *et al.*, 1971), in contrast to the systems where there is electron microscopic and/or biochemical evidence for a human tumor virus (Gallagher and Gallo, 1975; McGrath *et al.*, 1974, Morton *et al.*, 1969), but the nature of the candidate particles is uncertain.

The tumor system which continues to merit the most attention as a model for other potentially virus-induced tumors is BL, where epidemiological evidence for a horizontally transmitted etiological agent is strong (Burkitt, 1962; Morrow *et al.*, 1971) and where laboratory studies continue to implicate a particular virus with oncogenic properties (EBV) as the responsible agent. (For recent reviews, see W. Henle and G. Henle, 1973*a*; Klein, 1973; Miller, 1974.) Regarding the role of an infectious agent in the etiology of BL, the initial epidemiological evidence [geographic variation (Burkitt, 1962) and time-space clustering (Morrow *et al.*, 1971)] has been bolstered by reports of seasonal variation (Williams *et al.*, 1974) and the observation that migrants to an endemic BL area have an appreciable incidence of disease at an older age (Morrow *et al.*, 1976*b*). The mounting evidence for an infectious etiology has naturally focused attention on EBV for the following reasons:

1. EBV was initially identified in a culture derived from a BL specimen (Epstein *et al.*, 1964) and has regularly been identified in every BL tumor placed in tissue culture.
2. African BL patients are invariably EBV antibody-positive and have higher antibody titers than matched controls (G. Henle *et al.*, 1969); furthermore, the antibody patterns frequently parallel the course of disease (G. Henle *et al.*, 1971*b*; W. Henle *et al.*, 1973*a*; Klein *et al.*, 1969).
3. EBV has been shown to transform normal human lymphocytes and to produce lymphomas in subhuman primates (Epstein *et al.*, 1973; Shope *et al.*, 1973).
4. Viral genome has been reported in fresh human tumor cells obtained from BL and NPC patients (Huang *et al.*, 1974; Reedman *et al.*, 1974); a variety of normal tissues or other tumors have not revealed evidence of EBV infection.
5. Viruses similar to EBV regularly produce lymphomas in their own

species of origin (Churchill and Biggs, 1968; Hinze, 1971) or in other animals (Ablashi and Pearson, 1974; Melendez *et al.*, 1968).

The massive data linking EBV to BL are, by necessity, indirect; and yet, as already stated, it is difficult to conceive of a means for proving that EBV causes BL without utilizing a highly specific vaccine that eliminates the tumor whereas a control vaccine is shown to be ineffective. For reasons outlined later (Klein *et al.*, 1976), such a study does not appear to be possible in the near future. The immunological methods that continue to implicate EBV as the cause of BL (W. Henle and G. Henle, 1973*a*; Klein, 1973; Miller, 1974) have obvious application to other tumors, however. It will be of great value for investigators evaluating other candidate oncogenic viruses to learn from the experience of those studying EBV.

The immunological evidence for a specific virus's oncogenicity would be greatly enhanced if the virus were highly oncogenic with a high rate of tumor production. One would therefore have a clear-cut antibody incidence and titer differential in patients and close contacts as compared to the normal population. Seroepidemiology continues to be the first means of approaching problems of etiology, with particular attention to the close contacts so that the disease process itself cannot be implicated as affecting the antibody pattern. Such studies have been unrewarding in the herpesvirus field, particularly because detectable antibodies to the relevant viruses are so widespread in the tumor-free population (Kessler, 1974; Tischendorf *et al.*, 1970), but the possibility of finding a pattern of specificity in family members is raised by studies in other human tumor systems (see below).

Another seroepidemiological approach which has been proven to be costly and difficult, but which has been strongly encouraged because it permits the possibility of a definitive answer, is the prospective study, a technique which has been successful in proving that EBV is the major cause of infectious mononucleosis (IM) (Evans *et al.*, 1968; W. Henle and G. Henle, 1972). In the West Nile region of Uganda, 30,000 African children have been bled and are being followed for the subsequent occurrence of BL (Geser and de The, 1972). Cases of Burkitt's tumor in this cohort are now being identified; but because of the likelihood that the incubation period for this tumor is longer than that for IM it will not be possible to make a final conclusion until a large number of cases are identified that have had several years between the initial bleeding and the development of a tumor.

The three human DNA viruses (EBV, HSV-2, and the papovaviruses) most closely associated with human tumors give a pattern of widespread infection, and if cancer is indeed a result of infection with any of these viruses, it is a relatively infrequent event. In such a setting, where viral infection results only rarely in malignancy, seroepidemiological studies must measure more than simply viral infection. More recent leads in viral oncology are therefore being developed to study immunity to virus-associated antigens that are more restricted to cancer patients and relatively infrequent in normal individuals. Examples of such antibodies are the antibodies to the EBV-associated early antigens (EA) (G. Henle *et al.*, 1971*a*), rarely found in high titer in normal individuals, but frequently found in patients with severe IM (W. Henle *et al.*, 1971), the only disease which has been proven to be caused by EBV. The discovery of these virus-induced antigens, named "early" antigens (EA) because of their appearance shortly after the indicator cells were infected by EBV and prior to the appearance of the viral capsid antigen (VCA), was of great importance because of their correlation with disease progression (W. Henle *et al.*, 1971, 1973*a,b*). In addition, initial studies indicated a disease specificity, with antibody to the "D" (diffuse) EA prominent in severe IM and NPC while the "R" (restricted) EA antibody was more closely associated with BL and Hodgkin's disease (HD) (W. Henle and G. Henle, 1973*b*). Although more recent studies have shown that the association of D and R antibodies with these diseases is not specific, the correlation of the different EBV antibodies to prognosis, their potential value as an indicator of an occult abnormality possibly related to cancer susceptibility (Levine *et al.*, 1974), and their diagnostic value in acute IM (W. Henle *et al.*, 1974) indicate the importance of developing a number of assays to monitor the immune response to viral infection.

The need for a battery of serological assays has also been apparent in the studies on the possible role of HSV-2 in cervical cancer. The presence of cross-reacting antigens between HSV-1 and HSV-2 has made interpretation of seroepidemiological studies exceedingly difficult, but the serological association between HSV-2 and cervical cancer appears to be as strong as the one between EBV and BL. As in the EBV field, the report of a more specific disease-related antibody to virus-induced nonvirion antigens (Hollinshead *et al.*, 1971, 1973; Tarro and Sabin, 1970, 1973; Aurelian *et al.*, 1973*a,b*, 1974) provided the possibility of tightening a link between HSV-2 and cervical cancer that had first been proposed on epidemiological grounds (Nahmias *et al.*, 1970). The significance of these nonvirion antibodies is, at present, the subject of considerable debate (Sabin, 1974; Hollinshead *et al.*, 1976). Future studies in this area will be followed with great interest.

As particles similar to oncogenic RNA viruses have been detected in cell lines obtained from human tumors (Gallagher and Gallo, 1975; Morton *et al.*, 1969; Priori *et al.*, 1971*a*; McGrath *et al.*, 1974), an early immunological approach to determine the nature of these particles has included the testing of these lines with sera obtained from patients with similar diseases and their family members (Eilber and Morton, 1970; Priori *et al.*, 1972; Priori and Dmochowski, 1974). In addition, comparable studies have been performed using fresh tumor cells from patients with leukemia (Bias *et al.*, 1972), melanoma (Morton *et al.*, 1968; Bowen *et al.*, 1976), sarcoma (Morton and Malmgren, 1968; Priori *et al.*, 1971c), and breast cancer (Priori *et al.*, 1971b, 1972) in order to avoid the possible artifacts induced by adventitious agents or tissue culture contamination. These studies have been based on the observation that tumors which are induced by any specific virus have common antigens that are directly identifiable as being related to that virus, whereas chemically induced tumors do not share antigens. Attention to sorting out the numerous antigen—antibody reactions has demonstrated potentially significant information, particularly in the human sarcoma system (Eilber and Morton, 1970; Hirshaut *et al.*, 1974; Mukherji and Hirshaut, 1973), but more sophisticated assays will be needed to separate the viral, embryonic, fetal, and irrelevant antigens that may be detected in these studies. It is apparent that seroepidemiology can be valuable in identifying specimens which are most likely to harbor oncogenic viruses, but the ultimate determination of whether or not these particles are indeed human oncogenic viruses must be decided by other means.

The attempt to translate these serological findings to the area of cellular immunology was obvious in view of the importance of cell-mediated immunity (CMI) to tumor rejection. The Hellströms were the first to apply CMI assays to immunoepidemiology by demonstrating that relatives of neuroblastoma patients appeared to have specific immunity against cultured neuroblastoma cells, whereas family members of Wilms' tumor patients appeared to react specifically against Wilms' tumor cells (Hellström *et al.*, 1968). Other investigators have shown family-related immunity against fresh and cultured tumor cells as well. In one study designed to avoid false positive results secondary to HL-A incompatibilities or neoantigens appearing in the course of tissue culture passage, we concentrated on identical twins, one with cancer and one without, and used fresh cells as a source of antigen. We evaluated 12 sets of identical twins with a number of CMI assays (Levine *et al.*, 1972a) and demonstrated that the cytotoxicity assay, which had been successful in detecting specific antigens in the Hellströms' hands, also appeared to indicate specific immunity against leukemia-associated antigens in the family members of leukemic patients (Levine *et al.*, 1972a; Rosenberg *et al.*, 1972). The relationship of these antigens to viruses has not been demonstrated as of this time, and it has also become apparent that individuals outside of the immediate family react against the same or similar antigens (Anderson *et al.*, 1974). Since these immunoepidemiological studies can only provide, at best, indirect evidence for a viral etiology for these tumors, a major effort is now being made to characterize the specific antigens involved in these reactions and to develop assays to detect specific immunity to these antigens.

In summary, two basic approaches have been utilized in the attempt to detect human oncogenic viruses. When a well-characterized human virus has been linked to a specific tumor, the key approach has been to identify viral antigen or viral nucleic acid in the tumor. The reproducible detection of EBV-induced nuclear antigen in fresh BL and NPC tumor cells (Huang *et al.*, 1974; Reedman *et al.*, 1974) provides the strongest evidence to date for EBV's etiological role in these two tumor systems. The detection of HSV-2-related antigen in exfoliated cervical cancer cells has been reported (Royston and Aurelian, 1970; Pasca *et al.*, 1975) and strengthens the possibility that HSV-2 is the etiological agent for this tumor.

The second approach, attempting to detect oncogenic viruses in fresh and cultured tumor cells by utilizing specific immune responses localized to patients and their close contacts, has yielded many suggestive findings but has not resulted in the isolation of any proven oncogenic viruses.

III. PREVENTION

As noted previously, the application of immunological techniques to the prevention of virus-associated tumors has classically meant the development of vaccines. Not only do vaccines have the obvious virtue of disease control, but also in the field of viral oncology there has been the additional hope that a successful specific vaccine would provide the ultimate proof that a certain virus was actually the cause of the associated tumor. In the use of any biological material in normal individuals, however, the first decision that must be made is whether the potential benefit in receiving this material outweighs the risk (Meyer and Ennis, 1976), and all other considerations are secondary. Deliberations as to benefit/risk involve detailed knowledge about the individual's susceptibility to the disease, the likelihood of his acting as a carrier, the likelihood that the specific vaccine to be utilized will not cause the disease or any other disease, etc. A great deal of relevant information on pathogenic viruses has been accumulating in recent years which cannot be ignored when considering the preparation of antiviral cancer vaccines.

In considering the use of a vaccine for a human tumor, attention should be given to the epidemiology of the disease and the selection of appropriate animal models in order to have an idea of the form of vaccine preparation that would be most useful for the particular virus under consideration. Some of the questions that are most relevant to vaccines are the following:

1. Is the human tumor more frequently a result of horizontal viral transmission, or vertical transmission. If there is horizontal transmission, at what age is there the greatest risk?
2. What is the risk of developing cancer from infection with the virus?
3. How many diseases are caused by the candidate agent?

In regard to the question of horizontal or vertical transmission, the two human tumors that provide the most information are BL and cervical cancer. There is little doubt that environmental factors of an infectious nature are responsible for BL, as noted before, although the relative importance of malaria versus the postulated viral factor (EBV?) remains uncertain (O'Conor, 1970). Cervical cancer most certainly appears to be a venereal disease (Kessler, 1976). In both of these tumors, it has been possible to identify periods of increasing risk as a natural concomitant of demonstrating probable horizontal transmission. While environmental factors clearly influence a number of other human tumors, such as HD (Cole *et al.,* 1968; Correa and O'Conor, 1971; Levine, 1974) and breast cancer (Buell, 1973), the data accumulated to date do not reveal how a putative, infectious agent is transmitted. Only in HD has a testable hypothesis been presented that is relevant to this question (Vianna *et al.,* 1971), and this is now being actively evaluated (Smith and Pike, 1976).

The second question, involving the risk of developing cancer after infection with a particular virus, can be answered when a specific agent is identified. It is apparent that the general risk of developing BL after infection with EBV is quite small, with an appreciable risk occurring only in areas of holoendemic malaria. Similar data on the maximum risk of developing NPC after EBV infection or cervical cancer after HSV-2 infection are being gathered and can be closely estimated without having the certainty that the particular tumor necessarily results from the particular virus with which it has been associated.

It is important to recognize that more than one disease may be affected by control of infection with a specific virus, particularly since this adds to the potential importance of a vaccine. Gardner *et al.* (1976) have suggested that neurological as well as hematological diseases may occur as a result of horizontal transmission of leukemia viruses, and EBV infection has clearly been associated with several nononcogenic diseases (Grose *et al.,* 1975; Hirshaut *et al.,* 1970), as well as being associated with several human tumors (Johansson *et al.,* 1970, 1971; Levine *et al.,* 1971*a,b,* 1972*b*). Infection with feline leukemia virus (FeLV) has been shown to result in a number of severe and frequently fatal diseases; abortion, anemia, glomerulonephritis, and an immunosuppression syndrome are only a few (Anderson *et al.,* 1971; Anderson and Jarrett, 1971; Mackey, 1975). Whether the disease is a direct result of the action of FeLV on the target organ or an indirect result of the immunosuppressive effect of the virus is irrelevant; the fact remains that increasing control of FeLV infection in cats will significantly reduce the number of deaths due to a variety of diseases.

As more information is gained about the natural history of human cancer and the viruses associated with cancer, the choice of appropriate animal models for vaccine studies becomes critical. Multiple model systems exist for both leukemia and lymphoma, and in spite of the intensive efforts in these systems over the past decade, it has not been possible to determine which is the best model (if indeed there is one best model) for the prevention of human disease. In the herpes-lymphoma field, years of comparative studies in humans, monkeys, and chickens have failed to produce agreement as to the best model for a human vaccine. The first and most successful large-scale vaccine programs for naturally occurring lymphoma have been those initiated for Marek's disease (MD) of chickens. Several vaccines have been utilized, including an apathogenic strain, a live-attenuated pathogenic strain, and a live turkey herpesvirus (Biggs *et al.*, 1970; Churchill *et al.*, 1969; Purchase, 1976). Concern regarding the application of a similar technique to humans (such as vaccination with a related simian herpesvirus) has been raised because of a number of other precedents, such as simian B-virus, which is highly dangerous to humans although nonpathogenic in the host of origin and the herpesvirus saimiri (HVS), which causes lymphoma in owl monkeys and marmosets, but apparently fails to harm its natural host, the squirrel monkey (Ablashi and Pearson, 1974; Melendez *et al.*, 1968). Since the transmission of herpesvirus across species barriers has been shown to prevent tumors under natural conditions in birds (Biggs *et al.*, 1970; Purchase, 1976) and to cause tumors under controlled but almost natural conditions in monkeys (Hunt *et al.*, 1973; Rabin *et al.*, 1975), the safest course at the present time appears to be the development of several models until more is known about the biology of the apparently different isolates of EBV that are now being identified (Gerber *et al.*, 1976).

The desire to understand the mechanisms of viral oncogenesis and the need to have the tools to distinguish oncogenic virions from nononcogenic virions has not prevented serious consideration of testing an EBV vaccine for the prevention of BL (Epstein, 1976). As the tumor-virus system which has provided the most relevant clinical data, BL can be considered the prototype for a disease in which a specific successful vaccine would prove the oncogenicity of a human virus. Epstein has discussed the rationale for utilizing an EBV vaccine to prevent IM and BL as a preliminary step in the preparation of a vaccine for NPC, a disease with a significant mortality rate in high-risk individuals. Although an EBV vaccine eventually may be possible, and even practical, a number of concerns remain. In the first place, the possibility that EBV is oncogenic for humans makes it highly unlikely that a live vaccine can be utilized in normal individuals as long as we lack the means of measuring viral attenuation. A killed whole-virus vaccine also poses problems in that present technology does not permit the use of such vaccines that can be guaranteed to be effective while free of occasional viable particles and/or infectious nucleic acid.

Noting the recent developments in the preparation of effective nucleic acid-free vaccines for MD (Kaaden and Dietzschold, 1974; Lesnik and Ross, 1975), Epstein has suggested that similar preparations be used in man. Such preparations could perhaps allow an individual to get through a period of disease susceptibility into a relatively refractory period, but, in such a situation, the epidemiology of the disease must be carefully considered to determine if a vaccine with a noninfectious antigen, which will probably provide a more temporary immunity, is practical. Morrow *et al.* (1976*a*) have reviewed the possible temporal relationships between EBV and malaria infection that might lead to BL, and in the situation where EBV infection must precede the maximal host response to malaria, a vaccine could prove to be successful. Since information regarding the temporal relationship between EBV infection and BL may be forthcoming through the prospective study in Uganda (Geser and de The, 1972), further planning regarding the feasibility of an EBV vaccine for BL should be postponed. One consideration that requires caution regarding any form of vaccine in BL is that the tumor, which in most cases appears to be monoclonal in origin (Fialkow *et al.*, 1970), could be the result of the escape of one cell from immune surveillance, and this event may be initiated by multiple antigenic assaults. A vaccine might therefore increase the number of assaults and have a detrimental rather than a beneficial effect on BL incidence.

In addition to the uncertainties about which model to use for a vaccine [it is fortunate that a successful killed vaccine exists for simian (Laufs and Steinke, 1975) as well as avian (Kaaden and Dietzschold, 1974; Lesnik and Ross, 1975) herpes-induced lymphomas], the selection of a study group and an appropriate protocol for the prevention of BL poses formidable problems. For example, there are sufficient uncertainties about the natural history of BL that would make evaluation of an EBV vaccine difficult. There appears to be a declining incidence of Burkitt's tumor in the West Nile region of Uganda (Morrow *et al.*, 1976*b*), perhaps related to general improvement in health standards or greater use of antimalarial drugs. Other relevant factors must also be considered, and since malaria control may have more general beneficial effects and lower risk in relationship to the control of BL, the impetus for an EBV vaccine in the highly endemic Burkitt's tumor area may be practically nonexistent.

When the possibility of a vaccine to prevent virus-induced tumors was first transplanted into an organized effort by an act of Congress (Baker *et al.*, 1966), the disease that was foremost in consideration was acute leukemia. It has been discouraging to many to find that in spite of abundant leads in a number of animal systems, previous reports of human leukemia isolates have not been confirmed, and it has only been in recent months that the repeated isolation of an oncornavirus from the leukemia cells of a patient with acute myelogenous leukemia (Gallagher and Gallo, 1975) has been followed by reports of similar or identical isolates in other laboratories (Nooter *et al.*, 1975; Panem *et al.*, 1975; Teich *et al.*, 1975). Immunological and biochemical techniques suggest that these isolates are similar or identical to a virus isolated from a woolly monkey sarcoma (Theilen *et al.*, 1971). Since this tumor-bearing animal was a house-raised pet which belonged to a leukemia patient who carried this virus (or one closely related), the possibility of horizontal transmission of leukemia viruses and preventive vaccines has again become a relevant and exciting area.

The C-type RNA viruses, or oncornaviruses, provide an interesting contrast to the herpesviruses because of the evidence in the carefully studied murine system that leukemia is a result of vertically transmitted oncogenic material (Huebner and Todaro, 1969). Endogenous "oncornaviruses" have also been shown in other animal systems, but their classification in the oncogenic group may be misleading since their ability to cause cancer has not yet been proven (Essex, 1975). In view of the recent evidence that horizontally transmitted P-30 antigen of mice correlates with subsequent appearance of cancer (Gardner *et al.*, 1976), and the now-well accepted data that it is the horizontally transferred FeLV, not the endogenous "oncornavirus," that causes most naturally occurring feline leukemia/lymphosarcoma (Essex, 1975), model systems for the prevention of horizontally transmitted human leukemia are again being studied. As with the EBV-BL system, however, the question of benefit/risk indicates that the exciting new leads in the area of leukemia research may not be translatable as a leukemia vaccine, particularly in view of the relatively small and constantly diminishing mortality rate (Holland, 1976) from this disease.

It is important that these considerations weighing against the implementation of EBV vaccines for BL and acute leukemia not cast a pall over the general area of vaccine development for prevention of virus-induced tumors in general. While the risk/benefit ratio may be too high in diseases that are being controlled with increasing effectiveness by conventional therapy, such as BL, ALL, and HD, there are other malignancies such as breast cancer, cervical cancer, and NPC that have an unacceptable mortality in certain parts of the world and show no promise of being more effectively controlled by methods now available.

Of these "high-impact" malignancies, cervical cancer is a prime candidate for a preventive vaccine because of several factors. As already discussed, the epidemiology of cervical cancer and its associated herpesvirus suggest that both are transmitted by sexual contact (Nahmias *et al.*, 1970; Kessler, 1974, 1976). In a recent review of the status of HSV-2 as a possible cause of cervical cancer, Roizman and Frenkel (1975) concluded that elimination of genital herpes might be the only means of demonstrating the etiological role of HSV-2 in this tumor. The arguments for an HSV-2 vaccine have a relative advantage over those for EBV—genital herpes is a more debilitating and chronic problem than IM, elimination may be needed to protect the newborn, and the associated malignancy, cervical cancer, has a higher incidence and mortality than BL. However, the dangers of vaccinating with a potentially oncogenic virus and the apparently prolonged latent period between infection and cancer remain formidable obstacles to an HSV-2 vaccine trial demonstrating the etiological role of this herpesvirus in human cancer.

At the present time, therefore, the application of immunity to oncogenic viruses in the form of a preventive vaccine does not appear to be an immediate prospect, but the long-term possibility for vaccines having an impact on the prevention of a number of human tumors remains. Further definition of high-risk groups and identification of specific individuals at increased risk will be necessary before it is possible to identify a specific cohort with the lowest risk/benefit ratio of vaccination.

IV. IMMUNODIAGNOSIS

The application of immunological principles to the early diagnosis of cancer, both as a screening technique in high-risk populations and as a tool for detecting early relapse in a patient with previously treated cancer, has great potential in the area of virus-induced tumors. A number of approaches to detect viral antigens, virus-induced tumor antigens, and non-virus-associated tumor antigens are being developed, and it has already been possible to utilize some of these assays in the clinical field without determining the precise nature of the antigens involved.

In transplanting the immunological principles of immunodiagnosis from animal to man, leukemia has provided a useful model because of the relative ease of obtaining tumor cells throughout all phases of disease. A practical technique for early identification of FeLV (the FOCMA assay to detect "feline oncorna-virus membrane antigen") has been used effectively in the early diagnosis of feline leukemia, and has proved to be important in decreasing the incidence of feline leukemia/lymphoma by permitting the diagnosis of virus carriers, often in the preleukemic state (Hardy et al., 1976). The detection of leukemia-associated antigens in humans, a potentially important tool in immunodiagnosis, is being undertaken in patients who are already diagnosed because of the importance of detecting early relapse in attempts at curative chemotherapy. There is a marked difference between using an assay as a diagnostic tool on a population basis and using it in monitoring the treatment of a patient that has already been diagnosed, but experience with the carcinoembryonic antigen (CEA) (Gold and Freedman, 1965a,b) has demonstrated that the clinical studies correlating prognosis and antigen detection are a necessary and valuable first step in determining whether a specific technique has potential value in immunodiagnosis.

A number of investigators have reported the detection of leukemia-associated antigens using heterologous sera prepared against animal oncorna-viruses (Bates et al., 1966; Fink et al., 1965; Ioannides et al., 1968), lymphoid cell line antigens (Mann et al., 1974), and fresh leukemic cells (Metzgar et al., 1972; Mohanakumar et al., 1974). Others have used naturally occurring sera

(Bias *et al.,* 1972) or CMI assays directed against apparent leukemia-related antigens (Gutterman *et al.,* 1974) to detect leukemic cells present in small numbers. Although the problem of antigen specificity has already been discussed previously in the context of etiology, the nature of the antigen is of less concern in immunodiagnosis as long as the assay is easily performed and reasonably specific. Thus the early controversy regarding the nature of the virus-associated leukemia antigens (Fink *et al.,* 1965; Yohn *et al.,* 1968; Mann *et al.,* 1974), while important to resolve in terms of viral etiology, becomes of less concern if the techniques continue to demonstrate clinical relevance.

As studies with CEA have demonstrated, antigen detection can be an important means of diagnosing tumors not readily accessible to the clinician at an early stage. Possible areas of future development in the viral immunodiagnosis of breast cancer are being evaluated on the model provided by Van Blitterswijk *et al.* (1975), who has been able to predict the incidence of murine breast cancer by detecting a viral antigen designated as ML. Similar approaches will undoubtedly be tried in other animal and human tumors as the techniques for antigen detection become more sensitive.

The ability to detect a variety of antibodies to virus-associated antigens has been used to detect susceptibility to disease, as well as early disease in both animals and man. In the herpesvirus system, neutralizing and membrane-associated antibodies against HSV have been shown to protect against viral infection and lymphoma, while antibodies to antigens similar to the EBV-associated early antigens have correlated with disease progression. The diagnosis of one EBV-induced disease, IM, has been greatly enhanced by recent advances in EBV serology. Whereas initial documentation of primary EBV infection required a predisease antibody-negative serum and subsequent seroconversion, it is now possible to diagnose early infection by demonstrating the presence of antiviral antibodies directed against the capsid antigen in the absence of antibodies to the EBV-nuclear antigen (EBNA), which arise several weeks later than VCA but persist, as does VCA, for life in most normal individuals (Henle *et al.,* 1974). As noted before in regard to detection of antigen, it is possible to consider the potential value of assays in the detection of new tumors by evaluating their patterns in patients who already have disease. In the EBV-BL system as noted previously, high titers of antibody to the soluble complement-fixing antigen and the virus-induced early antigen have been shown to be higher in short-term survivors with BL than long-term survivors (G. Henle *et al.,* 1971*b*; W. Henle *et al.,* 1973*a*; Sohier and de The, 1972). Similar findings in NPC have now led to attempts to predict early relapse in these two tumors on the basis of the EA findings. The membrane-associated antibody, an antibody that is associated with a more favorable clinical course in BL, has been reported to decline approximately 6 months prior to relapse in a BL patient who was followed through a 4-year remission (Klein *et al.,* 1969). The biological reason for these serological changes has been difficult to define, but the development of a number of longitudinal studies to determine the usefulness of these assays in predicting tumor relapse will be of great interest, particularly since BL and NPC are so responsive to treatment when detected at an early stage.

As serological assays are shown to relate to the prognosis of the patients under observation, their extension to field trials for early diagnosis is inevitable. Since each particular serological assay appears to have its own biological variation and, as with the CMI, in assays utilized in the monitoring of cancer patients discordant results rather than concordant results appear to be the rule, it is important to apply every possible technique to these prospective immuno-diagnostic and longitudinal patient studies in order to be able to select the most useful assays. Studies in Africa are currently in progress to determine if EBV antibody titers are predictive of subsequent BL development (Geser and de The, 1972), and in view of the elevated antibody levels in normal individuals within certain multiple-case cancer families (Levine et al., 1974; Li et al., 1974) prospective studies should also be considered in the United States to determine if individuals with high EBV antibody titers subsequently have a higher incidence of cancer.

In the avian (Crittenden, 1976) and the feline (Hardy et al., 1976) leukemia systems, detection of virus as well as neutralizing antibody has permitted the identification of individual animals in respect to their carrier state, their chance of developing leukemia, and their status as a hazard to other animals. In both systems, high levels of neutralizing antibody correlate with resistance to the virus, but in the cat the extra data provided by the antibody to the FOCMA antigen indicate that the protection of this antibody against leukemia/lympho-sarcoma operates independently from the neutralizing antibody's antiviral effect (Hardy, 1976). Because of the comparable serological patterns in animals and man in regard to lymphotropic herpesvirus infection, it is likely that a similar comparability will be noted for oncornavirus-induced immunity as well.

V. THERAPY

The utilization of viral vaccines in the treatment of cancer has far greater potential than in prevention at the present time because one is dealing with a patient who already has cancer and the opportunity for a beneficial effect greatly outweighs the risk of a harmful effect from the treatment. The principle for vaccine treatment of patients would be, as in immunotherapy directed against tumor antigens, to identify immunocompetent patients, generally in remission, and utilize the vaccine to prevent viral reinduction of tumor. The recurrence of disease in patients with leukemia, BL, and breast cancer following long-term remission has suggested that reinduction of tumor rather than recurrence of temporarily suppressed disease is occurring. Since genetic susceptibility is considered a major factor in viral oncogenesis, it would not be surprising if the factors that combined to cause cancer in an individual were present to cause another tumor at some future time. Thus a "therapeutic vaccine" in this sense could actually be a preventive one. Clinical observations providing the rationale for such a vaccine include the multifocal appearance of NPC and breast cancer, the latter being more susceptible to preventive measures by removal of the target organ than the former. The best case for viral reinduction of disease has been made in patients with acute leukemia who have had their disease controlled by the transplantation of donor cells only to have the disease occur in the donor cells (Thomas et al., 1972). These findings suggest that control of the oncogenic agent is as important as control of the malignancy itself, and detailed experimental studies to investigate this suggestion have been developed by Bekesi and his colleagues. Working in the AKR-Gross leukemia virus (GLV) system, Bekesi et al. (1976) have shown that chemotherapy alone increases survival in AKR mice but does not reduce viral titers, while antiviral therapy that is associated with successful reduction of circulating GLV is accompanied by a significant extension of remission. These same investigators have developed comparative studies in mice and humans which demonstrate a multifaceted attack on the disease with apparent success (Bekesi et al., 1974, 1975; Holland and Bekesi, 1976). Following chemotherapy to reduce the tumor burden, augmentation of the antitumor response has been provided by intradermal inoculation of neuraminidase-treated tumor cells, and control of the oncogenic virus (or putative oncogenic virus, in the case of the human studies) is attempted by using antiviral drugs, such as interferon inducers. Significantly prolonged survival in the mice appears to parallel longer remissions in the patients.

Hersh et al. (1974a,b) also have evaluated the feasibility of a combined antiviral–antitumor approach by immunizing leukemia patients in chemotherapy-induced remissions with a formalinized preparation of Rauscher leukemia virus. By stimulating humoral and cell-associated immunity to virus-associated antigens in the leukemia patients, these workers have demonstrated that immunological tolerance should not be a major problem in a clinical trial utilizing viral vaccines as part of an immunotherapy program.

EBV vaccines may have a place in the treatment of cancer as well. Ziegler et al. (1972) have observed that late relapses in BL occur in sites other than those initially involved by tumor, whereas early relapses occur at the same sites. Noting also that patients with late relapse are more likely to respond to the same chemotherapy as they originally received in achieving clinical remission, Ziegler suggested that the late relapses were the result of viral reinduction. If further studies indicate that this conclusion is valid, a vaccine trial in BL patients early in the course of remission may be appropriate.

Attempts to transfer antiviral immunity have been more successful in infectious diseases, such as disseminated varicella, than they have been in cancer immunotherapy, but recent advances utilizing materials such as transfer factor have evoked new attempts to develop more effective treatment regimens. Goldenberg and Brandes (1976) have tried to use transfer factor to treat NPC based on the indirect evidence implicating EBV as a cause of NPC. The source of the transfer factor has been the leukocytes of IM patients, who would be expected to have active immunity against EBV. Because of the paucity of effective treatment programs for metastatic NPC, it is understandable that less-conventional therapeutic trials would be undertaken. The potential value of such trials is great, since it may be possible to learn more about the role of EBV in NPC as a by-product, but it is unfortunate that the limited methods available for measuring cellular immunity to EBV make evaluation of such a study very difficult.

VI. SUMMARY AND CONCLUSIONS

The development of more varied and sophisticated methods of measuring immunity to oncogenic viruses has improved our understanding of the pathogenesis of virus-induced tumors in animals. As epidemiological and laboratory studies begin to identify human tumors that are apparently caused by viruses, applications of the animal data to clinical problems need to be considered. Four general areas can be identified where immune mechanisms can be utilized in clinical studies: etiology, prevention, diagnosis, and therapy.

Etiological studies continue to be a focus of attention since specific control measures cannot be applied until one has the etiological agent well characterized, but the data have been insufficient to prove causality. The strongest evidence to date for EBV's etiological role in BL and NPC has been the identification of viral antigens in fresh tumor cells; similar data have been reported linking herpes simplex II to cervical carcinoma. Seroepidemiological studies, while initially linking these viruses to their respective tumors, have not been sufficient to prove causality because of the widespread pattern of immunity to EBV and HSV-2 in the general population. The attempts to localize specific immune responses to cancer patients and close contacts have suggested a viral etiology for human leukemia, sarcoma, and breast cancer, but this type of approach has, as yet, failed to isolate any proven oncogenic viruses.

The application of immunological techniques to the prevention of virus-associated tumors has classically meant the development of vaccines. Consideration of the benefit/risk ratio is necessary before a vaccine can be utilized in normal individuals. Pertinent animal models for the prevention of herpesvirus-induced lymphomas have been successful, but further information is needed regarding the epidemiology of candidate oncogenic viruses and their respective tumors before a human tumor virus vaccine can be seriously considered.

The application of immunological principles to the early diagnosis of cancer, both as a screening technique in high-risk populations and as a tool for detecting early relapse in a patient with previously treated cancer, has great potential in the area of virus-induced tumors. Tumor-associated antigens have been utilized in the management of colon cancer, and some studies have reported the use of leukemia antigens to diagnose relapse. Identification of relevant tumor- and/or virus-associated antigens is particularly important since clinical correlation can lead to practical usage even before the specificity of the antigen is fully determined. Studies in avian and feline leukemia have demonstrated patterns of immunity that lead to the identification of individuals who are resistant or susceptible to oncogenic viruses, as well as carriers who pose hazards to unprotected animals. Studies to characterize the immune response to EBV in humans as a means of detecting susceptibility to cancer have been reported, but their value still remains unconfirmed.

Utilization of the immune response as part of a therapeutic program has particular potential in leukemia, BL, and breast cancer, where late relapse suggests reinduction of disease is occurring. Since the therapist is dealing with a cancer patient, greater risks are permissible because the potential benefit of immunomanipulation is greater than in a normal individual. Clinical application of immunotherapeutic studies in control of virus-induced murine leukemia has yielded promising results in human leukemia as well.

In summary, it is likely that humans are not tolerant to oncogenic viruses, and promising ways of utilizing these responses must now be considered.

ACKNOWLEDGMENTS

The author wishes to thank Dr. Alan Rabson, NCI, for his helpful comments and suggestions. The bibliographic assistance of Miss Marie Purdy and the secretarial assistance of Miss Rebecca Duvall are gratefully acknowledged.

VII. REFERENCES

Ablashi, D. V., and Pearson, G. R., 1974, Animal models: *Herpesvirus saimiri,* a nonhuman primate model for herpesvirus-associated neoplasia of man, *Cancer Res.* 34:1232.
Anderson, L. J., and Jarrett, W. F., 1971, Membranous glomerulonephritis associated with leukemia in cats, *Res. Vet. Sci.* 12:179.

Anderson, L. J., Jarrett, W. F. H., Jarrett, O., and Laird, H. M., 1971, Feline leukemia-virus infection of kittens: Mortality associated with atrophy of the thymus and lymphoid depletion, *J. Natl. Cancer Inst.* **47**:807.

Anderson, P. N., Klein, D. L., Bias, W. B., Mullins, G. M., Burke, P. J., and Santos, G. W., 1974, Cell-mediated immunological reactivity of patients and siblings to blast cells from adult acute leukemias, *Isr. J. Med. Sci.* **10**:1033.

Aurelian, L., Schumann, B., Marcus, R. L., and Davis, H. J., 1973*a*, Antibody to HSV-2 induced tumor specific antigens in serums from patients with cervical carcinoma, *Science* **181**:161.

Aurelian, L., Davis, H. J., and Julian, C. G., 1973*b*, Herpesvirus type-2 induced tumor specific antigen in cervical carcinoma. *Am. J. Epidemiol.* **98**:1.

Aurelian, L., Strandberg, J. D., and Marcus, R. L., 1974, Neutralization, immunofluorescence and complement fixation tests in identification of antibody to a herpesvirus type-2 induced tumor specific antigen in sera from squamous cervical carcinoma, *Prog. Exp. Tumor Res.* **19**:165.

Baker, C. G., Carrese, L. M., and Rauscher, F., 1966, The special virus leukemia program of the National Cancer Institute: Scientific aspects and program logic, *Proc. Zool. Soc. London* **17**:259.

Bates, H. A., Bankole, R. O., and Swaim, W. R., 1966, Immunofluorescent studies in human leukemia, *Blood* **34**:430.

Bekesi, J. G., Roboz, J. P., Walter, L., and Holland, J. F., 1974, Stimulation of specific immunity against cancer by neuraminidase-treated tumor cells, *Behring Inst. Mitt.* **55**:309.

Bekesi, J. G., Holland, J. F., Yates, J. W., Henderson, E., and Fleminger, R., 1975, Chemotherapy of acute myelogenous leukemia with neuraminidase treated allogeneic leukemia cells, *Proc. Am. Assoc. Cancer Res.* **16**:121.

Bekesi, J. G., Roboz, J. P., Zimmerman, E., and Holland, J. F., 1976, Treatment of spontaneous leukemia in AKR mice with chemotherapy, immunotherapy, or interferon, *Cancer Res.* **36**:631.

Bias, W. B., Santos, G. W., Burke, P. J., Mullins, G. M., and Humphrey, R. L., 1972, Cytologic antibody in normal human serums reactive with tumor cells from acute lymphocytic leukemia, *Science* **178**:304.

Biggs, P. M., Payne, L. N., Milne, B. S., Churchill, A. E., Chubb, R. C., Powell, D. G., and Harris, A. H., 1970, Field trials with an attenuated cell associated vaccine for Marek's disease, *Vet. Rec.* **87**:704.

Bittner, J. J., 1952, Tumor-inducing properties of the mammary tumor agent in young and adult mice, *Cancer Res.* **12**:510.

Bittner, J. J., 1960, Influence of the mammary-tumor agent on the genesis of mammary cancer in agent-free mice after milk transmission, *J. Natl. Cancer Inst.* **25**:177.

Blair, P. B., and Lane, M-A., 1974, Immunologic evidence for horizontal transmission of MTV, *J. Immunol.* **113**:1446.

Bowen, J. M., McBride, C. M., Miller, M. S., and Dmochowski, I., 1976, Relationship of nucleolar antigens in malignant melanoma cells to disease prognosis, *Proc. 9th Int. Pigment Cell Conf.* (in press).

Bryan, W. R., 1962, The search for causative viruses in human cancer: A discussion of the problem, *J. Natl. Cancer Inst.* **29**:1027.

Bryan, W. R., Dalton, A. J., and Rauscher, F. J., 1967, The viral approach to human leukemia and lymphoma: Its current status, *Prog. Hematol.* **5**:137.

Buell, P., 1973, Changing incidence of breast cancer in Japanese-American women, *J. Natl. Cancer Inst.* **51**:1479.

Burkitt, D., 1962, A "tumour safari" in East and Central Africa, *Br. J. Cancer* **16**:17.

Chopra, H. C., and Mason, M. M., 1970, A new virus in a spontaneous mammary tumor of a Rhesus monkey, *Cancer Res.* **30**:2081.

Churchill, A. E., and Biggs, P. M., 1968, Herpes-type virus isolated in cell culture from tumors of chickens with Marek's disease. II. Studies *in viivo, J. Natl. Cancer Inst.* **49**:951.

Churchill, A. E., Payne, L. N., and Chubb, R. C., 1969, Immunization against Marek's disease using a live attenuated virus, *Nature (London)* **221**:744.

Cole, P., MacMahon, B., and Aisenberg, A., 1968, Mortality from Hodgkin's disease in the United States, *Lancet* **11**:1371.

Correa, P., and O'Conor, G. T., 1971, Epidemiologic patterns of Hodgkin's disease, *Int. J. Cancer* **8**:192.

Crittenden, L. B., 1976, The epidemiology of avian lymphoid leukosis, *Cancer Res.* **36**:570.

Eilber, F. R., and Morton, D. L., 1970, Immunologic studies of human sarcomas: Additional evidence suggesting an association sarcoma virus, *Cancer* **26**:588.

Epstein, M. A., 1976, Implications of a vaccine for the prevention of Epstein-Barr virus infection: Ethical and logistic considerations, *Cancer Res.* **36**:711.

Epstein, M. A., Achong, B. G., and Barr, Y. M., 1964, Virus particles in cultured lymphoblasts from Burkitt's lymphoma, *Lancet* **1**:702.

Epstein, M. A., Rabin, H., Ball, G., Rickinson, A. B., Jarvis, J., and Melendez, L. V., 1973, Pilot experiments with EB virus in owl monkeys (*Aotus Trivirgatus*). II. EB virus in a cell line from an animal with reticuloproliferative disease, *Int. J. Cancer* **12**:319.

Essex, M., 1975, Horizontally and vertically transmitted oncornaviruses of cats, *Adv. Cancer Res.* **21**:175.

Evans, A. S., Niederman, J. C., and McCollum, R. W., 1968, Seroepidemiologic studies of infectious mononucleosis with EB virus, *N. Engl. J. Med.* **279**:1121.

Fialkow, P. J., Klein, G., Gartler, S. M., and Clifford, P., 1970, Clonal origin for individual Burkitt tumours, *Lancet* **1**:384.

Fink, M. A., Karon, M., Rauscher, F. J., Malmgren, R. A., and Orr, H. C., 1965, Further observations on the immunofluorescence of cells in human leukemia, *Cancer* **18**:1317.

Gallagher, R. E., and Gallo, R. C., 1975, Type C RNA tumor virus isolated from cultured human acute myelogenous leukemia cells, *Science* **187**:350.

Gardner, M. B., Henderson, B. E., Estes, J. D., Rongey, R. W., Casagrande, J., Pike, M., and Huebner, R. J., 1976, The epidemiology and virology of C-type virus-associated hematological cancers and related diseases in wild mice, *Cancer Res.* **36**:574.

Gerber, P., Nkrumah, F. K., Prichett, R., and Kieff, E., 1976, Comparative studies of Epstein-Barr virus strains from Ghana and the United States, *Int. J. Cancer* **17**:71.

Geser, A., and de The, G., 1972, Does the Epstein-Barr virus play an aetiological role in Burkitt's lymphoma? in: *Oncogenesis and Herpesviruses* (P. M. Biggs, G. de The, and L. N. Payne, eds.), p. 372, International Agency for Research on Cancer, Lyon, France.

Gold, P., and Freedman, S. O., 1965*a*, Demonstration of tumor-specific antigens in human colonic carcinomata by immunological tolerance and absorption techniques, *J. Exp. Med.* **121**:439.

Gold, P., and Freedman, S. O., 1965*b*, Specific carcinoembryonic antigens of the human digestive system. *J. Exp. Med.* **122**:467.

Goldenberg, G. J., and Brandes, L. J., 1976, *In vivo* and *in vitro* studies of immunotherapy of nasopharyngeal carcinoma with transfer factor, *Cancer Res.* **36**:720.

Grose, C., Henle, W., Henle, G., and Feorino, P. M., 1975, Primary Epstein-Barr virus infections in acute neurologic diseases, *N. Engl. J. Med.* **292**:392.

Gross, L., 1951, Pathogenic properties and "vertical" transmission of mouse leukemia agent, *Proc. Soc. Exp. Biol.* **78:***342.*

Gutterman, J. U., Mvligit, G., Burgess, M. A., McCredie, K. B., Hunter, C., Freireich, E. J., and Hersh, E. M., 1974, Brief Communication: Immunodiagnosis of acute leukemia: Detection of residual disease, *J. Natl. Cancer Inst.* **53:**389.

Hardy, W. D., Jr., Hess, P. W., MacEwen, E. G., McClelland, A. J., Zuckerman, E. E., Essex, M., Cotter, S. M., and Jarrett, O., 1976, Biology of feline leukemia virus in the natural environment, *Cancer Res.* **36:**582.

Heath, C. W., Jr., and Hasterlik, R. J., 1963, Leukemia among children in a suburban community, *Am. J. Med.* **34:**796.

Hellström, I. E., Hellström, K. E., Pierce, G. E., and Bill, A. H., 1968, Demonstration of cell-bound and humoral immunity against neuroblastoma cells, *Proc. Natl. Acad. Sci. U.S.A.* **60:**1231.

Henle, G., Henle, W., Clifford, P., Diehl, V., Kafuko, G. W., Kirya, B. G., Klein, G., Morrow, R. H., Munube, G. M. R., Pike, P., Tukei, P. M., and Ziegler, J. L., 1969, Antibodies to Epstein-Barr virus in Burkitt's lymphoma and control groups, *J. Natl. Cancer Inst.* **43:**1147.

Henle, G., Henle, W., and Klein, G., 1971*a,* Demonstration of two distinct components in the early antigen complex of Epstein-Barr virus-infected cells, *Int. J. Cancer* **8:**272.

Henle, G., Henle, W., Klein, G., Gunven, P., Clifford, P., Morrow, R. H., and Ziegler, J. L., 1971*b,* Antibodies to early Epstein-Barr virus-induced antigens in Burkitt's lymphoma, *J. Natl. Cancer Inst.* **46:**861.

Henle, W., and Henle, G., 1972, Epstein-Barr virus: The cause of infectious mononucleosis— A review, in: *Oncogenesis and Herpesviruses* (P. M. Biggs, G. de The, and L. N. Payne, eds.), p. 269, International Agency for Research on Cancer, Lyon, France.

Henle, W., and Henle, G., 1973*a,* Evidence for an oncogenic potential of the Epstein-Barr virus, *Cancer Res.* **33:**1419.

Henle, W., and Henle, G., 1973*b,* Epstein-Barr virus-related serology in Hodgkin's disease, *J. Natl. Cancer Inst. Monogr.* **36:**79.

Henle, W., Henle, G., Niederman, J. C., Klemola, E., and Haltia, K., 1971, Antibodies to early antigens induced by Epstein-Barr virus in infectious mononucleosis, *J. Infect. Dis.* **124:**58.

Henle, W., Henle, G., Gunven, P., Klein, G., Clifford, P., and Singh, S., 1973*a,* Patterns of antibodies to Epstein-Barr virus-induced early antigens in Burkitt's lymphoma. Comparison of dying patients with long-term survivors, *J. Natl. Cancer Inst.* **50:**1163.

Henle, W., Ho, H.-C., Henle, G., and Kwan, H. C., 1973*b,* Antibodies to Epstein-Barr virus-related antigens in nasopharyngeal carcinoma. Comparison of active cases with long-term survivors, *J. Natl. Cancer Inst.* **51:**361.

Henle, W., Henle, G. E., and Horwitz, C. A., 1974, Epstein-Barr virus specific diagnostic tests in infectious mononucleosis, *Hum. Pathol.* **5:**551.

Hersh, E. M., Gutterman, J. U., Mavligit, G., Gschwind, C. R., Freireich, E. J., Levine, P. H., and Plata, E. J., 1974*a,* Human immune response to active immunization with Rauscher leukemia virus. I. Cell-mediated and cell-associated immunity, *J. Natl. Cancer Inst.* **53:**317.

Hersh, E. M., Hanna, M. G., Jr., Gutterman, J. U., Mavligit, G., Yurconic, M., Jr., and Gschwind, C. R., 1974*b,* Human immune response to active immunization with Rauscher leukemia virus. II. Humoral immunity, *J. Natl. Cancer Inst.* **53:**327.

Hinze, H. C., 1971, New member of the herpesvirus group isolated from wild cottontail rabbits, *Infect. Immun.* **3:**350.

Hirshaut, Y., Glade, P., Viera, L. O. B. D., Ainbender, E., Dvorak, B., and Siltzbach, L. F.,

1970, Sarcoidosis, another disease associated with serologic evidence for herpes-like virus infection, *New Engl. J. Med.* 283:502.

Hirshaut, Y., Pei, D. T., Marcove, R. C., Mukherji, B., Spielvogel, A. R., and Essner, E., 1974, Seroepidemiology of human sarcoma antigen (S1), *New Engl. J. Med.* 291:1103.

Holland, J. F., 1976, Immunological control of human leukemia: Discussion, *Cancer Res.* 36:657.

Holland, J. F., and Bekesi, J. G., 1976, Immunotherapy of human leukemia with neuraminidase modified cells, in: *Symposium on immunotherapy in malignant diseases, Medical Clinics of North America,* Vol. 60 (W. Terry, ed.), pp. 539–549.

Hollinshead, A. C., Melnick, J. L., and Rawls, W. E., 1971, Reactivity between herpesvirus type 2-related soluble membrane antigens in cells from carcinoma of the cervix, vulva, and vagina and matched cancer and control sera, *Int. Virol.* 2:105.

Hollinshead, A. C., Lee, O., Chretien, P. B., Tarpley, J. L., Rawls, W. E., and Adam, E., 1973, Antibodies to herpesvirus nonvirion antigens in squamous carcinomas, *Science* 182:713.

Hollinshead, A. C., Chretien, P. B., Lee, O., Tarpley, J. L., Kerney, S. E., Silverman, N. A., and Alexander, J. C., 1976, *In vivo* and *in vitro* measurements of the relationship of human squamous carcinomas to herpes simplex virus tumor-associated antigens, *Cancer Res.* 36:821.

Huang, D. O., Ho, J. H. C., Henle, W., and Henle, G., 1974, Demonstration of Epstein-Barr virus-associated nuclear antigen in nasopharyngeal carcinoma cells from fresh biopsies, *Int. J. Cancer* 14:580.

Huebner, R. J., and Todaro, G. J., 1969, Oncogenes of RNA tumor viruses as determinants of cancer, *Proc. Natl. Acad. Sci. U.S.A.* 19:1087.

Hunt, R. D., Garcia, F. G., Barahona, H. H., King, N. W., Fraser, C. E. O., and Melendez, L. V., 1973, Spontaneous herpesvirus saimiri lymphoma in an owl monkey, *J. Infect. Dis.* 127:723.

Ioannides, A. K., Rosner, F., Brenner, M., and Lee, S. L., 1968, Immunofluorescent studies of human leukemic cells with antiserum to a murine leukemic virus (Rauscher strain), *Blood* 31:381.

Jarrett, W., Jarrett, O., Mackey, L., Laird, H., Hardy, W., Jr., and Essex, M., 1973, Horizontal transmission of leukemia virus and leukemia in the cat, *J. Natl. Cancer Inst.* 51:833.

Johansson, B., Klein, G., Henle, W., and Henle, G., 1970, Epstein-Barr virus (EBV)-associated antibody patterns in malignant lymphoma and leukemia. I. Hodgkin's disease, *Int. J. Cancer* 6:450.

Johansson, B., Klein, G., Henle, W., and Henle, G., 1971, Epstein-Barr virus (EBV)-associated antibody patterns in malignant lymphoma and leukemia. II. Chronic lymphocytic leukemia and lymphocytic lymphoma, *Int. J. Cancer* 8:475.

Kaaden, O. R., and Dietzschold, B., 1974, Alterations of the immunological specificity of plasma membranes of cells infected with Marek's disease and turkey herpes viruses, *J. Gen. Virol.* 25:1.

Kessler, I. I., 1974, Perspectives on the epidemiology of cervical cancer with specific reference to the herpesvirus hypothesis, *Cancer Res* 34:1091.

Kessler, I. I., 1976, Human cervical cancer as a venereal disease, *Cancer Res.* 36:783.

Klein, E., Klein, G., and Levine, P. H., 1976, Immunological control of human lymphoma: Discussion, *Cancer Res.* 36:724.

Klein, G., 1973, The Epstein-Barr virus, in: *The Herpesviruses* (A. S. Kaplan, ed.), p. 521, Academic Press, New York.

Klein, G., Clifford, P., Henle, G., Henle, W., Geering, G., and Old, L. J., 1969, EBV-associated serological patterns in a Burkitt lymphoma patient during regression and recurrence, *Int. J. Cancer* **4**:416.

Laufs, R., and Steinke, H., 1975, Vaccination of non-human primates against malignant lymphoma, *Nature (London)* **53**:71.

Lesnick, F., and Ross, L. J. N., 1975, Immunization against Marek's disease using Marek's disease virus-specific antigens free from infectious virus, *Int. J. Cancer* **16**:153.

Levine, P. H., 1974, The etiology of Hodgkin's disease, *Pathobiol. Annu.* **64**:143.

Levine, P. H., and Gravell, M., 1975, The viral etiology of leukemia, *Mod. Probl. Paediatr.* **16**:137.

Levine, P. H., Ablashi, D. V., Berard, C. W., Carbone, P. P., Waggoner, D. E., and Malan, L., 1971a, Elevated antibody titers to Epstein-Barr virus in Hodgkin's disease, *Cancer* **27**:416.

Levine, P. H., Merrill, D. A., Bethlenfalvay, N. C., Dabich, L., Stevens, D. A., and Waggoner, D. E., 1971b, A longitudinal comparison of antibodies to Epstein-Barr virus and clinical parameters in chronic lymphocytic leukemia and chronic myelocytic leukemia, *Blood* **38**:479.

Levine, P. H., Herberman, R. B., Rosenberg, E. B., McClure, P. D., Roland, A., Pienta, R. J., and Ting, R. C. Y., 1972a, Acute leukemia in identical twins: Search for viral and leukemia-associated antigens, *J. Natl. Cancer Inst.* **49**:943.

Levine, P. H., O'Conor, G. T., and Berard, C. W., 1972b, Antibodies to Epstein-Barr virus (EBV) in American patients with Burkitt's lymphoma, *Cancer* **30**:610.

Levine, P. H., Fraumeni, J. F., Jr., Reisher, J. I., and Waggoner, D. E., 1974, Antibodies to Epstein-Barr virus-associated antigens in relatives of cancer patients, *J. Natl. Cancer Inst.* **52**:1037.

Li, F. P., Melvin, K. E. W., Tashjian, A. H., Jr., Levine, P. H., and Fraumeni, J. F., Jr., 1974, Brief communication: Familial medullary thyroid carcinoma and pheochromocytoma: Epidemiologic investigations, *J. Natl. Cancer Inst.* **52**:285.

Mackey, L., 1975, Feline leukaemia virus and its clinical effects in cats, *Vet. Rec.* **96**:5.

Mann, D. L., Halterman, R., and Leventhal, B., 1974, Acute leukemia associated antigens, *Cancer* **34**:1446.

McGrath, C. M., Grant, P. M., Soule, H. D., Glancy, T., and Rich, M. A., 1974, Replication of oncornavirus-like particle in human breast carcinoma cell line, MCF-7, *Nature (London)* **252**:247.

Melendez, L. V., Daniel, M. D., Hunt, R. D., and Garcia, F. G., 1968. An apparently new herpesvirus from primary kidney cultures of the squirrel monkey (*saimiri sciureus*), *Lab. Anim. Care* **18**:374.

Metzgar, R. S., Mohankumar, T., and Miller, D. S., 1972, Antigens specific for human lymphocytic and myeloid leukemia cells: Detection by nonhuman primate antiserums, *Science* **178**:986.

Meyer, H. M., Jr., and Ennis, F. A., 1976, Regulatory approach toward vaccines against cancer: The benefit/risk ratio, *Cancer Res.* **36**:865.

Miller, G., 1974, The oncogenicity of Epstein-Barr virus, *J. Infect. Dis.* **130**:187.

Mohanakumar, T., Metzgar, R. S., and Miller, D. S., 1974, Human leukemia cell antigens: Serologic characterization with xenoantisera, *J. Natl. Cancer Inst.* **52**:1435.

Morrow, R. H., Pike, M. C., Smith, P. G., Ziegler, J. L., and Kisuule, A., 1971, Burkitt's lymphoma: A time-space cluster of cases in Bwamba County of Uganda, *Br. Med. J.* **2**:491.

Morrow, R. H., Gutensohn, N., and Smith, P. G., 1976a, Epstein-Barr virus-malaria interaction models for Burkitt's lymphoma: Implications for preventive trials, *Cancer Res.* **36**:667.

Morrow, R. H., Kisuule, A., Pike, M. C., and Smith, P. G., 1976b, Burkitt's lymphoma in the Mengo District of Uganda: Epidemiological features and their relationship to malaria, *J. Natl. Cancer Inst.* **56**:479.

Morton, D. L., and Malmgren, R. A., 1968, Human osteosarcomas: Immunologic evidence suggesting an associated infectious agent, *Science* **162**:1279.

Morton, D. L., Malmgren, R. A., Holmes, E. C., and Ketcham, A. S., 1968, Demonstration of antibodies against human malignant melanoma by immunofluorescence, *Surgery* **64**:233.

Morton, D. L., Hall, W. T., and Malmgren, R. A., 1969, Human liposarcomas: Tissue cultures containing foci of transformed cells with viral particles, *Science* **165**:813.

Mukherji, B., and Hirshaut, Y., 1973, Evidence for fetal antigen in human sarcoma, *Science* **181**:440.

Nahmias, A. J., Josey, W. E., Naib, Z. M., Luce, C., and Duffey, C., 1970, Antibodies to herpesvirus hominis type 1 and 2 in humans. I. Patients with genital herpetic infections, *Am. J. Epidemiol.* **91**:539.

Nooter, K., Aarssen, A. M., Bentvelzen, P., Degroot, F. G., and Van Pelt, F. G., 1975, Isolation of infectious C-type oncornavirus from human leukaemic bone marrow cells, *Nature (London)* **256**:595.

O'Conor, G. T., 1970, Persistent immunologic stimulation as a factor in oncogenesis, with special reference to Burkitt's Tumor, *Am. J. Med.* **48**:279.

Padgett, B. L., Walker, D. L., Zurhein, G. M., Eckroade, R. J., and Dessel, B. H., 1971, Cultivation of Papova-like virus from human brain with progressive multifocal leucoencephalopathy, *Lancet* **1**:1257.

Panem, S., Prochownik, E. V., Reale, F. R., and Kirsten, W. H., 1975, Isolation of Type-C virions from a normal human fibroblast strain, *Science* **189**:297.

Pasca, A. S., Kummerlander, L., Pejtsik, B., and Pali, K., 1975, Herpesvirus antibodies and antigens in patients with cervical anaplasia and in controls, *J. Natl. Cancer Inst.* **55**:775.

Priori, E. S., and Dmochowski, L., 1974, Immunofluorescence antibodies in human sera to antigens in cells of a type C virus producing human culture of tumor origin, *Prog. Exp. Tumor Res.* **19**:182.

Priori, E. S., Dmochowski, L., Myers, B., and Wilbur, J. R., 1971a, Continuous type C virus production in a tissue culture of human origin (Burkitt lymphoma), *29th Ann. Proc. Electron Microsc. Soc.*, p. 376.

Priori, E. S., Seman, G., Dmochowski, L., Gallager, H. S., and Anderson, D. E., 1971b, Immunofluorescence studies on sera of patients with breast carcinoma, *Cancer* **28**:1462.

Priori, E. S., Wilbur, J. R., and Dmochowski, L., 1971c, Immunofluorescence tests on sera of patients with osteogenic sarcoma, *J. Natl. Cancer Inst.* **46**:1299.

Priori, E. S., Anderson, D. E., Williams, W. C., and Dmochowski, L., 1972, Immunological studies on human breast carcinoma and mouse mammary tumors, *J. Natl. Cancer Inst.* **48**:1131.

Purchase, H. G., 1976, Prevention of Marek's disease: A review, *Cancer Res.* **36**:696.

Rabin, H., Neubauer, R. H., Pearson, G. R., Cicmanec, J. L., Wallen, W. C., Loeb, W. F., and Valerio, M. G., 1975, Spontaneous lymphoma associated with herpesvirus saimiri in owl monkeys, *J. Natl. Cancer Inst.* **54**:499.

Reedman, B. M., Klein, G., Pope, J. H., Walters, M. K., Hilgers, J., Singh, S., and Johansson, B., 1974, Epstein-Barr virus-associated complement-fixing and nuclear antigens in Burkitt lymphoma biopsies, *Int. J. Cancer* **13**:755.

Roizman, B., and Frenkel, N., 1975, Does genital herpes cause cancer? A midway assessment, in: *Sexually Transmitted Diseases* (R. D. Catterrall and C. S. Nicol, eds.), p. 151, Academic Press, New York.

Rosenberg, E. B., Herberman, R. B., Levine, P. H., Halterman, R. H., McCoy, J. L., and Wunderlich, J. R., 1972, Lymphocyte cytotoxicity reactions to leukemia-associated antigens in identical twins, *Int. J. Cancer* 9:648.

Royston, I., and Aurelian, L., 1970, Immunofluorescent detection of herpesvirus antigens in exfoliated cells from human cervical carcinoma, *Proc. Natl. Acad. Sci. U.S.A.* 67:204.

Sabin, A. B., 1974, Herpes simplex-genitalis virus nonvirion antigens and their implication in certain human cancers: unconfirmed, *Proc. Natl. Acad. Sci. U.S.A.* 71:3248.

Shope, T., Dechairo, D., and Miller, G., 1973, Malignant lymphoma in cottontip marmosets after inoculation with Epstein-Barr virus, *Proc. Nat. Acad. Sci. U.S.A.* 70:2487.

Smith, P. G., and Pike, M. C., 1976, Current epidemiological evidence for transmission of Hodgkin's disease, *Cancer Res.* 36:660.

Sohier, R., and de The, G., 1972, Evolution of complement-fixing antibody titers with the development of Burkitt's lymphoma, *Int. J. Cancer* 9:524.

Tarro, G., and Sabin, A. B., 1970, Virus-specific, labile, non-virion antigen in herpesvirus-infected cells, *Proc. Natl. Acad. Sci. U.S.A.* 65:753.

Tarro, G., and Sabin, A. B., 1973, Nonvirion antigens produced by herpes simplex viruses 1 and 2, *Proc. Natl. Acad. Sci. U.S.A.* 70:1032.

Teich, N. M., Weiss, R. A., Salahuddin, S. Z., Gallagher, R. E., Gillespie, D. H., and Gallo, R. C., 1975, Infective transmission and characterisation of a C-type virus released by cultured human myeloid leukaemia cells, *Nature (London)* 256:551.

Theilen, G. H., Gould, D., Fowler, M., and Dungworth, D. L., 1971, C-type virus in tumor tissue of a woolly monkey (Logothrix spp.) with fibrosarcoma, *J. Natl. Cancer Inst.* 47:881.

Thomas, E. D., Bryant, J. I., Buckner, C. D., Clift, R. A., Fefer, A., Johnson, F. L., Neiman, P., Ramberg, R. E., and Storb, R., 1972, Leukaemic transformation of engrafted human marrow cells in vivo, *Lancet* 1:1310.

Tischendorf, P., Shramek, G. J., Balagtas, R. C., Deinhardt, F., Knospe, W. H., Noble, G. R., and Maynard, J. E., 1970, Development and Persistence of Immunity to Epstein-Barr virus in man, *J. Infect. Dis.* 122:401.

Van Blitterswijk, W. J., Emmelot, P., Hilgers, J., Kamlag, D., Nusse, R., Feltkamp, C. A., 1975, Quantitation of virus induced (MLr) and normal (THY.1.2) cell surface antigens in isolated plasma membranes and the extracellular ascites fluid of mouse leukemia cells, *Cancer Res.* 35:2743.

Vianna, N. J., Greenwald, P., and Davies, J. N. P., 1971, Nature of Hodgkin's disease agent, *Lancet* 1:733.

Williams, E. H., Day, N. E., and Geser, A. G., 1974, Seasonal variation in onset of Burkitt's lymphoma in the West Nile district of Uganda, *Lancet* 11:19.

Witter, R. L., 1976, Natural mechanisms of controlling lymphotropic herpesvirus infection (Marek's disease) in the chicken, *Cancer Res.* 36:681.

Yohn, D. S., Horoszewicz, J. S., Ellison, R. R., Mittelman, A., Chai, L. S., and Grace, J. T., Jr., 1968, Immunofluorescent studies in human leukemia, *Cancer Res.* 28:1692.

Ziegler, J. L., Bluming, A. Z., Fass, L., and Morrow, R. H., Jr., 1972, Relapse patterns in Burkitt's lymphoma, *Cancer Res.* 32:1267.

Index